The National Medical Series Questions and Answers for Independent Study

family medicine

David R. Rudy, M.D., M.P.H.

Professor and Chairman
Department of Family Medicine
Finch University of Health Sciences
The Chicago Medical School
North Chicago, Illinois

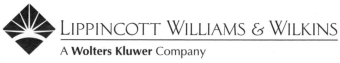

LIPPINCOTT WILLIAMS & WILKINS
A **Wolters Kluwer** Company

Philadelphia • Baltimore • New York • London
Buenos Aires • Hong Kong • Sydney • Tokyo

Dedication

This work is dedicated to my wife, Rose Mary S. Rudy, M.A.; our children Douglas David Rudy, Steven William Rudy, Katharine Rudy Hoffer, and Hunter Ashley Elam; and to our five grandchildren in descending order of age: Elizabeth Lynn Rudy, Michael Robert Rudy, Steven Douglas Rudy, Jacob Rudy Hoffer, and Molly Nicole Hoffer; and last, but far from least, to my father, Robert Sale Rudy, CPA (ret.), who is turning 92 years of age as this is being written.

SECTION VIII Problems Unique to Males   129

SECTION IX Musculoskeletal and Connective Tissue Problems   137

SECTION X Sports Medicine   171

SECTION XI Other Infectious Diseases Encountered in Primary Care   177

SECTION XII Endocrinology in Primary Care   191

SECTION XIII Allergies   221

SECTION XIV Preventive Care, Health, and Efficiency   229

SECTION XV Behavior and Psychology in Family Practice   293

Contents

Foreword

Family medicine was the first specialty to require recertification to ensure that family physicians remain current with advances in medicine. We are continually challenging ourselves with questions of the type presented in this book. These questions help us remain abreast of new information and prepare for written examinations, whether they be the in-training exams given in the medical clerkships, to family practice residents, or the certification and recertification exams taken by physicians in practice.

The questions in this book focus on practical issues also presented in *Family Medicine: The House Officer Series*. The answers not only give the preferred course of action, but also discuss why other options are incorrect. New information is added, supplementing that provided in *Family Medicine: The House Officer Series*. These questions and the discussion of the answers give the reader insight into the problem-solving process in primary care, which often differs from that in the consulting specialties.

Dr. Rudy has, through *Family Medicine: The House Officer Series* and *NMS Q&A for Family Medicine*, provided the reader with an excellent overview of our discipline, reflecting the variety of problems encountered in practice. It is this variety that keeps us perpetually challenged. These books let us keep pace with modern advances and help us sustain the excitement and satisfaction of primary care.

Robert E. Rakel, M.D.

Preface

This book, the first for Family Medicine in the respected NMS series, is intended to provide study material for students in preparation for USMLE Step 2 and for residents in preparation for USMLE Step 3 and Family Practice board certification. *NMS Q&A Family Medicine* is also a useful adjunct for Family Medicine clerkships. This book is formulated to complement *Family Medicine: The House Officer Series,* 1997, by Williams & Wilkins. Nevertheless, we hope that this work will stand on its own due to the comprehensiveness of the answer and explanation section. In preparing this book, I discovered first hand the exacting standards of Lippincott Williams & Wilkins, the publisher, that have earned the NMS series the respect that it holds among medical students and residents. As with the House Officer series book, the project itself has been engrossing and fulfilling. I hope that the reader will receive a fair measure of these benefits as well.

David R. Rudy, M.D., M.P.H.

Acknowledgments

For the material contained in this book, I wish to acknowledge a great debt owed to the authors of *Family Medicine: The House Officer Series*. Included among those in great measure is my co-editor for that work and generous contributor, Kurt Kurowski, M.D., who is also my Vice Chairman at Chicago Medical School. The team at Williams & Wilkins, which during the publishing process for this book became Lippincott Williams & Wilkins, were crucial to the success of this work. My first contact, with the idea for the book, was with Elizabeth Nieginski, Senior Acquisitions Editor. She put me in contact with Julie Scardiglia, Editorial Director, and ultimately the Senior Managing Editor on the project, Amy Dinkel. These wonderful people, through their professionalism and their personal winning ways, put a competent and human face on the publishing process. It is with a measure of pride that this work will take its place in the successful NMS series.

Problems of the Head, Eyes, Ears, Nose, and Throat

Test 1

Problems of the Ears, Throat, and Sinuses

DIRECTIONS (Items 1–23): Each of the numbered items or incomplete statements in this section is followed by answers or by completions of the statement. Select the ONE lettered answer or completion that is BEST in each case.

1. A 24-year-old man complains of a stuffy nose in the aftermath of a viral cold of 5 days duration. He has taken a proprietary nasal spray for self-treatment of this symptom for the past 3 days and has noted that the stuffiness has become bilateral and has now interfered seriously with his sleep. An accepted treatment approach to his condition is

- (A) Discontinuance of the medication, followed by inhaled glucocorticoids for a brief period, and humidification
- (B) Discontinuance of the present spray, followed by prescription of more potent vasoconstrictors in a topical preparation
- (C) Discontinuance of the present spray in favor of longer-acting nasal decongestants
- (D) Skin testing and desensitization
- (E) Topical application of a basophile-stabilizing agent, such as cromolyn

2. A 15-year-old, white male patient is experiencing a "nosebleed," one of many within a month. The current grouping of epistaxes is similar to one his mother reports he experienced approximately 1 year ago. She says that this group of nosebleeds have occurred solely on the left side, and, untreated, they have lasted approximately 5–10 minutes each, unless the boy remains active during the bout. She reports she has controlled the nosebleeds by tampanading the naris from the side toward the septum. Last week an episode was severe enough to require an emergency-room physician to stop the bleeding with a cotton pledget soaked in phenylephrine. At this time, which of the following measures is most appropriate?

- (A) Arrange a consultation with an otolaryngologist to ascertain the general bleeding site.
- (B) Give the patient a 10-mg capsule of fast-acting nifedipine, and instruct him to bite down on it for rapid release and absorption across the buccal mucosa.
- (C) Identify the bleeding site by examination with a head mirror, and cauterize with silver nitrate.
- (D) Tamponade the side of bleeding with a catheter balloon.
- (E) Sedate the patient with meperidine to bring the blood pressure under control.

3. A 3-year-old boy has had an earache since the previous night. He has a temperature of 38.3°C (101°F). He has had five bouts of middle-ear infection during the past year, three of which were in the past 6 months. It is the month of March. A likely underlying factor in the recurrence of his condition is

- (A) Atopic constitution
- (B) African-American ancestry
- (C) Exposure to cold winds
- (D) Tonsillar hypertrophy and/or tonsillitis
- (E) Anterior attached frenulum

4. Which viral cause of upper respiratory infection is associated with the greatest risk of otitis media?

- (A) Influenza A/B
- (B) Rhinoviruses
- (C) Respiratory syncytial viruses
- (D) Enteroviruses
- (E) Adenoviruses

5. The three most frequent bacterial causes of otitis media (in descending order) are

- (A) *Streptococcus pyogenes, Staphylococcus aureus, Klebsiella pneumoniae*
- (B) *Streptococcus pneumoniae, Haemophilus influenzae, Moraxella catarrhalis*
- (C) *Moraxella catarrhalis, Pseudomonas species, Haemophilus influenzae*
- (D) *Haemophilus influenzae, Streptococcus pyogenes, Staphylococcus aureus*
- (E) *Moraxella catarrhalis, Streptococcus pyogenes, Staphylococcus aureus*

6. Among organisms involved in otitis media, approximately which proportion would be expected to be resistant to penicillin and ampicillin?

- (A) 10%–20%
- (B) 20%–30%
- (C) 30%–40%
- (D) 40%–50%
- (E) 50%–75%

7. To justify a diagnosis of otitis media, which is the symptom that MUST be present?

  (A) Pain in the area of the ear without external tenderness
  (B) Temperature greater than 101°F (38.3°C)
  (C) Fiery-red tympanic membrane
  (D) Local tenderness of the tragus
  (E) Conductive hearing loss in the affected ear

8. After treatment of otitis media, what is the upper limit of time that is acceptable for resolution of effusion in the middle ear?

  (A) 10 days
  (B) 3 weeks
  (C) 6 weeks
  (D) 2 months
  (E) 16 weeks

9. The defining characteristic of malignant otitis externa is

  (A) Conductive hearing loss
  (B) *Pseudomonas* species
  (C) Associated diabetes mellitus
  (D) Osteomyelitis of the bony canal or mastoid
  (E) Requirement of intravenous antibiotics

10. A 35-year-old woman's routine audiogram at her place of employment found a conductive hearing loss on the left. She is vaguely aware of an increasing tendency to turn her right ear toward conversation and to use that ear on the telephone. She denies pain, recent upper-respiratory infection, atopic constitution, or allergic symptoms. Both eardrums are normal in appearance and move briskly when she performs a modified Valsalva maneuver. What is the most likely diagnosis?

  (A) Cholesteatoma
  (B) Temporomandibular joint (TMJ) syndrome
  (C) Secretory otitis media
  (D) Purulent otitis media
  (E) Otosclerosis

11. Which is most characteristic of the condition described in question 10?

  (A) African-Americans and Asians are particularly susceptible to the condition.
  (B) A conductive loss occurs in the face of a completely normal physical examination, including mobile tympanic membrane.
  (C) It constitutes a classic form of sensorineural hearing loss.
  (D) It is acquired secondary to noise exposure.
  (E) Pregnancy remediates the process.

12. A 55-year-old man complains of gradually increasing tinnitus over the past 2 years and two incidences of sudden drop in right-side hearing acuity. The first instance lasted 2 days; the second, 12 hours. With the first attack, the patient noted vertigo and was treated with a meclizine-containing prescription drug, by another physician. A Weber test lateralizes to the left ear. Which is an acceptable characterization of the pathophysiology of this patient's disease?

  (A) This disease is caused by recurrent otitis media in childhood.
  (B) The pathophysiology may involve an increased permeability of Reissner's membrane.
  (C) The condition is autoimmune based and responds in many cases to glucocorticoid administration.
  (D) Vertigo is rarely present.
  (E) The ossicles become adherent to one another.

13. Which pattern is most characteristic of noise-induced hearing loss?

  (A) Flat audiogram testing multiple frequencies
  (B) Low-frequency hearing loss
  (C) Early complaint of difficulty hearing at a conversational level
  (D) Early and deep involvement of the 4000 cycles-per-second frequency
  (E) Crisp response to a hearing aid

14. A 45-year-old man is sent to you for follow-up. Two days earlier the hospital emergency department diagnosed the hearing loss about which he had complained as left otitis media, for which amoxicillin was prescribed. You examine him and find that his tympanic membrane is mobile, and the color of the drum is normal. He denies previous coryza. The Weber test confirms sensorineural loss on the left (i.e., lateralizes to the right). Which statement characterizes his disease?

  (A) His disease is synonymous with cerebellopontine angle tumors.
  (B) Males are involved more than females in a ratio of 3:2.
  (C) Advanced cases can cause trigeminal nerve and visual dysfunction through space occupation.
  (D) Patients with this disease always present with sensorineural hearing loss.
  (E) The disease is a rapidly growing tumor that assumes malignant characteristics.

15. Which is associated with vertigo of peripheral origin (i.e., from the labyrinth rather than the central nervous system)?

    (A) Observable nystagmus, violent nausea, and vertigo begin immediately with the Hallpike maneuver.

    (B) Motion of the head is followed by violent symptoms that occur after a latent period.

    (C) Basilar artery insufficiency is among the causes.

    (D) Associated nystagmus exhibits pendular motion.

    (E) An associated conductive hearing loss occurs.

16. A 3-year-old girl presents with a foul-smelling post-nasal drip, a temperature of 102°F (38.8°C), and perceptible swelling of the face. Which is the most important reason to diagnose and treat this child's disease in a timely fashion?

    (A) It is associated with a malodorous discharge.

    (B) It is probably caused by maxillary sinusitis.

    (C) It may be caused by lactamase-producing organisms.

    (D) Orbital cellulitis is a feared complication.

    (E) Treatment must be carried out for 3 weeks.

17. Sore throat is one of the most common complaints encountered in a primary care setting. Which organism may be a cause of bacterial pharyngitis?

    (A) *Neisseria meningitidis*

    (B) *Staphylococcus aureus*

    (C) *Moraxella catarrhalis*

    (D) Beta-hemolytic *Streptococcus pyogenes*

    (E) All of the above

18. Which agent causes the majority of cases of symptomatic infectious pharyngitis (i.e., with sore throat)?

    (A) *Corynebacterium diphtheriae*

    (B) *Neisseria gonorrheae*

    (C) *Haemophilus influenzae*

    (D) Viruses

    (E) Beta-hemolytic *Streptococcus pyogenes*

19. In order to prevent rheumatic fever in children infected with beta-hemolytic *Streptococcus pyogenes,* treatment must begin within how many days after onset?

    (A) 2 days

    (B) 5 days

    (C) 9 days

    (D) 15 days

    (E) 20 days

20. Of the following conditions, which can present a clinical picture most like infectious mononucleosis?

    (A) Streptococcal pharyngitis

    (B) Non-Hodgkin's lymphoma

    (C) Cytomegalovirus infection

    (D) Influenza virus infection

    (E) Coxsackie virus infection

21. A 20-year-old, male medical student complains of severe sore throat for 3 days and of inability to ingest solid foods for the past 2 days. He appears moderately ill, and in pain, with his head held in a "sniffing"-type position, lips slightly parted, grimacing while swallowing saliva. His temperature is 101°F (38.3°C). His cervical lymph nodes are visibly and palpably enlarged; his tonsils are present and show a mixed white and yellowish exudate against an erythematous and edematous background. The rim of the epiglottis, visible above the base of the tongue, appears normal in color and size. A survey for other adenopathy yields nothing of note, and an abdominal examination is negative for masses and organomegaly. A rapid streptococcal screen is negative; therefore, you order a stat spot test for mononucleosis, which is also negative. Despite the negative findings, and because of the patient's state of illness, you decide to prescribe penicillin V K+, 250 mg, 4 times daily, for 10 days. The patient returns in 4 days complaining of no improvement; he appears just as uncomfortable as before, and the cervical adenopathy has not abated. Which is the most logical measure you should take at this time?

    (A) Change the antibiotic to ampicillin 500 mg, 3 times a day, for the balance of 10 days, and instruct the patient to return in 48–72 hours.

    (B) Consult a general surgeon in anticipation of cervical node biopsy.

    (C) Change the antibiotic to a newer macrolide (e.g., clarithromycin) for the balance of 10 days.

    (D) Repeat the monospot test.

    (E) Hospitalize the patient and consult an infectious disease specialist.

22. Which of the following sinuses are most frequently infected as complications of viral upper respiratory infections?

(A) Frontal
(B) Maxillary
(C) Anterior ethmoid
(D) Posterior ethmoid
(E) Sphenoid

23. A 27-year old woman, who says she has "hay fever" in the spring and fall of the year, complains of recurrence of symptoms present with colds and sometimes without preceding coryza. She complains she awoke with pain in the left cheek area as well as in the center of her head and left frontal area. Upon examination, you find tenderness over the left medial zygomatic arch, but no tenderness over the frontal area. Which structures are involved in this disease?

(A) Left medial turbinate and left otitis media
(B) Left frontal sinus and left temporomandibular joint
(C) Left maxillary and frontal sinuses
(D) Left maxillary and sphenoid sinuses
(E) Left anterior ethmoid and left frontal sinuses

DIRECTIONS (Item 24): The numbered item in this section is negatively phrased, as indicated by the capitalized word, NOT. Select the ONE lettered answer that is BEST in this case.

24. A 56-year-old patient complains of hearing loss on both sides, on the fifth day of taking a drug you prescribed for him for the first time last week. The Rinné test shows air conduction better than bone conduction in both ears. Which drug would NOT be associated with this patient's hearing loss?

(A) Doxycycline
(B) Kanamycin
(C) Neomycin
(D) Ethacrynic acid
(E) Streptomycin

DIRECTIONS (Items 25–29): The matching questions in this section consist of a list of five lettered options, followed by several numbered items that represent throat conditions. For each numbered item, select the ONE lettered option that is most closely associated with it. Each lettered option may be selected once, more than once, or not at all.

(A) Rhinovirus
(B) Infectious mononucleosis
(C) Thumb sign
(D) *Staphylococcus aureus*
(E) Beta-hemolytic *Streptococcus pyogenes*

25. Incidental finding on culture for sore throat

26. Sore throat that is worse in the morning and is present 2 days

27. Severe sore throat throughout the day for 7 days. Tonsillar membrane; painful to swallow saliva. Cervical lymph nodes are enlarged but not tender.

28. Epiglottiditis

29. Coryza and cough associated with sore throat

ANSWERS AND EXPLANATIONS

1. The answer is A. An accepted, rational approach to the treatment of rhinitis medicamentosa (the condition indicated by the symptoms) is immediate withdrawal from the spray, followed by inhaled glucocorticoids for a brief period to aid in withdrawal, combined with the use of mist or warm, moist towels for nasal inhalation. Another approach is short-term, systemic glucocorticoid. Prescription of longer-lasting, topical decongestants is not a solution to this problem, which has been brought on by the overuse of such medications. Rhinitis medicamentosa is the condition of rebound bogginess caused by local tissue refractoriness to the effects of a topical decongestant. It may be viewed as addiction at a local level, so that withdrawal of the medication, as between doses, produces an effect opposite to that of the medication itself. (This is analogous to the occurrence of seizures upon withdrawal of a sedative/anticonvulsant such as diazepam.) When topical decongestants are prescribed, they should be used only intermittently, most likely on only one side of the nose, at bedtime.

2. The answer is C. Because the setting is classic for an anterior epistaxis, which is venous in origin, the bleeding site should be identified and cauterized with silver nitrate. Many cases of anterior epistaxes resolve without treatment after a few bouts; others cease for a time after topical applications of phenylephrine; those that still recur almost always respond to cauterization of the site. Anterior epistaxes occur at all ages; they may be associated with allergic rhinitis or with drying by indoor heat during the winter, and they are often precipitated by digital agitation by the patient. The measures represented in the other answer choices (consulting with an otolaryngologist, giving the patient a 10-mg capsule of fast-acting nifedipine, tamponading the side of bleeding with a catheter balloon, and sedating the patient with meperidine) are useful in cases of *posterior* epistaxes, in the setting of uncontrolled hypertension, almost always in individuals of middle age or older. Posterior epistaxes, which may also occur in the elderly in the absence of hypertension, are likely to appear from both nares, and are very difficult to control by external measures.

3. The answer is A. Atopic constitution is the most prevalent underlying factor in recurrent otitis media; food allergies alone account for 78%. An atopic constitution, which possesses an inherent tendency for atopic allergies, gives the individual a tendency for mucosa membrane reactivity as a nonspecific response to numerous assaults besides exposure to an allergen (e.g., viral infection, changes in temperature or humidity). Native American race, but not African-American race, is a factor in recurrent otitis media. Contrary to earlier teaching, tonsillar hypertrophy and tonsillitis are not factors; however, adenoidal hypertrophy is the second most prevalent underlying risk factor. Another risk factor is congenital palatal deformity. Exposure to a population with increased incidence of viral upper-respiratory infection (URI) is also an underlying risk factor, because the most common precipitating insult is viral URI superimposed on one of the foregoing risks. Anterior attached frenulum ("tongue tied" state) is not a risk factor for recurrent otitis media.

4. The answer is C. Respiratory syncytial viruses carry an approximate 33% risk of otitis media as a sequela. Adenoviruses and influenza viruses are associated with a 28% incidence each. The others mentioned, along with parainfluenza viruses, are associated with a significantly lower incidence.

5. The answer is B. *Streptococcus pneumoniae,* *Haemophilus influenzae,* and *Moraxella catarrhalis* are the three most frequent bacterial causes of otitis media. *Streptococcus pyogenes,* the cause of "strep" pharyngitis and tonsillitis, is the agent of otitis media in just 5% of cases.

6. The answer is B. Among organisms involved in otitis media, a proportion approximating 20%–30% would be expected to be resistant to penicillin, ampicillin, and amoxicillin. *Haemophilus influenzae* causes 19% of otitis media cases; one third of these (responsible for about 6% of all cases) are highly lactamase producing. *Moraxella catarrhalis* causes about 22% of cases; 80%–90% of these bacteria (about 20% of the total) are "low grade" producers (i.e., are relatively resistant).

7. The answer is E. Conductive hearing loss in the affected ear (assuming it is a hearing ear) is a *sine qua non* for otitis media. A common mistake is over-interpreting a perceived color change in the eardrum, without finding out whether a conductive hearing loss is present before making the diagnosis. Color changes associated with otitis media vary from fiery red through purple, as well as the creamy hue of pus. On the other hand, apparent color change may be the stable state of an eardrum overlain with vascular ectasia.

8. The answer is E. While most children show a nearly normal middle ear within 3–4 weeks after the start of treatment (or, often, even without treatment), otolaryngologists define a case in which effusion persists as "failure-to-respond" only when 16 weeks have passed.

9. The answer is D. By definition, osteomyelitis of the bony canal or mastoid is present in malignant otitis externa. The characteristics listed in the other answer choices are true of malignant otitis media, but only osteomyelitis of the bony canal or mastoid is defining. Although a conductive hearing loss is often present in external otitis secondary to debris blocking the canal, it is not necessary for the diagnosis and not necessarily present in either uncomplicated or malignant external otitis. Pseudomonas species remains the most common pathogen. Associated diabetes mellitus is the most common underlying condition rendering the patient susceptible, and intravenous antibiotics are virtually always required.

10. The answer is E. The most likely diagnosis is otosclerosis. Cholesteatoma is a chronic granulomatous complication of chronic or recurrent otitis media with a perforated eardrum. Physical findings show the eardrum and middle ear are grossly abnormal, with the anatomy greatly distorted. Both secretory and purulent otitis media show immobile eardrums, the former with sterile fluid or hemorrhage visible behind the drum, and the latter with pus visible along with annular erythema. Temporomandibular joint (TMJ) syndrome causes pain in the area of the ear, but without hearing loss.

11. The answer is B. In otosclerosis, a conductive loss occurs in the face of a completely normal physical examination, including the finding of a mobile tympanic membrane. In all other forms of conductive hearing loss, either the external canal is occluded on examination, or the tympanic membrane is immobile or nearly immobile (as a result of purulent or serous exudate) or nonfunctional (as a result of perforation). A conductive loss is the first clinical manifestation; the loss is curable through surgery. Only in advanced, complicated cases may sensorineural loss result (from erosion into the labyrinth). Otosclerosis is inherited as an incompletely penetrant, Mendelian dominant trait, and its progress is accelerated by pregnancy. Asians are virtually without risk of this condition.

12. The answer is B. The pathophysiology of Meniere's disease (to which the symptoms point) may involve an increased permeability of Reissner's membrane. None of the other statements is true regarding Meniere's disease, a condition that can cause a sensorineural hearing loss, tinnitus, and vertigo. Although severe vertigo is the trademark of Meniere's disease, it does not occur in a significant minority of cases. The condition responds in many cases to dietary salt restriction and to judicious use of diuretics. Ablative surgery may be required.

13. The answer is D. The 4000 cycles per second (cps) is the first and most severely affected frequency (deepest loss on a tonal audiogram) involved in noise-induced hearing loss. (A standard audiogram tests a patient's threshold for hearing at 250–8000 cps. Spoken conversation occurs between 250 and 2000 cps.) Noise-induced hearing loss is sensorineural. A flat audiogram is more characteristic of a conductive than of a sensorineural loss. Early involvement of conversational frequencies is not a strong characteristic of noise-induced loss, because most conversation occurs at lower frequencies. Noise-induced, sensorineural hearing loss is not as amenable to correction by a hearing aid as is conductive loss.

14. The answer is C. Advanced cases of acoustic neuromas (also called acoustic neurinomas), the disease to which the symptoms point, can cause trigeminal nerve and visual dysfunction as a result of space occupation. Little more than 50% of patients with acoustic neuromas present with hearing loss (sensorineural); others present with tinnitus (16%), vertigo (9%), or unsteadiness. Acoustic neurinoma makes up 78% of cerebellopontine angle tumors, so it is not synonymous with that group. Females are involved more than males in a ratio of 3:2. When acoustic neuroma is bilateral (2%–3% of cases), it may be a manifestation of Von Recklinghausen's disease. The tumor grows slowly and assumes benign characteristics.

15. The answer is B. Motion of the head that affects the semicircular canals, followed by violent symptoms that occur after a latent period of 3–60 seconds (most often 15–20 seconds), characterizes vertigo of peripheral origin (labyrinth rather than CNS). (Symptoms that begin immediately upon motion of the head, rather than after a period of latency, are characteristic of centrally based vertigo.) Vertigo of peripheral origin manifests a positive Hallpike maneuver, characterized by typical nystagmus (whipping or fast motion, alternating with a slower recovery phase), after a latency period. It is caused by vestibular neuronitis, benign positional vertigo, and Meniere's disease, among others. It tends to be relieved by fixation of gaze upon a fixed point. It is seldom associated with hearing loss.

16. The answer is D. The feared complication, orbital cellulitis, is the *most important* reason to diagnose ethmoid sinusitis (ethmoiditis) in timely fashion. Maxillary sinusitis does not occur until preadolescence. Ethmoid sinusitis is associated with a malodorous discharge, and it may be caused by lactamase-producing organisms. In cases diagnosed early, treatment may be completed within 10 days instead of an otherwise mandatory 3 weeks.

17. The answer is D. Beta-hemolytic *Streptococcus pyogenes* causes more than 95% of bacterial pharyngitis. Other bacterial causes are rare; they include *Corynebac-*

terium diphtheriae, Neisseria gonorrhoeae, and, if epiglottitis is included as pharyngitis, *Haemophilus influenzae.*

18. The answer is D. Viral infections account for 62%–90% of pharyngitis cases. All the other answer choices are bacterial causes. (See answer to question 16.)

19. The answer is C. Children infected with beta-hemolytic *Streptococcus pyogenes* must be treated within 7–9 days to assure prevention of rheumatic fever.

20. The answer is C. Cytomegalovirus infection tends to present a clinical picture similar to that of infectious mononucleosis (i.e., the patient may present with severe exudative pharyngitis, enlarged, nontender cervical adenopathy, and generalized lymphadenopathy). Along with infectious mononucleosis and toxoplasmosis, cytomegalovirus infection constitutes one of "seronegative mononucleosis" syndromes. The characteristics that differentiate these diseases from streptococcal pharyngitis are the surprising lack of tenderness in the otherwise impressive adenopathy, and the systemic symptoms devoid of significant fever.

21. The answer is D. The most logical measure in this situation is to repeat the Monospot test. Considering the description and the severity of symptoms in the absence of tenderness, the clinical picture is classic for infectious mononucleosis. The immunologic screens and the heterophile agglutination test are known to require 5–7 days of illness before they become positive. Nevertheless, despite the negative strep screen, the decision to treat the disease as streptococcal is justified in light of the degree of illness. Rapid screening tests are only 80%–87% sensitive. Generalized adenopathy, despite the pathophysiology of infectious mononucleosis, is often not appreciable. The cervical adenopathy is frequently notable posteriorly in infectious mononucleosis and anteriorly in streptococcal disease, but the distinction is not dependable. If this patient has infectious mononucleosis, he has a greater than 90% chance of developing a morbilliform rash if he is given ampicillin (compared with a 5% chance without such treatment).

22. The answer is B. The maxillary sinuses are infected (usually not at clinically severe degrees) in 87% of upper respiratory infections. The ethmoids (anterior and posterior together) are involved in 65%; the sphenoids in 39%; and the frontals in 32%. These infections are clinically significant in only 0.5%–5% of cases.

23. The answer is D. The left maxillary and sphenoid sinuses are involved in this disease. The patient has the setting of acute sinusitis (on this occasion in the absence of a preceding viral upper respiratory infection) in an atopic individual. The referral patterns and tenderness are those of the left sphenoid sinus (pain in the center of the head and frontal areas, without the frontal tenderness that accompanies frontal sinusitis) and left maxillary sinus (pain located over the maxilla, with associated local tenderness). [See Table 1.5 (p. 23) in *Family Medicine* (House Officer Series) for pain and tenderness patterns associated with various sinuses.]

24. The answer is A. Doxycycline is NOT associated with sensorineural hearing loss (VIII nerve damage). Kanamycin, neomycin, ethacrynic acid, and streptomycin are each associated with such loss.

25. The answer is D. *Staphylococcus aureus* is an incidental finding on throat cultures done for symptomatic sore throat. The only bacterial pathogens that cause symptomatic pharyngitis are *Streptococcus pyogenes, Corynebacterium diphtheriae,* and *Neisseria gonorrhoeae.*

26. The answer is A. Rhinovirus, the most common cause of the common cold, produces a sore throat that is typically worse in the morning than later in the day, unlike streptococcal pharyngitis which tends to be worse toward the end of the day when fatigue begins to occur. The 2-day sore throat may be followed by coryza, which helps to identify the condition as a viral "cold."

27. The answer is B. In infectious mononucleosis, nontender enlarged cervical lymph nodes are the rule (as distinguished from cases of streptococcal disease with notable adenopathy, in which the nodes are almost always tender). The tonsillar membrane is often present and takes on a yellowish hue after the first few days. Epiglottiditis does not cause such a membrane.

28. The answer is C. The thumb sign is a radiographic sign virtually pathognomonic for epiglottiditis in the presence of the symptoms of sore throat and inspiratory stridor. The lateral view of the neck on x-ray shows edema of the epiglottis in the shape of a lateral view of an extended thumb.

29. The answer is A. The cause is rhinovirus when coryza and a cough are associated with a sore throat. Neither streptococcus sore throat nor any of the other answer choices cause this combination of symptoms.

BIBLIOGRAPHY

Rudy, DR: Problems of the ears, nose and throat. In *Family Medicine* (House Officer Series). Edited by Rudy DR, Kurowski K. Baltimore, Williams & Wilkins, 1997, pp 1–26.

Test 2

Problems of the Oral Cavity

DIRECTIONS (Items 1–11): Each of the numbered items or incomplete statements in this section is followed by answers or by completions of the statement. Select the ONE lettered answer or completion that is BEST in each case.

1. One of the most frequently asked questions of the family physician or pediatrician has to do with the time at which deciduous teeth are expected to erupt. What is the mean age of children at the eruption of the last of the deciduous dentition?

(A) 4 months
(B) 6 months
(C) 18 months
(D) 27 months
(E) 4 years

2. The first permanent tooth eruptions occur when children are at which age?

(A) 4–5 years
(B) 6–7 years
(C) 9–10 years
(D) 12–13 years
(E) 17–22 years

3. At which age range does the peak period of eruption of the third molars (wisdom teeth) occur?

(A) 6–7 years
(B) 11–11.5 years
(C) 15–15.5 years
(D) 20–20.5 years
(E) 22–24 years

4. A male teenager complains of having severe mouth soreness for 10 days. Examination discloses a fetid odor and fibrous pseudomembrane on many gingival crests. The name of his condition is

(A) Necrotizing gingivitis
(B) Periodontal abscess
(C) Dentigerous cyst
(D) Herpes labialis
(E) Molar impaction

5. A homeless, 42-year-old male with a history of poor dental hygiene complains of pain and swelling in the floor of his mouth. Physical examination shows edema of the area of the anterior neck as it merges with the tissue between the two mandibles. What is this form of infection?

(A) Caseous scrofula
(B) Lymph node infection secondary to dental caries
(C) Coronary insufficiency
(D) Ludwig's angina
(E) Mucosal epidermolysis

6. A 4-year-old boy suffered trauma to the mouth (today) that resulted in the loss of his upper left incisor. The mother says the child fell. Examination reveals a contusion of the upper lip, a fresh 1-cm laceration on the buccal surface of the upper lip, and a contusion, of blue, brown, and yellowish hues, on the buttock. What is the most likely cause of the traumatic loss of the tooth?

(A) A fall
(B) Chemical ingestion
(C) Electrical burns
(D) Dog bites
(E) Child abuse

7. A 34-year-old woman complains of bilateral jaw swelling which is found to result from parotid gland swelling. She exhibits cheilitis at the corners of the mouth. The most likely cause of this enlargement is

(A) Mumps
(B) Staphylococcal infection
(C) Sialolithiasis
(D) Pernicious anemia
(E) Sjögren's syndrome

8. During a routine periodic evaluation, gingival hypertrophy is found in a 25-year-old male patient who has a history of cerebral palsy and seizures. The most likely cause is

(A) Heredity
(B) Medication
(C) Ascorbic acid deficiency
(D) Poor oral hygiene
(E) Mycotic overgrowth

9. Which organism is virtually the sole cause of cellulitis seeded by caries in the United States?

(A) *Haemophilus influenza*
(B) Beta-hemolytic *Streptococcus pyogenes*
(C) *Streptococcus pneumoniae*
(D) *Moraxella catarrhalis*
(E) *Staphylococcus aureus*

10. Which are the most commonly impacted (chronically unerupted or partially erupted) teeth in the adult?

    (A) Third molars
    (B) First premolars
    (C) Second molars
    (D) Upper central incisors
    (E) Lower cuspids

11. Petechiae of the mucosa overlying the hard palate are associated with which nonbacterial disease?

    (A) Herpes simplex I
    (B) Infectious mononucleosis
    (C) Herpes simplex II
    (D) *Haemophilus influenzae* infection
    (E) Rhinovirus infection

DIRECTIONS (Items 12–15): Each of the numbered items or incomplete statements in this section is negatively phrased, as indicated by a capitalized word such as NOT, LEAST, or EXCEPT. Select the ONE lettered answer or completion that is BEST in each case.

---

12. Despite the protection afforded by lifelong exposure to fluoridated drinking water, dental caries may form in children's teeth. The risk factors include all of the following EXCEPT

    (A) A diet rich in refined carbohydrates
    (B) Poor oral hygiene
    (C) Tetracycline exposure before the eruption of deciduous teeth
    (D) Xerostomia
    (E) Radiation therapy

13. A 35-year-old man complains of irritation of the tongue for 2 weeks. Examination shows fiery redness of the entire dorsum of the tongue. The causes of his condition could include any of the following EXCEPT

    (A) Pernicious anemia
    (B) Riboflavin deficiency
    (C) Iron deficiency
    (D) Excessive smoking
    (E) Rubeola

14. A 23-year-old woman complains of a nonhealing "canker" sore of the mouth. In considering the many possible causes of gingival stomatitis, which one of the following etiologies would you NOT consider in the differential diagnosis of this finding?

    (A) Odontogenesis imperfecta
    (B) Herpes simplex I
    (C) Herpes simplex II
    (D) Cytomegalovirus
    (E) Streptococcal periodontitis

15. A 4-year-old boy has been slow to reach expected milestones in speech although all other developmental milestones have been met on schedule. Your examination reveals that he is unable to touch the upper anterior dental arch with the tip of his tongue. He has a mandibular lingual frenum. All of the following are true of this condition EXCEPT

    (A) It is called "ankyloglossia."
    (B) It is called "tongue-tie."
    (C) Surgical intervention is rarely required in uncomplicated cases.
    (D) It may compromise periodontal status, an indication for frenotomy or frenectomy.
    (E) The speech impediment is likely to be a functional one.

ANSWERS AND EXPLANATIONS

1. The answer is D. Children's mean age at the eruption of the last of the deciduous teeth is approximately 27 months. Deciduous dentition is completed in a mesiolateral gradient; the first eruptions occur at approximately 7.5 months and the last by 30 months. Children's peak ages at the eruption of teeth are as follows: Maxillary and mandibular incisors, 7.5–9.3 months; mandibular and maxillary lateral incisors, 11.0–13.2 months; mandibular and maxillary cuspids, 15.6–16.0 months; mandibular and maxillary first molars, 19.5–19.6 months; mandibular and maxillary second molars 26.5–28.0 months.

2. The answer is B. The first permanent tooth eruptions occur in children of 6–7 years of age.

3. The answer is D. The peak period for the eruption of the third molars (the last permanent teeth to erupt) is in the age range of 20–20.5 years. The peak times for eruptions of earlier permanent dentition are as follows: first premolars, 6.0–6.3 years; central and lateral mandibular incisors, 7.2 years; central and lateral maxillary incisors, 8.5 years; mandibular cuspids ("canines"), 9.7 years; maxillary cuspids, 11.6 years; first premolars 10.0–10.7 years; second premolars (maxillary before mandibular), 10.7–11.5 years; first molars, 6–7 years; second molars, 10.7–11.5 years; and third molars ("wisdom teeth"), 20–20.5 years.

4. The answer is A. The patient's condition is necrotizing gingivitis. Gingivitis progresses to periodontitis, which, if untreated and severe, leads to acute necrotizing gingivitis (trench mouth). A periodontal abscess generally involves only a single tooth and occurs as acute, localized, severe pain. A dentigerous cyst is an expanding cyst that contains an unerupted tooth, usually a third molar. Herpes labialis is herpes simplex, usually type I, involving the lips. An impacted molar is a partially erupted molar, thus subject to infection.

5. The answer is D. This form of oral cavity infection is Ludwig's angina, which is cellulitis of the submandibular space by extension from the sublingual area. It usually results from the infection of a dental site, such as the site of an extraction or root canal therapy, or from an abscessed third molar. Caseous scrofula is tuberculous cervical lymph nodes. Infectious lymphadenopathy (the result, for example, of dental caries) presents as palpable nodules rather than cellulitis of the floor of the mouth. Coronary insufficiency may cause pain referred to the jaw or neck, but would result in no local physical findings.

6. The answer is E. Child abuse is the probable cause of this child's loss of a tooth. The finding of two sites of trauma of different ages reinforces that likelihood. Child abuse is officially the leading cause of injury to children's teeth.

7. The answer is E. Sjögren's syndrome, an autoimmune disease that occurs more commonly in women than in men, is characterized by parotid gland swelling, angular cheilitis, and xerostomia. Mumps is not characterized by cheilitis (nor xerostomia). Neither staphylococcal infection nor sialolithiasis is likely to be bilateral, as was this woman's swelling. Pernicious anemia is not a cause of parotid or other salivary gland enlargement.

8. The answer is B. The most likely cause of gingival hypertrophy in this patient is drug related. Drug-induced gingival overgrowth is usually caused by phenytoin, cyclosporin, nifedipine, or nitrendipine. In this case, phenytoin is the likely cause if the patient (who is subject to seizures) is on that anticonvulsant. Hereditary gingival hyperplasia is the cause in only a small percentage of cases. The differential diagnosis does not include vitamin deficiency, but the bleeding that accompanies vitamin C deficiency may be confused with hyperplasia. Oral hygiene is preventative. Surgery is a viable option. Fluoridation prevents progression of this disease. Candida overgrowth may cause a membranous stomatitis, but not gingival hyperplasia.

9. The answer is B. Beta-hemolytic *Streptococcus* is virtually the only bacterial cause of cellulitis seeded by caries in the United States. In fact, *Streptococcus pyogenes* group A, along with groups C, G, and B (group B being generally less virulent than group A) account for most bacterial infection in the oral cavity. In pharyngitis, after diphtheria and gonorrhea, groups C and G *Streptococcus pyogenes, Francisella tularensis, Corynebacterium haemolyticum,* and fusospirochetal organisms (seen in Vincent's angina) make up a minority of bacterial causes. (However, missing from serious treatises on the subject are *Streptococcus pneumoniae, Moraxella catarrhalis,* and *Staphylococcus aureus.*)

10. The answer is A. In the adult, the third molars ("wisdom teeth") are commonly only partially erupted. In that state, they are the foci of frequent abscesses, caused by beta-hemolytic *Streptococcus pyogenes.* Third molars that remain totally unerupted may form dentigerous cysts that grow slowly over time, taking on the characteristics of benign tumors, dislodging other teeth, and eroding the maxillary or mandibular arch.

11. The answer is B. Infectious mononucleosis is a nonbacterial cause of petechiae over the hard palate. (Streptococcal pharyngitis is a bacterial cause.)

12. The answer is C. Tetracycline exposure that occurs before eruption of the deciduous teeth does NOT constitute a risk for formation of dental caries, although it does constitutes a high risk for mottling of the teeth. Poor hygiene permits culturing of bacteria in vulnerable niches. A diet high in carbohydrates assists in rapid acid formation against the teeth. Xerostomia (dryness of the mouth from salivary gland dysfunction) probably deprives the mouth of antibacterial defenses present in saliva. The same may be true of radiation therapy.

13. The answer is E. Rubeola ("hard measles") does NOT cause glossitis (inflammation of the tongue). It produces the classic, buccal Koplik spot. Pernicious anemia, riboflavin deficiency, iron deficiency, and excessive smoking may cause glossitis.

14. The answer is A. You would NOT consider odontogenesis imperfecta (congenitally fragile dentition) in the differential diagnosis of gingival stomatitis. Herpes simplex I and II, cytomegalovirus, and streptococcal periodontitis (the cause of acute necrotizing gingivitis) are well-known causes of gingival stomatitis.

15. The answer is E. A speech impediment is NOT likely to be of functional origin in a child with lingual immobility caused by a mandibular lingual frenum. All of the other answer choices are true. The abnormality is also called ankyloglossia. Another name, "tongue-tie," refers to the effects the condition has on speech, one of the indications for correction. Compromise of periodontal status may occur and constitute another indication for frenotomy (incision of the frenum) or frenectomy (excision of the frenum). Although the case presented in this question is likely an exception, surgical intervention is rarely required.

BIBLIOGRAPHY

Tryon AF, Stechfus CF: Problems of the oral cavity. In *Family Medicine* (House Officer Series). Edited by Rudy DR, Kurowski K. Baltimore, Williams & Wilkins, 1997, pp 27–42.

Test 3

Headache

DIRECTIONS (Items 1–14): Each of the numbered items or incomplete statements in this section is followed by answers or by completions of the statement. Select the ONE lettered answer or completion that is BEST in each case.

1. Approximately what percentage of adult women experience at least one migraine headache per year?

(A) 5%
(B) 10%
(C) 15–20%
(D) 25–30%
(E) 40–50%

2. A 30-year-old woman complains of a 10-year history of headaches. The headaches encircle her head, are noted only at the end of work days, and have always been quickly relieved by acetaminophen. The patient notes an increase in her headaches when she is under stress. Which of the following characteristics is most commonly associated with this type of headache?

(A) An aura experienced about 30 minutes before the onset of the headache
(B) Nausea with several episodes of emesis during the headache
(C) A gradual, often not precisely noticed, start and end to the headache
(D) An incidence approximately three times higher in men than in women
(E) An occurrence frequently caused by oral contraceptive usage

3. Which symptom is commonly associated with tension headaches?

(A) Flashing lights
(B) Homonymous scotomas
(C) Retro-orbital location of headache pain
(D) Facial flushing
(E) Sleep pattern disturbance

4. A 27-year-old woman describes right-side, throbbing, parietal headaches which began to occur in her high school years. Her headaches last about 24 hours and are associated with some nausea and photophobia. They are often brought on by stressful events. No trauma has occurred. She notes no focal neurologic symptoms before the headache, but senses fatigue a few minutes beforehand. The diagnosis that best fits this pattern is

(A) Migraine headache without aura
(B) Migraine headache with aura
(C) Cluster headache
(D) Status migrainosus
(E) Tension headache

5. You are examining a 42-year-old woman who describes a very severe headache that developed abruptly, 45 minutes earlier, in her occipital area and upper neck. She says the intensity of the pain was worse than labor pains. She denies any history of chronic headache, any drug use, or use of any prescription medication. She has no allergies. Her temperature = 99.9°F (37.7°C); blood pressure = 150/90; respiratory rate = 16; pulse = 100 and regular. She has no ecchymoma, no bruits. Her pupils are equal and reactive; fundi appear normal; extraocular movements are normal. She has no cervical spine tenderness, but resistance to flexing and rotation is present. The patient is sleepy but arousable. She can respond to questions, but frequently they must be repeated. She can move all extremities, and sensation to touch is intact to all extremities. Deep tendon reflexes are 2+ on a 4-point scale (DTR 2/4) at biceps, knee, and ankle. Which would you order FIRST to evaluate this patient?

(A) Computed tomography (CT) scan of head without contrast
(B) CT scan of head with contrast
(C) Magnetic resonance imaging (MRI) of the brain
(D) Cerebrospinal fluid examination (CSF)
(E) Erythrocyte sedimentation rate (ESR)

6. A 60-year-old man complains of a 1-week history of generalized, mild headaches, accompanied by pain in his jaw muscles with chewing. He denies any history of trauma or of past chronic headaches. He does not drink alcohol, takes no medication, and denies any drug use. He denies any visual changes. His temperature = 99.5°F (37.5°C); blood pressure = 130/80; respiratory rate = 16; heart rate = 70 and regular. No ecchymosis, no swelling are present. His pupils are equal and reactive to light; extraocular movements are normal; discs are clear. In the pharynx, no erythema, no exudate, no peritonsillar swelling are found. The neck is supple, with no adenopathy, no bruits. The patient is oriented "times 3" (i.e., in three spheres; oriented with respect to person, time, and space), is alert, and is communicating well. Motor strength is normal; all extremities are normal; sensation to pin prick is intact in all extremities; DTR 2/4 in biceps, knee, and ankle; gross visual field by confrontation is normal. Which would you order FIRST to evaluate this patient?

(A) A CT scan of the head without contrast
(B) A CT scan of the head with contrast
(C) An MRI of the brain
(D) A sedimentation rate
(E) A temporal artery biopsy

7. What is the most common presenting sign or symptom of an intracerebral arteriovenous malformation?

(A) Focal neurologic deficits
(B) Intracranial hemorrhage
(C) New onset of seizures
(D) Headache
(E) Photophobia

8. A 32-year-old man hit his head against the windshield during a motor-vehicle accident. The windshield did not crack and the patient did not lose consciousness. In the emergency room, examination of the man's head showed some tenderness and swelling of the mid-frontal scalp. He was alert and oriented times 3, and the results of his ear examination were normal. He had full strength and sensation in all extremities, and normal deep tendon reflexes. Cervical spine x-rays were negative, and a CT scan of the head without contrast showed no skull fractures and no areas of hemorrhage. Now, 1 week since the injury, he has no residual scalp or frontal tenderness, but he continues to complain of headaches. A repeat CT scan of the head without contrast continues to show no evidence of hemorrhage. He denies a prior history of headaches. Which is characteristic of patients with this type of headache?

(A) Headaches last for only a few days to a week after the injury.
(B) Patients report no associated symptoms, such as visual changes, vertigo, or light-headedness.
(C) Headaches are typically very severe.
(D) Headaches are more likely if the patient's head trauma was accompanied by a concussion.
(E) Areas of contusion would usually be visible with a CT scan of the head with contrast or with an MRI.

9. Which headache patient would be appropriately treated with oral sumatriptan? (Assume that treatment will start immediately and that no other interventions or precautions are exercised.)

(A) A 58-year-old man who has hypertension, hypercholesterolemia, and type II diabetes mellitus, but no history of angina
(B) A 40-year-old woman with cluster headaches and no significant, past medical history
(C) A 30-year-old woman, pregnant, at 10 weeks gestation
(D) A 28-year-old man with basilar migraine
(E) A 32-year-old woman whose migraine did not respond to a sublingual ergotamine tablet taken 4 hours earlier

10. A 32-year-old woman complains of a 2-year history of chronic headaches which causes her to miss several days of work each month. Every week she gets 2–3 attacks, each lasting about 20 hours and each preceded by a visual distortion that ends when the headache starts. Her past medical history is otherwise unremarkable. An agent shown to be effective in prophylaxis against this type of headache is

(A) Amitriptyline
(B) Sumatriptan
(C) Fiorinal®
(D) Midrin®
(E) Codeine

11. Which treatment option is beneficial in cluster headaches but not in other types of primary headaches?

(A) Sumatriptan
(B) Verapamil
(C) Sublingual ergotamine
(D) Oxygen inhalation
(E) Analgesia

12. A youth of 8–10 years has been experiencing bouts of weekly headaches for 2 years. What is the most common cause of such headaches in a person of this age?

(A) Migraine, tension, or other primary headache
(B) Carbon monoxide exposure
(C) Child abuse
(D) Side effects of a medication
(E) Lead poisoning

13. You are interpreting the results of the sedimentation rate of a 60-year-old patient. In a patient of this age, which factor produces a higher "normal range" for this test?

(A) Renal failure
(B) Polymyalgia rheumatica (PMR)
(C) Liver failure
(D) Sepsis
(E) Female sex

14. A 22-year-old male patient complains of a 1-month history of headaches in the right temporal area which he notices all day, every day, at varying degrees of severity. He reports that the headaches are present when he awakens in the morning and increase when he sits up or gets out of bed. He is seeking treatment because the headaches, which are generally mild in intensity, are persistent and seem to be increasing in intensity. He denies any head or neck trauma; any numbness, weakness, or vision changes; any cough; and any history of headaches (except for a day or two during "colds"). His family and friends report that he seems more labile emotionally. He was diagnosed with mitral valve prolapse 3 years ago, but has otherwise been healthy. He has not traveled within the last year, and an HIV test a year ago was negative. No one in his family or in his household has experienced headaches, and he has no potential carbon monoxide exposure at his workplace. His temperature is 98.9°F (37.2°C); blood pressure is 117/83; respiratory rate is 16 and regular; and pulse is 80. No bruising or swelling is evident on his face or skull; he is fully alert; his pupils are equal and reactive. Fundoscopic examination shows sharp disc margins. No tenderness is exhibited over the frontal or maxillary sinuses. Motor and sensory examinations are normal on the face and in all extremities. The right frontal and maxillary sinuses transilluminate normally. You do not appreciate any cranial bruits. The neck is supple, and no cervical adenopathy is evident. Which of the following is the most appropriate next step in this patient's evaluation and management?

(A) A sedimentation rate
(B) Sinus x-rays
(C) A CT scan of the head without contrast
(D) A CBC with differential
(E) A magnetic resonance (MR) study of the head

DIRECTIONS (Items 15–16): Each of the numbered items or incomplete statements in this section is negatively phrased, as indicated by a capitalized word such as NOT, LEAST, or EXCEPT. Select the ONE lettered answer or completion that is BEST in each case.

---

15. All of the following are associated with temporal arteritis EXCEPT

(A) Pain in the hip and shoulder girdle
(B) A loss of unilateral vision
(C) Pain in the jaw muscles during mastication
(D) A photosensitive, macular rash over the facial cheeks
(E) A fever

16. Which is NOT a common side effect of, or contraindication for, dihydroergotamine mesylate (DHE)?

(A) It can cause nausea and emesis.
(B) It can cause ischemic heart disease.
(C) It is contraindicated in patients on monoamine oxidase inhibitors.
(D) It is contraindicated in patients with Prinzmetal's angina.
(E) It is contraindicated in pregnancy.

ANSWERS AND EXPLANATIONS

1. The answer is C. About 17% of adult females and 5% of adult males experience one or more migraines per year.

2. The answer is C. This patient is describing a tension headache, which is typically associated with a gradual, often not precisely noticed, start and end. This slower, more insidious onset distinguishes it from a migraine headache. The presence of an aura and the exacerbation by menstruation, pregnancy, and oral contraceptives, are characteristics of migraine headaches. Nausea and emesis are associated with migraine headaches rather than with tension or cluster headaches. Both tension and migraine headaches are more common in women than in men.

3. The answer is E. The only associated symptoms for patients with tension headache are those of depression and anxiety, such as sleep-pattern disturbance, weight gain or loss, and a hyposensitive or hypersensitive motor state. Flashing lights are associated with migraine headaches. Other auras, such as those preceding homonymous scotomas (island-like blind gaps in the visual field, experienced on the same side as the headache), are also associated with migraine headache. Retro-orbital headache and facial flushing, as well as coryza (profuse nasal discharge) are characteristic of cluster headaches.

4. The answer is A. This woman's symptoms suggest migraine headache without aura. Migraine sufferers sometimes notice a sense of euphoria, thirst, fatigue, or irritability, which predict the onset of this headache but this prodrome is distinct from the focal symptoms of an aura. Both tension and migraine headaches are aggravated by stress.

5. The answer is A. For this patient, you would order a computed tomography (CT) scan of the head without contrast, the correct first test for a suspected subarachnoid hemorrhage (SAH), which this clinical description suggests. A CT scan of the head without contrast is 90% sensitive in detecting SAH. The contrast agent and magnetic resonance imaging (MRI) take more time and cost more, but they are no more sensitive. A cerebrospinal fluid (CSF) examination is not necessary if blood is visible in the ventricles on the CT scan; however, it should follow a negative study where SAH is still suspected, to avoid brain stem herniation. Sedimentation rate elevation is sensitive for temporal arteritis (unusual before age 50), rather than SAH.

6. The answer is D. You would first order a sedimentation rate. The clinical history is consistent with temporal arteritis, especially given the patient's age (>50) and the jaw claudication. (Only a minority of temporal arteritis patients present with visual loss.) With this history and examination, a markedly elevated sedimentation rate (usually > 80) would be sufficient to begin therapy with prednisone and to make arrangements for a temporal artery biopsy in the near future. This patient demonstrates no focal neurologic defects to suggest a mass lesion and thus a CT scan with contrast or an MRI is not initially indicated. He is fully alert and communicating and has no history of trauma, so looking for a hemorrhage (with a CT scan of the head without contrast) is not the first diagnostic concern. A temporal artery biopsy may be indicated, but it is invasive. In a patient in whom temporal arteritis is clinically suspected, such a biopsy is performed only after a sedimentation rate is found to be markedly elevated.

7. The answer is B. Intracranial hemorrhage is the most common presenting symptom of an intracerebral arteriovenous malformation. A malformation may present with headache, seizures, or focal neurologic symptoms, but hemorrhage is most common. Photophobia, a symptom commonly associated with migraine headaches, including those without auras, is not commonly associated with intracerebral arteriovenous malformations.

8. The answer is D. Posttraumatic headaches are more likely if the patient's head trauma was accompanied by a concussion. Patients with posttraumatic headache may have mid-intensity headaches for months after the head injury. No changes in these patients are visible on a CT or MRI of the brain.

9. The answer is B. A 40-year-old woman with cluster headaches would be appropriately treated with oral sumatriptan, which can be used for migraine or cluster headaches, but is contraindicated in basilar or hemiplegic migraine headaches. Extra caution is warranted in prescribing sumatriptan to older patients, especially older men, with cluster headaches, because these patients are more likely to have recognized or unrecognized coronary artery disease. Sumatriptan cannot be given within 24 hours of a dose of any ergot preparation. Also, sumatriptan and vasoconstrictors like it are contraindicated in pregnancy, because they may compromise the fetal circulation.

10. The answer is A. Among these choices, only amitriptyline is used in prophylaxis against migraine headaches, although all the other listed agents can be used to abort migraines. Many other agents are also effective in prophylaxis, including other tricyclic antidepressants, selective serotonin reuptake inhibitors, beta blockers, valporic acid, as well as aspirin and certain NSAIDs (such as naproxen and ketoprofen).

11. The answer is D. Oxygen inhalation is used for cluster headaches and is not used for the other types of primary headaches. Sumatriptan, verapamil, sublingual ergotamine, and analgesia are all sometimes used to treat cluster headaches, but are used also to treat migraine headaches with or without auras.

12. The answer is A. Primary headaches, such as migraine or tension headaches, are the most common reason for recurring headaches in the age group of 8–10 years, as well as in adolescents and young adults. Carbon monoxide exposure, child abuse, medication side effects, and lead poisoning need to be considered as potential secondary causes of headaches in children, but primary headaches are the most common cause, especially in older children.

13. The answer is E. The patient's female sex produces a higher normal range. The normal range of the sedimentation rate for women over 50 is higher than the normal range for men over 50; the upper limit of normal for these women must be calculated with the formula (age + 10)/2, whereas for men over 50, it is calculated with age/2. Only among patients older than 50 is the accepted range different for women than it is for men. Polymyalgia rheumatica and sepsis increase the sedimentary rate, but do not affect what is considered the normal range for that individual. Renal and liver failure do not alter the normal range for the sedimentation rate.

14. The answer is E. A magnetic resonance (MR) study of the head is the most appropriate next step in this case, in which the most likely diagnosis is intracranial mass lesion (despite the absence of papilledema on fundoscopic examination). This diagnosis is suggested by the slow progression of the intensity of the headache,

the lack of asymptomatic intervals, the aggravation of the headache with postural changes, and the possible personality changes. A CT scan of the head, especially without contrast, has much poorer sensitivity. The sedimentation rate study is not appropriate in this case, even though the headache is in the temporal area, because the patient is not in the age group in which temporal arteritis is seen (age over 50 years). Sinus x-rays are sometimes useful in diagnosing chronic or unresponsive sinusitis (although the CT scan has better sensitivity for this), but physical examination reveals no evidence of sinusitis in this patient. A CBC with differential is appropriate when a toxic headache, secondary to sepsis, or meningitis is suspected, but this patient presents with no fever and a fully clear sensorium.

15. The answer is D. A photosensitive, macular rash over the facial cheeks is NOT known to be associated with temporal arteritis. Temporal arteritis may be preceded by, or develop simultaneously with, the symptoms of polymyalgia rheumatica, including pain in the hip and shoulder girdle. Unilateral vision loss is present in only about 7% of temporal arteritis patients at the time of presentation, but will develop in about 44% of patients if they are not treated. Since temporal arteritis is really a cranial arteritis, pain in the jaw muscles with mastication is a common complaint. Temporal arteritis must be considered as a potential source of fever in patients over age 50.

16. The answer is C. Dihydroergotamine mesylate (DHE) is NOT contraindicated in patients on monoamine oxidase inhibitors. DHE is a vasoconstrictor like most abortive medications for migraines and can produce nausea and emesis and can provoke ischemic heart disease, severe hypertension, or claudication. It is not a sympathomimetic amine such as Midrin®. In patients with Prinzmetal's angina, it can elicit vasospasm that results in ischemic chest pain. In pregnancy, it can compromise fetal circulation.

BIBLIOGRAPHY

Kurowski K: Headache. In *Family Medicine* (House Officer Series). Edited by Rudy DR, Kurowski K. Baltimore, Williams & Wilkins, 1997, pp 43–56.

Test 4

Problems of the Eye

DIRECTIONS (Items 1–14): Each of the numbered items or incomplete statements in this section is followed by answers or by completions of the statement. Select the ONE lettered answer or completion that is BEST in each case.

1. A 5-year-old boy is brought to your office for the first time. The parents are concerned that the child has crossed eyes. As a permanent condition, crossed eyes are most often associated with which visual defect?

(A) Myopia
(B) Amblyopia
(C) Hyperopia
(D) Astigmatism
(E) Exotropia

2. Exotropia, or a squint in which the gaze falls laterally (sometimes called "cock-eye" or "walleye") is most often associated with which visual defect?

(A) Myopia
(B) Amblyopia
(C) Hyperopia
(D) Astigmatism
(E) Esotropia

3. A 4-month-old male infant has returned for routine well baby care. Your record shows that he first held his head at 45° at 7 weeks, and at 90° at 3 months. He held his hands together at 3.5 months, and has begun to smile in the past week. His arms and legs move symmetrically. On eye examination, the infant has nonparallel gaze, with the left eye falling laterally. If the eye condition continues, at what age can nonoperative correction begin with general good success?

(A) 6–9 months
(B) 12–18 months
(C) 18–24 months
(D) 3–4 years
(E) 5 years

4. With respect to infantile strabismus, what is the age after which nonoperative correction is not likely to be successful?

(A) 18–24 months
(B) 3–4 years
(C) 5 years
(D) 7 years
(E) 9 years

5. A parent brings a 6-week-old infant girl to you because the left eye shows crusting and matting of a conjunctival discharge for the past week. The infant is in no apparent distress. The rectal temperature is 99°F (37.2°C). The infant's birth weight was 6 pounds and 6 ounces (3 kilograms), and is now 8 pounds and 5 ounces (3.8 kilograms). Her formula intake remains 4 oz every 4 hours (5 times each 24 hours). Her bowel movements are pasty; they number 3–4 per 24 hours. Pupils are equal and reactive. What is the most logical disposition today?

(A) Prescribe sulfacetamide sodium eyedrops for bacterial conjunctivitis.
(B) Explain that this is a usual prodrome of a viral upper respiratory infection and invite the parent to check back with regard to progress within 48 hours.
(C) Consult an ophthalmologist with regard to probable iritis.
(D) Reassure the parent that this is conjunctival drainage of tears caused by a delayed opening of the lacrimal duct.
(E) Treat the infant for a foreign body in the eye.

6. With respect to the "red eye," speedy diagnosis is urgent because of the possibility that the cause is acute, angle-closure glaucoma. Which finding is most specific for acute, angle-closure glaucoma?

(A) An ipsilateral dilated pupil
(B) Fixed, dilated pupils
(C) An ipsilateral miotic pupil and photophobia
(D) Red, irritated conjunctiva on the affected side
(E) Ipsilateral pruritus

7. Iritis is a more common cause of the "red eye" than is acute, angle-closure glaucoma. Which finding is most specific for acute iritis?

(A) An ipsilateral dilated pupil
(B) Fixed, dilated pupils
(C) An ipsilateral miotic pupil and photophobia
(D) Red, irritated conjunctiva on the affected side
(E) Ipsilateral pruritus

8. A 45-year-old Caucasian woman notes the gradual onset of irritated eyes, alternately and intermittently, over the past several weeks. You find conjunctival irritation (OS > OD = left eye more than right). The Schirmer test is positive in both eyes. This condition is associated with which family of illnesses?

(A) Atherosclerosis
(B) Multiple endocrine neoplasia type I
(C) Multiple endocrine neoplasia type II
(D) Sialoadenitis
(E) Collagen vascular diseases

9. You have instituted screening for glaucoma in certain routine physical examinations. A risk factor for primary open-angle glaucoma is .

(A) Age > 35 years
(B) Male sex
(C) Asian race
(D) Excess exposure to sunlight
(E) African-American race

10. When you are asking a patient to count fingers so that you can ascertain visual fields, at what angle from the central visual axis should your fingers be held?

(A) 15 degrees
(B) 25 degrees
(C) 30 degrees
(D) 45 degrees
(E) 60 degrees

11. A 19-year-old male patient complains of irritation of both eyes. He says this irritation has also occurred for several weeks in each of the last 5 years, but not as severely as now. Examination shows both eyes (inside the lids) to be covered with velvety red, thickened conjunctivae that hide all but the corneas and irises. Which symptom or sign is most specific for the cause of this conjunctivitis?

(A) Redness
(B) Pruritus
(C) Decreased visual acuity
(D) Diplopia
(E) Sandy sensation

12. A 28-year-old man complains of photophobia in the left eye. Examination reveals a relatively miotic ipsilateral pupil and redness of that orb. The patient denies previous pupil inequality (anisocoria). Which disease or problem may be associated with this condition?

(A) Ankylosing spondylitis
(B) Atopic disease (hay fever, asthma, eczema)
(C) Eyestrain from visually close work
(D) Myopia
(E) Gouty arthritis

13. A 68-year-old woman complains of left-sided headache. You find a palpable, tender, nodular segment in the left temporal scalp. The patient describes, incidentally, proximal muscle aching in the neck, hips, and shoulder. Her sedimentation rate is 40 millimeters per hour. Which is true with regard to this woman's condition?

(A) Retinal vein occlusion may occur if polymyalgia rheumatica is also present.
(B) Retinal detachment is a complication.
(C) Loss of vision is likely if polymyalgia rheumatica is also present.
(D) Acute glaucoma is a likely complication if the sedimentation rate is more than 50 millimeters per hour.
(E) Suppression amblyopia is a frequent prior condition.

14. A 45-year-old mother of 5 children complains of headache. Her blood pressure is 120/75. Fundoscopy reveals papilledema. A lumbar tap reveals elevated cerebrospinal fluid (CSF) pressure, otherwise normal. Neurologic examination and CT scan of the central nervous system are both normal. Which is true with regard to this condition?

(A) It is a frequent cause of papilledema.
(B) It is a benign condition.
(C) It may be associated with use of vitamins D, E, and K.
(D) Females are less likely to be affected than males.
(E) Females, when affected, are more likely to be nulliparous.

15. A 65-year-old Caucasian man makes an urgent appointment to see you for sudden loss of vision in the right eye 3 hours earlier. He has a history of hypertension and type II diabetes mellitus and, cumulatively, has smoked 40 pack years. He denies any headache at present and in the previous days and weeks, but he admits to a history of frequent headaches, sometimes unilateral and sometimes frontooccipital, during the past 30 years. His present medication consists of metformin 500 milligrams twice a day and sustained-release verapamil 240 milligrams daily. His blood pressure is 155/95. In the right eye, he perceives only light. All of the following are reasonable possibilities in the differential diagnosis EXCEPT

    (A) An embolism from a carotid stenosis
    (B) Papillitis caused by giant cell arteritis
    (C) Central retinal artery occlusion
    (D) An embolism from an atrial thrombus
    (E) Ophthalmic migraine

16. A 25-year-old man has been in an accident in which he has suffered a blunt blow to the area of his right eye. Which is NOT a major consideration in the evaluation of an eye that has been involved in blunt trauma?

    (A) Hyphema
    (B) Presence of irregular pupil
    (C) Palpable irregularity of the ipsilateral orbital rim
    (D) Photophobia
    (E) Reduced range of motion of the involved eye

ANSWERS AND EXPLANATIONS

1. The answer is C. A "squint" (or condition of nonparallel gaze at distance), consisting of crossed-eyes (inward-turning of gaze or esotropia), is usually caused by hyperopia (farsightedness). In hyperopia, the basic defect is a shortened eyeball in relation to the focal distance of the lens and cornea. An individual whose point of convergence falls behind the retina at reading distances (or, in more severe cases, even at "infinity") continually attempts to accommodate for close vision, causing a strabismus in which the gaze is nonparallel and convergent. Myopia is nearsightedness. Amblyopia is impairment of vision without a detectable organic lesion of the eye; one form of amblyopia results from suppression of vision in one eye to avoid diplopia (double vision). Astigmatism is an unequal curvature of the refractive surfaces of the eye which results in a diffuse or fuzzy image.

2. The answer is A. Exotropia is most often associated with myopia (nearsightedness). In myopia, the eyeball is abnormally long in relation to the focal distance capability of the lens. Myopia causes the individual to attempt unsuccessfully to relax accommodation for distance; the efforts result in relaxation of convergence to a degree that goes beyond parallel and becomes divergent. The eye must relax accommodation of the ciliary apparatus even for reading (or, in the extreme, even unsuccessfully for reading). Accommodation and convergence are enervated together and act synchronously.

3. The answer is D. The age range of 3–4 years is best for nonoperative correction of the child's eye problem, strabismus. At this age, the child is old enough to cooperate in eye exercises and still young enough to avoid irreversible change. The corrective technique requires the intermittent masking of the weaker eye (to interdict amblyopia) and corrective lenses (to make accommodative and "de-accommodative" effort unnecessary for normal visual distances).

4. The answer is D. At the age of 7 years and beyond, amblyopia (present in about 50% of those with persistent strabismus) is irreversible, and strabismus requires operative correction. The form of amblyopia that is sometimes called suppression amblyopia (or strabismic amblyopia) is central suppression of the weaker eye that results from functional intolerance of diplopia, brought about by exotropia or esotropia. The result is severely decreased visual acuity, frequently to the degree of legal blindness. Surgery beyond the age of 7 results in pro-

gressively less remediation of vision; it is undertaken more for cosmetic effect.

5. The answer is D. An obstructed lacrimal duct (physiological) is a very common cause of conjunctival discharge after the first month of life. (An obstructed lacrimal duct can be expected to resolve physiologically at or about 6–9 months of age.) Bacterial conjunctivitis is statistically unlikely in this situation. However, if massage toward the nose does not produce clear fluid, or if it produces purulent fluid, sulfacetamide sodium drops, 1 or 2 four times a day (atypical choice) for a few days would be appropriate for either condition. Viral conjunctivitis, often preceding an upper respiratory infection, usually becomes bilateral rapidly, and coryza develops within a few days. Iritis would show unequal pupils. A foreign body would result in obvious distress and blepharospasm (inability to hold the eyelids open).

6. The answer is A. The most specific finding for angle-closure glaucoma is, upon luminous stimulation of each pupil, an ipsilateral (same side as pain and redness) fixed midposition pupil that shows as dilated, compared to the contralateral pupil. Acute angle-closure glaucoma, the third phase of angle-closure glaucoma, is a serious medical emergency: Increasing intraocular pressure causes great pain and can result in significant loss of visual field or in blindness. Fixed, dilated pupils are a presumptive sign of death. Ipsilateral miotic (constricted) pupil is a sign of iritis. Irritated conjunctiva occurs in bacterial, viral, and allergic forms of conjunctivitis. Pruritus is typical of allergic conjunctivitis.

7. The answer is C. The most specific finding for iritis is an ipsilateral miotic (constricted) pupil and photophobia. Ipsilateral iridospasm, assuming the miotic pupil is a change from the baseline state, is diagnostic of iritis (iridocyclitis, anterior uveitis). While photophobia is invariably present in all causes of red eye except conjunctivitis, it is a hallmark of iritis, because the iris, already in spasm, is stimulated by the light to contract further.

8. The answer is E. Keratoconjunctivitis sicca ("dry-eye"), the condition described in this question, is often associated with collagen vascular diseases, such as Sjögren's disease, and often coexists with rheumatoid arthritis and lupus erythematosus. The Schirmer test is positive when filter paper laid against the lower lid fails to conduct tears a distance of 5 millimeters in 5 minutes.

Multiple endocrine neoplasia type I (MEN I) is the association of parathyroid, pancreatic, and pituitary adenomas, while MEN II is the association of medullary carcinoma and pheochromocytoma. Sialoadenitis is inflammation of a salivary gland, which is often viral (as in mumps) and sometimes bacterial.

9. The answer is E. African-American race confers nearly a four-fold risk of primary open-angle glaucoma (4.7% prevalence versus 1.3% for whites). In addition, African-Americans are at risk much earlier in life and, therefore, warrant screening as early as 20 years of age. For others, age > 50 years is a risk factor (not >35 years). Open-angle glaucoma is chronic glaucoma, once called chronic simple glaucoma. The abnormal and destructive buildup of intraocular pressure occurs insidiously over a period of years, without causing pain, but eventually causing loss of vision, first in the peripheral fields, then involving central vision. Neither male sex nor Asian race is a risk factor. Exposure to sunlight is not a risk factor for primary open-angle glaucoma, but it is a risk factor for pterygium, a pinguecula that forms on the sclera and crosses the limbus to extend onto the cornea.

10. The answer is D. To ascertain visual fields, your fingers should be held 45 degrees from the central visual axis. In this version of confrontational field checking, the acuity with respect to the peripheral field is being tested as well as the range (i.e., discrimination adequate to count fingers). For detection of motion only, the angle from the central axis should be limited only by the anatomic barriers (i.e., the nose, brow, lateral orbit, and cheek).

11. The answer is B. Pruritus (itching) is the hallmark of this patient's condition, allergic conjunctivitis. A seasonal factor (e.g., pollen) is also virtually always present in allergic conjunctivitis, except when the allergen is an industrial or other focal environmental agent. Decreased visual acuity and diplopia are not characteristic of allergy (but they are serious findings that warrant an appropriate evaluation). Redness is present, but nonspecific. A sandy sensation is typical of bacterial conjunctivitis.

12. The answer is A. Ankylosing spondylitis is associated with iritis, the condition indicated by the patient's symptoms. Other conditions associated with iritis include systemic lupus erythematosus, Reiter's disease, rheumatoid arthritis, Crohn's disease, ulcerative colitis, and sarcoidosis. Atopic disease is associated with allergic conjunctivitis but not with iridospasm. Myopia, eyestrain, and gouty arthritis are not associated with iritis.

13. The answer is C. Because the symptoms indicate giant-cell arteritis affecting the temporal artery (temporal arteritis), and because the prior muscular aches suggest polymyalgia rheumatica (PMR), this woman is at risk for loss of vision in the presence of PMR. Loss of vision is even more likely if papillitis is present. (Papillitis is inflammation of the optic disk, without involving the optic nerve, and not caused by elevated intracranial pressure.) Temporal arteritis is known for its strikingly elevated sedimentation rates, and is also known for its dramatic responsiveness to systemic glucocorticoids, which not only produce rapid relief but also prevent sudden loss of vision. Retinal vein occlusion, retinal detachment, acute glaucoma, and suppression amblyopia are not complications of this condition.

14. The answer is A. This woman's condition, pseudotumor cerebri, is a frequent cause of papilledema. Despite the name "pseudotumor," the condition is not benign. The synonym, "benign intracranial hypertension," is also misleading. The condition is associated with visual disturbances in 35% of cases, and headache is a presenting symptom in 90% of cases. Pseudotumor cerebri may be associated with use of vitamin A, tetracycline, nalidixic acid, and oral contraceptives, but not with use of vitamins D, E and K. Females are more likely to be affected than males, and they are likely to be "fertile," not nulliparous.

15. The answer is E. Ophthalmic migraine is not a reasonable possibility in this case because its onset is unlikely in this patient's age group (the usual onset is in the teens or early twenties) and because 3 hours duration of loss of vision is rare in this condition. In addition, the visual loss in ophthalmic migraine is typically bilateral, consisting of homonymous arcuate scotomas. All of the other answer choices are reasonable initial considerations. The carotid arteries should be palpated and auscultated for pulse and bruit, to exclude stenosis and embolism; and more definitive duplex Doppler studies should follow. Carotid angiography is more sensitive and specific, but it carries a 1% risk of stroke during the procedure. Carotid artery stenosis can lead to unilateral blindness, either transiently through the mechanism of microembolism from an ulcerated plaque to the ophthalmic artery (amaurosis fugax) or permanently by larger embolization. Fundoscopy, with attention to the optic nerve head (optic disk), can quickly detect papillitis from giant cell arteritis or papilledema (the latter causes transient loss of vision). The retina and fovea would show the pale color of ischemia, along with a cherry-red macula. The temporal arteries should be palpated for nodularity, to rule out giant cell temporal arteritis (a possibility mostly because of the patient's history of vascular headaches for the past 30 years). If giant cell arteritis is the cause, a lack of headache at the time of visual loss would be highly atypical. However, if the diagnosis is giant cell arteritis, systemic glucocorticoids should be instituted rapidly.

16. The answer is D. Photophobia is NOT a major consideration in the evaluation of an eye that has been involved in blunt trauma. Photophobia is a nonspecific symptom of ophthalmic distress, usually denoting iridospasm, found particularly in iritis. Hyphema (blood in the anterior chamber) is a frequent sequela of blunt trauma; it may lead to secondary glaucoma as signaled by an elevated intraocular tension. An irregular pupil suggests a ruptured globe. A reduced limit of motion of the involved eye may be a clue to entrapment of one or more extraocular muscles in a fracture. An irregularity of the orbital rim may indicate a step-off fracture.

BIBLIOGRAPHY

Savory LM, Krasnow MA, Terry JE: Problems of the eye. In *Family Medicine* (House Officer Series). Edited by Rudy DR, Kurowski K. Baltimore, Williams & Wilkins, 1997, pp 57–70.

SECTION II

Cardiovascular Problems

Test 5

Common Cardiac Problems in Ambulatory Practice

DIRECTIONS (Items 1–19): Each of the numbered items or incomplete statements in this section is followed by answers or by completions of the statement. Select the ONE lettered answer or completion that is BEST in each case.

1. A diastolic murmur is the hallmark of

   (A) Aortic stenosis and aortic regurgitation
   (B) Mitral stenosis and aortic regurgitation
   (C) Hypertrophic cardiomyopathy and patent ductus arteriosus
   (D) Aortic stenosis and mitral stenosis
   (E) Ventricular septal defect and tricuspid regurgitation

2. Upon routine cardiac examination, an 18-year-old male patient manifests a systolic crescendo-decrescendo that is loudest over the left second interspace, near the left sternal border. The murmur radiates to both carotid arteries. The carotid pulse appears to be delayed and somewhat diminished. Pressure in the right arm is 150/90; in the left arm, 110/90. Which valve abnormality is commonly associated with this condition?

   (A) Mitral insufficiency
   (B) Bicuspid aortic valve
   (C) Mitral stenosis
   (D) Ventricular septal defect
   (E) Patent ductus arteriosus

3. In your attempt to distinguish among congenital, rheumatic, and calcific aortic stenosis, which epidemiologic information may be most helpful?

   (A) Sex
   (B) Race
   (C) Geographic area of residence
   (D) Occupation
   (E) Age at which the patient presents

4. A dentist's office calls to ask whether your 55-year-old female patient, scheduled for routine dental procedures, requires endocarditis antibiotic prophylaxis because of a history of mitral valve prolapse (MVP). Your record confirms MVP, whose evidence is an audible systolic click, without a murmur. Endocarditis antibiotic prophylaxis would be needed if her record included which additional circumstance?

   (A) Previous rheumatic fever without valvulitis
   (B) Previous Kawasaki disease without valvular dysfunction
   (C) Cardiac pacemaker and implanted defibrillator
   (D) Three-month status, postcoronary-bypass surgery
   (E) Prosthetic cardiac valves, including bioprosthetic and homograft valves

5. If the patient in Question 4 did have mitral regurgitation (mitral insufficiency), she would manifest a murmur that is holosystolic and radiates to

   (A) The left side of the neck
   (B) The right carotid area
   (C) The left sternal border
   (D) The left axilla
   (E) The aortic auscultatory area

6. You have followed the patient in Question 5 for 10 additional years. Now she has mitral regurgitation; she manifests fatigue; and three times per week, she manifests paroxysmal nocturnal dyspnea. These symptoms have responded to, and have eventually recurred after, successive institutions (additively) of furosemide and angiotensin-converting enzyme inhibitors. Which would be the next, most appropriate clinical action?

   (A) Add a calcium-channel blocker.
   (B) Recommend a reduction in the patient's work hours.
   (C) Recommend a program of aerobic exercise.
   (D) Refer the patient to an interventional cardiologist.
   (E) Prescribe a 4-gram salt diet.

7. Which valvular repair surgery is associated with the highest mortality?

   (A) Aortic valve replacement for aortic regurgitation
   (B) Aortic valve replacement for aortic stenosis
   (C) Mitral valve replacement
   (D) Patent ductus repair
   (E) Fracture of mitral valve leaflets for stenosis

8. On routine examination, a 59-year-old woman manifests a low-pitched, rumbling, diastolic murmur that, just before the first heart sound, is loudest at the apex. The cause of her condition is

   (A) Bacterial endocarditis
   (B) Congenital heart disease
   (C) Atrial thrombosis
   (D) Rheumatoid heart
   (E) Rheumatic heart disease

9. A frequent complication of mitral stenosis is

(A) Syncope
(B) Pulmonary embolism
(C) Peripheral edema
(D) Systemic embolism
(E) Papilledema

10. Which is the most potent risk factor for coronary artery disease (CAD) from the viewpoint of relative risk (rate of coronary disease in the person at risk, compared to the rate expected in the population)?

(A) Obesity
(B) Sedentary life style
(C) Hypertension
(D) Smoking
(E) HDL cholesterol less than 35 mg/dL

11. The most compelling reason for the development of a preventive program in CAD, besides its prodigious prevalence, is the mortality at the time of the first attack (myocardial infarction, coronary thrombosis). The mortality rate of first heart attacks is approximately

(A) 10%
(B) 35%
(C) 25%
(D) 50%
(E) 60%

12. Angina may be stable or unstable. The prognosis associated with unstable angina is poorer. What percentage of patients with unstable angina will have a myocardial infarction within 2 years?

(A) 5%
(B) 12%
(C) 25%
(D) 35%
(E) 50%

13. A 48-year-old patient has hypertension, controlled reasonably well on hydrochlorothiazide, and residual poliomyelitis that has left him with weakness of his left leg. He now complains of atypical chest pain, consisting of vague substernal pain lasting less than 1 minute, not associated with walking upstairs, but occasionally waking him during dream sleep. Which is the most reasonable direct method of evaluating this man's chest pain?

(A) Thallium treadmill stress test
(B) Minnesota Multiphasic Personality Inventory (MMPI)
(C) Dipyridamole thallium stress test
(D) Consultation with a cardiologist for coronary angiography
(E) 50 milligrams of atenolol four times daily

14. Which is a contraindication for coronary angiography?

(A) New onset angina
(B) Unstable angina
(C) Evaluation before major surgery, particularly vascular surgery
(D) Atypical chest pain
(E) Uncontrolled congestive heart failure

15. With regard to supraventricular tachycardias, which is simplest for differentiating paroxysmal atrial tachycardia with block from atrioventricular nodal reentry tachycardia?

(A) Osler's maneuver
(B) Orthostatic versus sedentary blood pressures
(C) Digoxin level
(D) Carotid sinus massage
(E) Presence or absence of anginal symptoms

16. A 55-year-old woman, who has a history of obesity and hypertension (with only fair control) for 15 years, presents with dyspnea. She complains she is easily fatigued and is unable to lie flat for more than 1 minute because of shortness of breath. No rales nor peripheral edema are found on physical examination. The multiple gated acquisition (MUGA) scan (a gated nucleotide study) shows an ejection fraction of 50%. Which of the following regimens is likely to be the most efficacious?

(A) Digoxin 0.125 mg per day
(B) Amlodipine 5 mg daily
(C) Captopril 25 mg four times per day
(D) Hydrochlorothiazide 50 mg daily
(E) Lisinopril 10 mg daily

17. A 55-year-old African-American man, who has uncontrolled hypertension (BP = 160/110) on verapamil 60 mg three times per day, complains that during each of the past 4 nights he has been awakened by dyspnea, for which he has gained relief by sitting up on the edge of his bed for 20 minutes. Examination reveals dilated neck veins; "late" venous emptying (peripheral veins of the arms do not empty when the arms are raised until they are 15 cm above the right atrium); cardiac percussible "shadow" enlarged to 2 cm left of the left mid-clavicular line; S3 gallop; 2+ bilateral ankle and pedal edema. Chest x-ray shows cardiomegaly with left ventricular dilatation. A MUGA reveals an ejection fraction of 30%. Which of the following regimens would be most appropriate?

(A) Digoxin 0.125 mg per day and triamterene/hydrochlorothiazide (25 mg hydrochlorothiazide) twice daily
(B) Amlodipine 5 mg daily
(C) Propranolol 20 mg four times per day
(D) An increase in verapamil to 60 mg four times a day
(E) A graduated increase in physical exercise

18. A 60-year-old man complains that for an hour he has been experiencing palpitations, a feeling of unease, and vague chest pains. The peripheral pulse is difficult to count because of the uneven amplitude and time span between beats; apical rate is 130 per minute, with only one heart sound evident in many of the beats; blood pressure (BP) is 115–130/60–75, imprecise because the Korotkoff sounds are inconsistent (his usual BP is 145/85). An EKG shows an electrical rate of 150, with clearly identifiable narrow QRS complexes, but an irregular baseline and no identifiable P waves. What is the first therapeutic goal in the treatment of this condition?

    (A) Achieve an increase in the BP
    (B) Obtain relief of chest pain
    (C) Convert the rhythm to regular sinus rhythm
    (D) Obtain reduced ventricular response
    (E) Ascertain state of oxygenation

19. With reference to the patient in Question 18, which of the following statements is true about anticoagulation?

    (A) It should commence immediately upon conversion to RSR.
    (B) It would be indicated if the atrial fibrillation had continued for 12 hours prior to conversion.
    (C) It would be indicated if the atrial fibrillation had continued for 24 hours prior to conversion.
    (D) It would be indicated if the atrial fibrillation had continued for 2 days prior to conversion.
    (E) It would be indicated if the atrial fibrillation had continued for 3 days prior to conversion.

DIRECTIONS (Items 20–22): Each of the numbered items or incomplete statements in this section is negatively phrased, as indicated by a capitalized word such as NOT, LEAST, or EXCEPT. Select the ONE lettered answer or completion that is BEST in each case.

---

20. A 55-year-old, male nonsmoker, who has type II diabetes, wants to begin a controlled exercise program. He has no history of chest pain nor diagnosed heart attacks, and no symptoms of heart failure. However, a routine EKG shows a QS configuration in leads II, III, and AVF (deep Q waves; no R wave). Which is NOT characteristic of this situation?

    (A) The prognosis is less favorable than in symptomatic cases.
    (B) It occurs more commonly in women, the aged, and diabetics.
    (C) If it were symptomatic, it might produce epigastric pain.
    (D) During the acute phase, it may be accompanied by sinus bradycardia.
    (E) During the acute phase, the EKG may have manifested ST elevation in II, III, and AVF.

21. The patient in Question 20 is 220 pounds (approximately 99.9 kilograms) in weight, 5 feet 11 inches (approximately 1.8 meters) in height, and has a blood pressure of 155/105. You fail to find popliteal, posterior tibial, and dorsalis pedis pulses in either lower extremity. The patient admits to symptoms of claudication of the legs (tightening calf pain with walking two blocks) and hopes for an exercise prescription that might improve his walking distance. He has been taking 5 milligrams of glyburide four times per day and hydrochlorothiazide/triamterene. The result of a glycochemoglobin test that you order is 9%. All of the following would be reasonable next measures EXCEPT

    (A) Placing the patient on a 1700 calorie American Diabetes Association (ADA) diet.
    (B) Adding metformin 500 milligrams twice daily to his drug regimen.
    (C) Ordering a treadmill thallium stress test.
    (D) Adding an angiotensin-converting enzyme blocking agent (ACE inhibitor) for blood pressure control and preservation of renal function; possibly withholding hydrochlorothiazide/triamterene.
    (E) Ordering a cardiology consultation to consider coronary angiography.

22. Systolic dysfunction as a basic mechanism of congestive heart failure is characterized by all of the following EXCEPT

(A) Left ventricular hypertrophy
(B) Reduced ejection fraction
(C) Elevated end diastolic pressure (increased preload)
(D) Increased resistance to flow from the heart (increased after-load)
(E) Cardiac dilatation

DIRECTIONS (Items 23–27): For each numbered heart lesion in these matching questions, select the letter of the identifying characteristic(s) of the heart murmur. Each lettered option may be selected once, more than once, or not at all.

(A) Holosystolic, low pitch, apex, radiating to axilla
(B) Diastolic decrescendo
(C) Crescendo-decrescendo, carotid
(D) Midsystolic, late systolic, or pansystolic; click
(E) Crescendo-decrescendo; decrease with squat

25. Hypertrophic cardiomyopathy

26. Mitral valve prolapse

27. Aortic regurgitation

23. Aortic stenosis

24. Mitral regurgitation

DIRECTIONS (Items 28–32): For each numbered maneuver in these matching questions, select the letter of the effect that may influence murmurs. Each lettered option may be selected once, more than once, or not at all.

(A) Decreases venous return
(B) Raises systemic vascular resistance, heart rate, and cardiac output
(C) Increases venous return
(D) Decreases arterial blood pressure
(E) Raises arterial blood pressure, bradycardia.

29. Expiration, standing

30. Valsalva, phase 3

31. Valsalva, phase 4

32. Handgrip

28. Inspiration, squatting

ANSWERS AND EXPLANATIONS

1. The answer is B. A diastolic murmur is the hallmark of both mitral stenosis (MS) and aortic regurgitation (AR). MS produces a rumbling diastolic murmur at the apex which, in its classic presentation, is associated with an "opening snap," marking the end of the murmur sound component until the next systolic cycle. AR produces a high-pitched diastolic murmur that starts immediately on the A2 second sound and falls off in a decrescendo, much like the sound of waves crashing on rocks. Aortic stenosis produces a systolic ejection-type murmur, loudest at the aortic auscultatory area (crescendo-decrescendo). Hypertrophic cardiomyopathy produces a harsh systolic ejection murmur, loudest at the apex. Patent ductus arteriosus classically produces a continuous murmur with both systolic and diastolic components. Ventricular septal defect produces a loud, harsh, systolic ejection murmur, loudest along the left sternal border at the third through sixth interspaces. Tricuspid regurgitation produces a high-pitched blowing systolic murmur, loudest along the lower left sternal border and subxiphoid area. The characteristics of these and other murmurs are listed in Table 5.1 in *Family Medicine*.

2. The answer is B. Bicuspid aortic valve is present in 46% of cases of coarctation of the aorta. This patient has typical findings of aortic stenosis with the systolic ejection murmur radiating to the carotid in which the pulse is "pulsus parvus et tardus" (a small, hard pulse that rises and falls slowly). The blood pressure findings are typical of coarctation at the most common location, in the arch opposite the attachment of the ligamentum arteriosum. The conditions listed in the other answer choices are not associated with congenital aortic stenosis.

3. The answer is E. The age at which the patient presents is the epidemiologic information that tends to be most helpful in distinguishing between the types of aortic stenosis (AS). With onset of symptoms before age 30, the cause is most likely congenital disease; during ages 30–60 years, the etiology may be congenital or rheumatic; after age 60, the cause is most likely calcific valvulitis. Information about sex, race, geographic area, and occupation do not help in making this distinction.

4. The answer is E. Prosthetic cardiac valves, including bioprosthetic and homograft valves, are indications for endocarditis antibiotic prophylaxis. Mitral valve prolapse (MVP) with demonstrable mitral insufficiency

(i.e., a murmur) is also an indication, but in this case no murmur was present. Other indications for prophylaxis include past history of bacterial endocarditis, history of rheumatic fever with valvular dysfunction, and surgical systemic pulmonary shunts. Table 5–4 in *Family Medicine* lists others. The table specifically excludes previous rheumatic fever without valvulitis, previous Kawasaki disease without valvular dysfunction, cardiac pacemaker and implanted defibrillator, and 3-month status postcoronary bypass surgery.

5. The answer is D. With mitral regurgitation (mitral insufficiency), the murmur radiates to the left axilla. The murmur is loudest at the apex.

6. The answer is D. This patient should be referred to an interventional cardiologist for evaluation and follow-up for left ventricular (LV) size and function. Salt reduction should have occurred before the institution of the medications. A calcium channel blocker may be helpful for further afterload reduction but would only delay the referral for an LV evaluation. Reduction of working hours at this point would come "too little and too late." An exercise program, which probably could not be performed by this patient, would aggravate the situation.

7. The answer is C. Mitral valve replacement (for mitral regurgitation) is the valve surgery associated with the highest mortality. Keeping a careful eye, by echocardiography, on the left ventricular size can help to limit the perioperative mortality. Thanks to improved technology, repair and preservation of the original anatomy, instead of replacement, is increasingly favored in cases such as the one followed in questions 4, 5, and 6.

8. The answer is E. The murmur is typical of mitral stenosis (MS), caused by rheumatic heart disease. MS is the most common valvular condition resulting from recurrent rheumatic fever; the second most common is aortic stenosis; and the third most common is combined aortic and mitral stenoses. No congenital lesion produces the murmur described in this case. Endocarditis produces changing murmurs and systemic febrile illness. Rheumatoid arthritis can be associated with pericarditis, which produces a typical friction rub.

9. The answer is D. Systemic thromboembolism is the most common of the listed complications in mitral stenosis. The left atrium is greatly enlarged in mitral stenosis, a situation greatly compounded by the presence of atrial fibrillation, a common complication of mitral stenosis. Coexistence of the two produces an 80% incidence of systemic embolism, compared to 20% in the absence of atrial fibrillation. Syncope is a hallmark of aortic stenosis. Pulmonary embolism, while not beyond risk in mitral stenosis, is not nearly as common as systemic embolism. Peripheral edema is a hallmark of right-sided congestive heart failure, while mitral stenosis mimics left heart failure more in producing pulmonary congestion. Papilledema does not occur with greater than expected frequency in mitral stenosis.

10. The answer is D. Smoking conveys a 3.5 relative risk of CAD while the next most powerful factor, family history, conveys 3.0. HDL cholesterol less than 35 mg/dL is associated with a 2.0 relative risk. (Table 5–2 in *Family Medicine* lists the risk factors and their relative risks.)

11. The answer is C. The mortality rate of first myocardial infarctions is approximately 25%.

12. The answer is B. At present, patients diagnosed as having unstable angina have a 12% risk of a heart attack within 2 years. By definition, unstable angina involves coronary circulation that is compromised to a segment of myocardium, but that does not culminate in an infarction (otherwise it would be crescendo angina). Therefore, it may be surprising that only 12% go on to infarction at a later date.

13. The answer is C. A dipyridamole thallium stress test is a valid non-exercise stress-test option for this patient, who is unable to exercise adequately as a result of his status post polio. Conversely, treadmill thallium stress testing is not workable because of his physical disability. Though his atypical chest pain may have a psychological basis, psychological testing would be inappropriate until organic possibilities are ruled out. Coronary angiography is too aggressive a step for this patient, because the chest pain is not typical of coronary disease. Finally, a trial of medical therapy may be appropriate, because the nocturnal bouts may signal a vasospastic cause (i.e., Prinzmetal's angina). However, a beta blocker is not the best choice because it may aggravate small vessel spasm. A calcium channel blocker or ACE inhibitor would be a better choice.

14. The answer is E. Uncontrolled congestive heart failure is a contraindication for coronary angiography.

15. The answer is D. Carotid sinus massage is simplest for differentiating paroxysmal atrial tachycardia (PAT) with block from atrioventricular nodal re-entry tachycardia (AVNRT). This maneuver has no effect on PAT ex-

cept to increase the block temporarily, while it may have the effect of converting AVNRT. Osler's maneuver consists of testing for palpability of a pulseless radial artery with the pressure of the blood pressure cuff raised above the systolic blood pressure. If present, Osler's maneuver explains systolic pseudohypertension. Digoxin level may be helpful in differentiating between the two, because digoxin toxicity is a cause of PAT; however, it is a "soft" association and serves only to rule out toxicity before further evaluation of the dysrhythmia. Orthostatic blood pressures have no particular value in differentiating between the two rhythms, but either may be associated with orthostatic symptoms: Circulation may be significantly compromised in either case because of the excessive rates involved. Anginal symptoms may occur with either mechanism (i.e., with any tachycardia) if the coronary circulation is compromised.

16. The answer is B. Amlodipine 5 mg daily (in a long-acting preparation) is likely to be the most efficacious in this case. The patient has left ventricular congestive heart failure with diastolic dysfunction (ejection fraction greater than 40%). Amlodipine is in the dihydropyridine class of calcium channel blockers. Calcium channel blockers are said to be the treatment of choice because of their anti-ischemic actions, preload reduction, blood pressure control, LVH regression potential, and heart rate control, which leads to increased coronary filling during prolonged diastolic relaxation. Beta blockers may also be helpful. Digoxin (form of digitalis) is most effective in cases of systolic dysfunction (ejection fraction < 40%). Lisinopril, as an ACE inhibitor, functions also to reduce afterload; thus it is indicated in systolic, rather than diastolic, dysfunction.

17. The answer is A. Digoxin (a form of digitalis) 0.125 mg per day and triamterene/hydrochlorothiazide (25 mg hydrochlorothiazide) twice daily is the most appropriate regimen at this time for this man. The patient has both symptoms (orthopnea) and signs (dilated neck veins, pedal edema, x-ray and MUGA scan findings) of congestive heart failure. In a patient such as this, who manifests systolic dysfunction (reduced ejection fraction, dilated heart) and hypertension with an S3 gallop, digitalis (a powerful, positive inotropic agent) is still an appropriate first step. Thiazide diuretic has a dual usefulness: as a diuretic in this fluid-overloaded patient, and as an antihypertensive in an African-American (whose race carries a two-thirds chance of being salt sensitive with low renin, and thus diuretic responsive). [See *Family Medicine* (House Officer Series), Chapter 9.] The triamterene in the combination counters the potassium-losing propensity of the thiazide. Although verapamil is a fair choice for treating hypertension in an African American, it may have become counter-productive in this man when he slipped into heart failure. Amlodipine and vera-pamil, as calcium channel-blocking agents, and propran-olol, as a beta-adrenergic blocking agent, are relatively contraindicated in systolic dysfunction because of their negative inotropism. Increased physical exercise is con-troversial and, most likely, counterproductive in a pa-tient with symptomatic heart failure. A person in heart failure is assumed to have a finite amount of cardiac re-serve that can be used up in foot-pounds of energy out-put on a daily basis, until the cause of failure is removed or the patient is brought into a compensated state.

18. The answer is D. Obtaining reduced ventricular re-sponse is the first therapeutic goal in the treatment of this man, who is having a typical attack of acute atrial fibrillation. The rapid ventricular response is the greatest threat at the outset. Conversion to regular sinus rhythm can await rate control. Agents that can achieve rate re-duction rapidly include digoxin, beta-blocking agents, and calcium channel-blocking agents. Calcium channel-blocking agents afford a fair chance of conversion to regular sinus rhythm; beta-blocking agents should be avoided if the ventricular rate is ≤ 80 per minute. If rate control is not established quickly, the criterion for hospi-talization in this case is met: The presenting rate is ≥ 110 in a patient with a disturbing complication (chest pain). Chest pain represents relative coronary insuffi-ciency, which exists as long as the excessive rate exists.

19. The answer is D. The clinical rule is that the patient should be anticoagulated if the atrial fibrillation has con-tinued longer than 2 days. Anticoagulation is necessary because fibrillating atria contain areas of stagnant, non-flowing blood prone to thrombus formation and subse-quent embolization.

20. The answer is A. A silent myocardial infarction (MI), which is asymptomatic and unrecognized, does NOT carry a worse prognosis than that of a recognized MI. This pa-tient's EKG shows an old inferior myocardial infarction by virtue of the QS pattern in II, III, and AVF. Because it was asymptomatic, it was a silent MI. As an inferior MI, it probably produced ST elevation in II, III, and AVF. The chest pain pattern may have included epigastric pain and sinus bradycardia, sequelae of injury to the right side of the heart, supplied by the right coronary artery.

21. The answer is C. A thallium treadmill (exercise) stress test is NOT a reasonable next measure to take in this case. This test may provide good information about cardiovascular exercise tolerance, but it gives no infor-mation about the operability of this patient's known coronary artery disease (given the EKG findings in the previous question). In addition, the patient's peripheral vascular insufficiency and claudication of the legs rule

out a treadmill test. Dipyridamole/thallium stress testing is a non-exercise option. The ADA diet and the possible elimination of chlorothiazide (which may aggravate dia-betes mellitus in 5% of cases) addresses the crucial need to refine the patient's diabetes control. Addition of an ACE inhibitor is a rational approach to renal preserva-tion and, because of its blood-pressure-lowering effect, may also help to control the hypertension. Coronary an-giography would be the "gold standard" for evaluating the operability of the patient's coronary disease.

22. The answer is A. Left ventricular hypertrophy does NOT characterize systolic dysfunction as a basic mecha-nism of congestive heart failure. Hypertrophy refers to myocardial thickening, a characteristic of diastolic dys-function, which occurs classically in infundibular hyper-trophic subaortic stenosis (IHSS), and often in untreated hypertension. Reduced ejection fraction, cardiac dilita-tion, increased end diastolic pressure, and increased resis-tance to flow are characteristics of systolic dysfunction.

23. The answer is C. With aortic stenosis, the identify-ing characteristic of the murmur is crescendo-de-crescendo, radiating to the carotid arteries. Other identi-fying aspects include diminishment with handgrip and accentuation with the squatting posture.

24. The answer is A. With mitral regurgitation, the identifying characteristic of the murmur is that it is holosystolic, without any appreciable rise or fall throughout the systole; low in pitch, best heard at the apex, radiating to the axilla.

25. The answer is E. With hypertrophic cardiomyopa-thy, the crescendo-decrescendo (i.e., ejection murmur) decreases when the patient squats.

26. The answer is D. With mitral valve prolapse, if re-gurgitation exists, the murmur is mid-, late, or pansys-tolic. Without regurgitation, there is no murmur (a sys-tolic click makes the diagnosis).

27. The answer is B. With aortic regurgitation, a dias-tolic decrescendo murmur starts immediately upon the second heart sound and falls off into diastole with a sound that mimics waves crashing on the rocks. Typi-cally, the pulse pressure is increased, a reflection of the increased diastolic "run-off" permitted by the "dump-ing" of a portion of the stroke volume back into the left ventricle. (See Table 5.1 in *Family Medicine*.)

28. The answer is C. Inspiration and squatting increase venous return. Squatting increases venous return into the right side of the heart in particular, and accentuates the murmur of mitral regurgitation.

29. The answer is A. Expiration and standing decrease venous return. Standing accentuates the click of mitral valve prolapse and the murmur of mitral regurgitation.

30. The answer is D. Valsalva phase 3 (the release phase) produces a rapid decline in arterial blood pressure.

31. The answer is E. Valsalva phase 4 (the rebound phase as the first inspiration occurs following the end of the expiratory release) produces a rise in arterial blood pressure, and a bradycardia.

32. The answer is B. The handgrip produces a rise in systemic vascular resistance, heart rate, and cardiac output. It also accentuates the murmurs of aortic regurgitation and of mitral regurgitation. (See Table 5.2 in *Family Medicine*.)

BIBLIOGRAPHY

Eaton CB and Cannistra AJ: Common cardiac problems in ambulatory practice. In *Family Medicine* (House Officer Series). Edited by Rudy DR, Kurowski K. Baltimore, Williams & Wilkins, 1997, pp 71–96.

Test 6

Peripheral Vascular Disease

DIRECTIONS (Items 1–13): Each of the numbered items or incomplete statements in this section is followed by answers or by completions of the statement. Select the ONE lettered answer or completion that is BEST in each case.

---

1. Besides atrial fibrillation, which condition is most likely to be associated with peripheral embolism?

- (A) Abdominal aortic aneurysm
- (B) Myocardial infarction
- (C) Superficial femoral artery atherosclerosis
- (D) Mitral stenosis
- (E) Aortic stenosis

2. A 63-year-old man complains that his right lower leg has been painful, numb, and cold since earlier that morning. Upon examining him, you note that the skin over the right lower leg appears normal, but feels colder than that of the left leg. No popliteal, posterior tibial, or dorsalis pedis pulses are found on the right, but they are all strongly felt on the left. With respect to these symptoms, which statement, if he reported it in his history, would lead you to believe that thrombosis is the etiology?

- (A) The patient had previously been experiencing claudication in one calf upon walking two blocks (approximately 0.25 kilometers).
- (B) The patient has atrial fibrillation.
- (C) The patient has mitral stenosis.
- (D) The patient has no collateral circulation around the occlusion and therefore suffers greater distal necrosis.
- (E) The patient was diagnosed with a 5.5-cm abdominal aortic aneurysm 1 year ago but refused surgical repair.

3. Which would be the MOST SENSITIVE indicator of chronic occlusive disease involving a patient's legs?

- (A) An audible bruit over the femoral artery
- (B) Symptoms of claudication after a brisk walk of approximately 0.25 kilometer, relieved by rest
- (C) A decrease to < 0.9 in the ankle/arm systolic blood-pressure ratio
- (D) The patient's 30-pack-per-year smoking history
- (E) Skin atrophy and hair loss over the dorsal part of the feet

4. A 40-year-old man complains of 3 days of anterior and posterior chest pains. His blood pressure is 138/84, pulse is 74 and bounding, temperature is 98.5°F (37°C), and respiratory rate is 16. His trachea is midline. His lungs are clear to auscultation and percussion. His cardiac examination reveals a new diastolic murmur over the right second intercostal space. A chest x-ray shows dilatation of the ascending aorta, and a CT scan of the chest confirms a 4-cm aneurysm of the ascending aorta. Which is the most likely cause of this patient's aneurysm?

- (A) Medial cystic necrosis
- (B) Cigarette smoking
- (C) Alcohol abuse
- (D) Atherosclerosis
- (E) Trauma

5. You are assessing a patient for atherosclerosis that involves arterial perfusion to the legs. You obtain a systolic blood-pressure (BP) reading on the posterior tibial artery and divide this by the systolic BP reading in the brachial artery. Which ratio would suggest SEVERE arterial occlusive disease at rest?

- (A) > 2.0
- (B) < 1.0
- (C) < 0.9
- (D) < 0.8
- (E) < 0.4

6. Which best describes pentoxifylline's mechanisms of benefit to patients with symptomatic, mild claudication?

- (A) Improvement in hemoglobin-oxygen saturation within the red blood cells
- (B) Reduction of peripheral atherosclerotic plaque
- (C) Decrease in the development of thrombi in partially occluded arteries
- (D) Improvement in venous return and cardiac output
- (E) Increase in red-blood-cell flexibility

7. In which symptomatic lesion would balloon angioplasty be likeliest to provide 5-year patency?

    (A) A stenosis of the aorta extending from the renal arteries to the bifurcation

    (B) A 2-cm distal occlusion of the distal right superficial femoral artery

    (C) A 4-cm lesion in the left common femoral artery

    (D) A 2-cm lesion in the left iliac vessel

    (E) A 1-cm lesion in the distal left dorsalis pedis artery

8. Of ascending aortic aneurysms smaller than 5 cm, what percentage rupture?

    (A) < 1%

    (B) 2%–3%

    (C) 5%–10%

    (D) 20%–40%

    (E) 50%–70%

9. During a general physical examination of a hypertensive male cigarette smoker, you palpate a pulsatile abdominal mass in the mid-supraumbilical region. This mass can be felt laterally as well as anteriorly. Which of the following would put this patient at increased risk of a catastrophic complication from your suspected diagnosis?

    (A) Diameter of mass less than 4 cm in diameter to palpation

    (B) Age of patient more than 65 years

    (C) Presence of chronic obstructive pulmonary disease

    (D) Presence of chronic hepatitis

    (E) Presence of diabetes mellitus

10. The patient in question 9 is now 1-week status after elective surgical repair of the condition you diagnosed. Which is most likely to cause his death within the next 5 years?

    (A) Aneurysm rupture

    (B) Wound infection

    (C) Stroke

    (D) Postsurgical pancreatitis

    (E) Coronary artery disease

11. Which is the correct statement about deep venous thrombosis (DVT)?

    (A) Almost all patients who develop DVT are eventually detected and treated with anticoagulants.

    (B) Most patients with DVT, if untreated, will die from pulmonary embolism.

    (C) Identification of DVT and treatment of the patient with therapeutic doses of anticoagulants almost always prevents pulmonary embolism.

    (D) Gangrene can be a complication of DVT.

    (E) Among fractures, those of the humerus carry the greatest risk for development of DVT.

12. What is the MOST COMMON genetic aberration found in patients with deep venous thrombosis?

    (A) Homocystinuria

    (B) A deficiency of antithrombin III

    (C) A deficiency of protein C

    (D) A mutation in factor V that causes a poor anticoagulant response to activated protein C

    (E) A deficiency of protein S

13. Assuming no extension into the deep venous system has occurred, which treatment is normally indicated in the management of patients with superficial thrombophlebitis?

    (A) Low-molecular-weight heparin

    (B) Topical heat application

    (C) Surgical division and ligation of the vein

    (D) Bed rest

    (E) Warfarin

DIRECTIONS (Items 14–15): Each of the numbered items or incomplete statements in this section is negatively phrased, as indicated by a capitalized word, such as NOT, LEAST, or EXCEPT. Select the ONE lettered answer or completion that is BEST in each case.

14. A 60-year-old man has a recurrence of symptomatic stenosis of the left iliac artery 6 months after undergoing successful balloon angioplasty of the lesion. Which is NOT indicated as a therapeutic intervention?

- (A) Cessation of smoking
- (B) Repeat balloon angioplasty
- (C) Mechanical atherectomy
- (D) Stent placement
- (E) Streptokinase infusion

15. Low-molecular-weight heparin, which has revolutionized management of venous thrombosis, has many advantages over traditional modalities. Which is NOT an advantage of low-molecular-weight-heparin in the treatment or prevention of deep venous thrombosis (DVT)?

- (A) It is less expensive to administer than an IV heparin drip.
- (B) It can be given even if the patient had a bleeding ulcer as recently as the last 1–2 days.
- (C) It does not require activated partial thromboplastin time (APTT) monitoring nor dose adjustment based on APTT results.
- (D) It is at least as effective as previous, standard heparin regimens
- (E) It permits earlier discharge from the hospital and, in some cases, even complete outpatient management.

DIRECTIONS (Items 16–20): For each numbered clinical situation in these matching questions, select the letter of the agent or therapy most appropriate for the treatment or prevention of thrombosis or embolism. (Assume the patient is not pregnant and has no allergies, no contraindications to any of the agents, and no recent spinal puncture.) Each lettered option may be selected once, more than once, or not at all.

- (A) Pneumatic compression boots
- (B) Warfarin
- (C) Low-molecular-weight heparin or adjusted-dose heparin (subcutaneous)
- (D) Low-dose heparin, without adjustment of dose, twice daily (subcutaneous)
- (E) Streptokinase

16. A 50-year-old man has chronic atrial fibrillation.

17. A 70-year-old man is at bed rest on his first postoperative day after a partial temporal lobectomy for a seizure disorder.

18. A 65-year-old woman who suffered a myocardial infarction 2 years ago is now hospitalized for an exacerbation of congestive heart failure.

19. A 39-year-old man has developed an extensive deep venous thrombosis in the left femoral vein which extends into the iliac vein.

20. A 69-year-old man is having difficulty walking because of incisional pain on the first postoperative day after radical prostatectomy.

ANSWERS AND EXPLANATIONS

1. The answer is B. Besides atrial fibrillation, myocardial infarction is most likely to be associated with peripheral embolism. Although only 5% of myocardial infarctions are complicated by systemic emboli, the relatively high incidence of infarctions makes them second to atrial fibrillation as an underlying source for emboli. Relatively more emboli originate from the heart (90%) than from aneurysms or peripheral atherosclerosis. Aortic stenosis is not usually associated with embolization. Mitral stenosis is associated with mural thrombi and embolization, particularly if associated left atrial enlargement exists, but with respect to atrial fibrillation and myocardial infarction, it is a much less common cause.

2. The answer is A. If this patient, who presents with signs and symptoms of acute arterial occlusion of the right lower leg, had experienced claudication in one calf upon walking two blocks (approximately 0.25 kilometer), the etiology suggested would be thrombosis. Without this additional information, the acute arterial occlusion could be secondary to either acute thrombosis or embolism. Patients with acute arterial thrombosis typically have some risk factors (including male gender) for atherosclerosis development and signs or symptoms of CHRONIC arterial occlusive disease (atherosclerotic occlusive disease) such as claudication. A history of atrial fibrillation, mitral stenosis, or left atrial enlargement all suggest embolism (originating in the cardiac atrium) and not thrombosis. Also, a known abdominal aneurysm could serve as a source of emboli to the legs. Patients with thrombosis as the cause typically have longstanding atherosclerosis of the arteries and, thus, have developed a collateral circulation which diminished ischemia (relative to embolism) if an acute occlusion occurs.

3. The answer is C. The earliest, most sensitive indicator of chronic occlusive disease is a decrease to less than 0.9 in the ankle/arm systolic blood pressure ratio. (A ratio of 0.4 represents very serious disease.) Cigarette smoking is the strongest risk factor for development of peripheral arterial occlusive disease, but it is not an indicator for it. Symptoms of claudication, bruits, skin changes, and loss of distal pulses occur later, as the occlusive disease progresses.

4. The answer is A. The likeliest cause of this person's aneurysm is medial cystic necrosis. DESCENDING aortic aneurysms are usually caused by atherosclerosis, although some are caused by trauma. ASCENDING aortic aneurysms, such as the one presented in this case, are usually secondary to cystic medial necrosis or syphilis. Alcohol abuse is not a risk factor for aortic aneurysm development.

5. The answer is E. The ratio < 0.4 would suggest *severe* arterial occlusive disease at rest. A ratio of > 1.0 is normal, because systolic blood pressure is normally slightly higher in the legs than in the arms. A ratio < 0.9 is consistent with some degree of arterial occlusive disease, and < 0.4 would indicate severe disease.

6. The answer is E. Pentoxifylline benefits patients who have mild claudication by increasing red-blood-cell flexibility. It improves tissue oxygenation in patients with chronic, peripheral-arterial occlusive disease by decreasing blood viscosity and increasing compliance in red blood cells. The other answer choices would tend to improve oxygen delivery to tissue, but they are not known responses to pentoxifylline therapy.

7. The answer is D. Five-year patency through balloon angioplasty would be likeliest to occur in a 2-cm lesion in the left iliac vessel. Five-year patency rates with balloon angioplasty improve with larger caliber vessels that have higher flow rates and that have shorter (< 3 cm) segments of occlusion. A 2-cm distal occlusion of the distal right superficial femoral artery, a 4-cm lesion in the left common femoral artery, or a 1-cm lesion in the distal left dorsalis pedis involve more distal arteries with poorer flow rates. A stenosis of the aorta extending from the renal arteries to the bifurcation or a 4-cm lesion in the left common femoral artery involve a longer occluded segment.

8. The answer is B. Of ascending aortic aneurysms smaller than 5 cm, 2%–3% rupture. Because of this relatively small risk of rupture versus the significant mortality (5%–10%) and morbidity risks of surgical repair, ascending aorta aneurysms smaller than 5 cm that are not expanding or symptomatic are often managed solely with aggressive blood-pressure control and observation.

9. The answer is C. Chronic obstructive pulmonary disease would put the patient at increased risk of rupture of his abdominal aortic aneurysm, which is the most likely clinical diagnosis. Such rupture is associated with larger diameter aneurysms, hypertension, and chronic obstructive pulmonary disease. Advanced age and, possibly, diabetes mellitus correlate with an increase in the incidence of abdominal aortic aneurysm, but are not identified risk factors for rupture. Chronic hepatitis is associated with portal hypertension and, rarely, pulmonary hypertension, but not systemic hypertension; chronic hepatitis is not associated with an increased rate of aneurysm rupture.

10. The answer is E. Coronary artery disease would be most likely to cause this patient's death within 5 years after elective surgical repair of his abdominal aortic aneurysm. An aggressive search for underlying coronary artery disease is necessary before the repair of the aneurysm. If a coronary artery bypass is indicated, it should be performed before the repair of the aneurysm. Aneurysm rupture, wound infection, stroke, and postsurgical pancreatitis are also potential postoperative complications in this patient, but are much less likely to be seen than coronary artery disease after the first postoperative week.

11. The answer is D. Venous gangrene can result from a particularly extreme DVT. Thrombolytic agents can be used for an extensive proximal DVT in an effort to prevent gangrene from developing. Most DVTs are not detected, but only about 30%–40% of patients with undetected DVT develop pulmonary embolism and only 10% of the patients who develop the pulmonary embolism die from it. DVT distal to the popliteal veins rarely embolizes. Distal DVT does not usually result in pulmonary embolism without extension of the clot into the proximal deep venous system. Treatment of DVT with anticoagulants decreases the risk of pulmonary embolism development by only about 50%. Among fractures, hip fractures carry the greatest risk for DVT, followed by knee fractures and other leg fractures.

12. The answer is D. A mutation in factor V that causes a poor anticoagulant response to activated protein C is the most common genetic aberration found in patients with DVT. This defect is not detected in standard activated partial thromboplastin time (APTT), prothrombin time, or protein-C assays. The most common method used now to assess factor V is a DNA analysis of the factor. Homocystinuria, and deficiencies of antithrombin III, protein C, and protein S are other potential causes of recurrent thromboembolism and must also be searched for in these patients, but they are much less common causes than the mutation in factor V.

13. The answer is B. Topical heat application and nonsteroidal anti-inflammation agents are usually all that are required for patients with superficial thrombophlebitis. Anticoagulants, such as heparin and warfarin, are not indicated unless extension into the deep venous system has occurred. Bed rest is not indicated because it may promote extension into the deep venous system. Surgical

division and ligation of veins is used rarely in the treatment of venous varicosities, but it is not used in the treatment of superficial thrombophlebitis.

14. The answer is E. Streptokinase infusion is NOT indicated for this patient. Thrombolytic agents are used in acute thrombosis, but not in chronic peripheral atherosclerosis. Smoking cessation reduces progression and recurrences of atherosclerotic stenoses. Recurrent iliac artery stenoses could be approached with stenting, atherectomy, or another trial of balloon angioplasty.

15. The answer is B. Low-molecular-weight heparin should NOT be given if the patient had a bleeding ulcer in the last 1–2 days. The absolute and relative contraindications to heparin therapy also apply to low-molecular-weight heparin, but the latter provides a more consistent anticoagulant response per dose to the degree that dosing can be done based solely on the patient's weight and without activated partial thromboplastin time (APTT) monitoring.

16. The answer is B. Warfarin is effective, and the agent of choice, in decreasing the incidence of embolic strokes in patients with atrial fibrillation. Heparin, both regular and low-molecular weight, can also be effective; however, because of a life-long indication for anticoagulation in patients such as this one, subcutaneous injections with heparin are too inconvenient and costly. Heparin is sometimes used when rapid reversal of coagulation may be necessary, such as perioperatively, but not for chronic treatment. The thrombus you are trying to prevent in this situation is a mural cardiac thrombus, so the pneumatic compression boots used to prevent deep venous thrombosis would not be effective. Thrombolytic agents, such as streptokinase, are also effective, but are much more prone to hemorrhagic complications (e.g., intracerebral hemorrhage) and also require continued intravenous access.

17. The answer is A. Pneumatic compression boots, while not as effective as anticoagulants, still significantly reduce the chance of development of deep venous thrombosis in surgical patients. In most surgical patients, the risk of hemorrhagic complications with prophylactic use of warfarin and heparin is very small (when dosing guidelines are followed). However, in patients who have had central nervous system surgery, hemorrhage is much more common, and anticoagulants are avoided. Thrombolytic agents (e.g., streptokinase) are even more likely to result in central nervous system hemorrhage, and their use is prohibited in this setting.

18. The answer is D. Prophylactic mini-dose heparin is appropriate for this patient, who is at moderate risk for deep venous thrombosis. Theoretically, low-molecular-weight heparin is effective as well, but it has not yet been subjected to clinical trials for this situation. (It has been tried in prophylaxis after hip surgery and in the treatment of known deep venous thrombosis and pulmonary embolism.) Warfarin treatment, which would take days to fully anticoagulate this patient, is not appropriate. Pneumatic compression boots would be better than no prophylaxis, but not as effective as heparin.

19. The answer is E. Streptokinase or other thrombolytic agent is appropriate for this patient who has an extensive, proximal vein deep venous thrombosis, and thus is at significant risk for fatal pulmonary embolism as well as phlebotic syndrome and venous gangrene. This is one of the few situations in which thrombolytic agents are warranted in the treatment of deep venous thrombosis. Heparin and warfarin are less likely to

avert these complications. Pneumatic compression boots do not produce resolution of a thrombus that has already formed.

20. The answer is D. Mini-dose heparin, given subcutaneously, is the preventative measure of choice for this patient who is at moderate risk for deep venous thrombosis. Achieving therapeutic anticoagulation with warfarin would take too long. The patient would have to be at higher risk to justify low-molecular-weight heparin or adjusted-dose heparin. Pneumatic compression boots would be effective, but not as effective as the heparin.

BIBLIOGRAPHY

Kurowski K: Peripheral vascular disease. In *Family Medicine* (House Officer Series). Edited by Rudy DR, Kurowski K. Baltimore, Williams & Wilkins, 1997, pp 97–121.

Test 7

Cerebrovascular Disease and Brain Injury

DIRECTIONS (Items 1–14): Each of the numbered items or incomplete statements in this section is followed by answers or by completions of the statement. Select the ONE lettered answer or completion that is BEST in each case.

1. Which is the major cause of intracerebral hemorrhage?

(A) Atrial fibrillation
(B) Hypertension
(C) Cigarette smoking
(D) Cerebral aneurysm
(E) Coagulopathy

2. Which patient most warrants an evaluation for vasculitis and the antiphospholipid antibody syndrome (as opposed to the more common atherosclerosis or embolism) as causes of a stroke?

(A) A 40-year-old woman with an ischemic stroke
(B) A 44-year-old man with known atherosclerosis of his iliac arteries who is status post two myocardial infarctions
(C) A 20-year-old patient who has had an intracerebral hemorrhage secondary to rupture of an arteriovenous malformation
(D) A 60-year-old diabetic with hypertension
(E) A 40-year-old patient with chronic atrial fibrillation

3. Which of the following features is most consistent with a hemorrhagic stroke?

(A) A slow development of hemiplegia
(B) Development of signs and symptoms of the stroke in a stuttering fashion
(C) A severe headache
(B) A fully clear sensorium
(E) A better prognosis relative to ischemic strokes

4. A 67-year-old male patient suffered an ischemic thrombotic stroke 2 hours earlier, and he has a pronounced left hemiparesis. A noncontrast CT scan of the head reveals no intracerebral hemorrhage. His blood pressure is 160/95. Which orders are most appropriate for him?

(A) Coumadin
(B) A low-salt, low-cholesterol diet
(C) Rapid reduction of blood pressure with labetalol until it is about 120/80
(D) Ticlopidine
(E) Intravenous tissue plasminogen activator

5. A 52-year-old man who has no previous history of headaches complains of a severe headache that developed 4 hours earlier, after weight lifting. No trauma has occurred. The patient denies any numbness or weakness. On examination, his temperature is 100° F (37.7°C), blood pressure is 150/90, pulse is 90 and regular, and respiratory rate is 16. He can answer questions, but he falls asleep after answering each one. He can move and has intact sensation to all extremities. Which of the following is the most likely diagnosis in this patient?

(A) Subarachnoid hemorrhage
(B) Migraine headache
(C) Tension headache
(D) Benign intracranial hypertension
(E) Temporal arteritis

6. With respect to the preceding question, which of the following complications is the greatest cause of morbidity in patients with this diagnosis?

(A) Vasospasm
(B) Rebleeding
(C) Communicating hydrocephalus
(D) Normal pressure hydrocephalus
(E) Seizures

7. Which is a characteristic change in a limb in a patient who has reflex sympathetic dystrophy after a stroke?

(A) Distal extremity edema
(B) Numbness in the distal extremity
(C) Paresthesias in the distal extremity
(D) Fasciculations in the involved limb
(E) Joint laxity in the involved limb

8. Which statement is correct with regard to the use of ticlopidine in a patient who has had a recent ischemic stroke?

(A) It is inexpensive.
(B) It is useful in preventing embolic strokes in patients with atrial fibrillation.
(C) It is used in the primary prevention of stroke.
(D) It can produce a severe neutropenia.
(E) It is the first-line agent in the secondary prevention of stroke.

9. In examining a 68-year-old male patient with hypertension and hypercholesterolemia, you detect a right carotid bruit. You obtain a carotid Doppler, which reveals a 70% stenosis of the right carotid and a 30% stenosis of the left. The patient denies ever having a stroke and has a normal neurologic examination. What is this patient's approximate stroke risk?

(A) < 0.5% per year
(B) 2% per year
(C) 5% per year
(D) 10% per year
(E) 20% per year

10. Chronic subdural hematomas are more likely to be seen in certain patient populations than in others. Which patient would be at increased risk for developing this type of hematoma?

(A) A cigarette smoker
(B) A patient with a generalized seizure disorder
(C) A patient on sublingual nitroglycerine as needed for stable angina pectoris
(D) A patient with a meningioma
(E) A patient younger than age 50

11. Which is a common sign or symptom in the presentation of a chronic subdural hematoma?

(A) Fully clear sensorium
(B) Headache which has been progressing in intensity for weeks
(C) Tonic pupil
(D) Bilateral symmetrical leg weakness with hyperactive deep tendon reflexes and Babinski signs (extensor plantar response)
(E) Unilateral, fixed numbness and weakness that is more prominent than the accompanying headache

12. You have a 24-year-old female patient who sustained significant head trauma with loss of consciousness a half-hour earlier. She is now alert and oriented, and her pupillary size and response, as well as her neurologic examination, are normal. If she were to develop an epidural hematoma, how long at most would it take to develop?

(A) Within the next 10 minutes
(B) Within the next hour
(C) Within 24 hours
(D) Within 3 days
(E) Within 10 days

13. Which feature suggests a better prognosis than others do in patients who require evacuation of acute subdural hematomas?

(A) Decerebrate posturing
(B) Age greater than 40 years
(C) Presence of a Hutchinson pupil
(D) A Glasgow Coma Scale score of 4
(E) Normal intracranial pressure

14. You suspect subarachnoid hemorrhage in a patient who shows confusion and has a new, extremely severe, brisk onset, occipital headache. The patient can speak and walk and is stable on cardiorespiratory assessment. Which test would you order first?

(A) A noncontrast CT scan of the head
(B) A CT scan of the head with contrast
(C) An MRI study of the brain
(D) Skull x-rays
(E) A lumbar puncture to look for red blood cells in the cerebrospinal fluid

---

DIRECTIONS (Item 15): The incomplete statement in this section is negatively phrased, as indicated by the capitalized word, NOT. Select the ONE lettered answer or completion that is BEST.

---

15. Clinically, you suspect an ischemic stroke in the region of the right anterior circulation in a 70-year-old male patient with hypertension, who has otherwise been healthy with no known illnesses. He presented with left hemiplegia. Which test would NOT be appropriate in the initial management of this patient?

(A) A noncontrast CT scan of the head
(B) A CBC
(C) A cardiac enzymes test
(D) An EEG
(E) A serum glucose test

ANSWERS AND EXPLANATIONS

1. The answer is B. Hypertension, which causes more than 50% of intracerebral hemorrhages, is the major cause of these hemorrhages. An even higher proportion of intracerebral hemorrhages within the basal ganglia is secondary to hypertension. Atrial fibrillation is associated with embolic stroke, but not with intracerebral hemorrhage. Cigarette smoking, cerebral aneurysm, and coagulopathy can be causes of intracerebral hemorrhage, but none of them is the major cause.

2. The answer is A. The 40-year-old female patient with an ischemic stroke is the one who most warrants an evaluation for vasculitis and the antiphospholipid antibody syndrome. A work-up for vasculitis or antiphospholipid antibodies is best reserved for patients who have other features of these disorders (e.g., evidence of systemic lupus), those who are on medications that are associated with these disorders (such as procainamide), and those who have suffered ischemic strokes at a young age (age < 45) with no risk factors for atherosclerosis and no other explanation (such as an AV malformation) for this stroke. The patient with chronic atrial fibrillation is at increased risk for embolic stroke and does not warrant a work-up for other causes.

3. The answer is C. A severe headache is most consistent with a hemorrhagic stroke. Headache is usually a prominent feature of hemorrhagic stroke and may be severe. The mechanism for this is the edema and swelling that develops in response to the hemorrhage and the resultant increase in intracranial pressure. Vomiting and a clouded sensorium are also typical features. Ischemic strokes do not produce this marked edema and produce either no headache or a very minimal headache. Hemorrhagic strokes are characterized by a more sudden onset and poorer prognosis than ischemic strokes. A stuttering, slower development of signs and symptoms is sometimes seen in ischemic strokes.

4. The answer is E. An order for intravenous tissue plasminogen activator would be most appropriate for this patient. Acute use of coumadin or ticlopidine has not been shown to be effective. Tissue plasminogen activator decreases the neurologic defect if it is given within the first 3 hours after ischemic stroke, but it increases the risk of hemorrhagic stroke development. An absolute contraindication to its use is any active internal bleeding. Relative contraindications include uncontrolled hypertension, recent (within less than 10 days) major trauma,

surgery, internal bleeding and coagulation disorders. Patients should initially be given nothing by mouth because of the frequency of associated swallowing difficulties and risk for aspiration. Rapid lowering of blood pressure in patients with acute ischemic stroke can cause worse neurologic deficits.

5. The answer is A. The most likely diagnosis in this patient is subarachnoid hemorrhage, which produces an abrupt, extremely severe headache, usually noted in the occipital area and frequently associated with a mild elevation in temperature. An altered sensorium or sleepiness are typical of subarachnoid hemorrhage, but not with tension or migraine headaches. Temporal arteritis is usually associated with an elevated temperature, but is not accompanied by an altered sensorium, and the headache is not as intense or acute as with subarachnoid hemorrhage. Patients who have benign intracranial hypertension, most commonly seen in young, overweight women, have papilledema and, rarely, visual defects, but they have clear sensoriums and are afebrile.

6. The answer is A. Seizures, communicating and normal pressure hydrocephalus, and rebleeding are all complications of subarachnoid hemorrhage, but the complication that carries the greatest morbidity is vasospasm. Prophylactic calcium channel blockers such as nimodipine are given to prevent this complication.

7. The answer is A. Distal extremity edema is a characteristic change in a limb in a patient who has reflex sympathetic dystrophy after a stroke. Reflex sympathetic dystrophy is most commonly seen after limb trauma, especially if immobilization or casting is necessary, but can also be seen after a stroke. The initial changes are burning pains, vasomotor skin changes, hyperesthesia, and edema in the affected limb. Atrophy can develop later, particularly if the reflex sympathetic dystrophy is not treated in its earlier stages.

8. The answer is D. A severe neutropenia can be produced by the use of ticlopidine in a patient who has had a recent ischemic stroke. Aspirin is the only recommended agent for the primary prevention of stroke, unless the patient has atrial fibrillation, in which case daily coumadin is recommended to achieve an INR of 2–3. Aspirin is also the first-line agent recommended for the secondary prevention of stroke. Ticlopidine, because of its risk of neutropenia and its high cost, is used only if the patient is aspirin intolerant or if ischemic strokes recur despite aspirin use.

9. The answer is B. This patient's approximate stroke risk is 2% per year. Carotid endarterectomy would reduce the risk by about 53%, but even in experienced centers and on patients in whom surgical risks are low, it carries a morbidity and mortality rate of 1%–3%.

10. The answer is B. A patient with a generalized seizure disorder would be at increased risk of developing a chronic subdural hematoma, secondary to head trauma that might occur during loss of consciousness. An atraumatic, chronic subdural hematoma is more commonly seen in alcoholics, the elderly, patients who have a seizure disorder, and patients on anticoagulants. Cigarette smoking increases the risk for ischemic strokes but not of subdural hematomas. (Alcohol use increases the risk for intracerebral bleeding and subdural hematomas.)

11. The answer is B. Progressive headache or confusion is more prominent than the often minimal and fluctuating neurologic defects in the typical presentation of a chronic subdural hematoma. Severe and fixed neurologic defects are not typical of chronic subdural hematomas and this feature often leads to a delay in its recognition. Hutchinson's pupil (ipsilateral pupil dilation secondary to a herniated temporal lobe impinging on the third cranial nerve) can be seen, but tonic pupil (a chronically large, rigid pupil that responds slowly to light and accommodation) is not seen.

12. The answer is C. If this patient were to develop an epidural hematoma, it would occur within 24 hours. Epidural hematomas accumulate rapidly, usually within minutes after the trauma, but sometimes development takes up to 24 hours.

13. The answer is E. Normal intracranial pressure suggests a better prognosis than do the other factors in patients who require evacuation of acute subdural hematomas. Elevated intracranial pressure is an adverse prognostic factor. A Glasgow Coma Scale score of 12–15 would suggest a likely full recovery; a score of less than 6 suggests severe brain injury, and is associated with a 75% mortality for subdural hematomas. Decerebrate posturing in a patient who requires evacuation of an acute subdural hematoma indicates that elevated intracranial pressure has produced a herniation against the upper brain stem; and the presence of the Hutchinson's pupillary sign indicates that increased pressure has herniated the temporal lobe against CN III. Both are adverse prognostic factors.

14. The answer is A. A noncontrast CT scan of the head should be ordered first in this patient. Ninety percent of SAH cases will show intraventricular blood on a noncontrast CT. Contrast adds nothing to the sensitivity of this study for SAH; in addition, it takes more time and is more expensive. Cerebrospinal fluid is obtained if SAH is suspected, but only when the CT is negative and shows no lesions that could cause herniation when the CSF is withdrawn. Skull x-rays do not detect subarachnoid hemorrhage. MRI is more expensive and more time-consuming, but no more sensitive, than a noncontrast CT scan in detecting SAH.

15. The answer is D. An EEG would NOT be appropriate in the initial management of this patient. It usually demonstrates abnormal wave forms in the affected lobe, but direct imaging studies are superior in localizing the lesion. A CBC, electrolytes, glucose, BUN, creatinine, prothrombin time, APTT, cholesterol, and liver function tests are typically ordered as baseline studies. The CBC is ordered to check for anemia that could exacerbate an ischemic stroke, and for leukemia or polycythemia, which (because of increased blood viscosity) could produce stroke. Serial cardiac enzymes are ordered because of the frequent concurrence of stroke and myocardial infarction. A noncontrast CT of the head is ordered at presentation to rule out a hemorrhagic stroke. If it is negative, a CT with contrast is performed in 2 days when thrombotic or embolic strokes can be demonstrated.

BIBLIOGRAPHY

Coletta EM: Cerebrovascular disease and brain injury. In: *Family Medicine* (House Officer Series). Edited by Rudy DR, Kurowski K. Baltimore, Williams & Wilkins, 1997, pp 123–132.

Test 8

Cardiovascular Problems in Children

DIRECTIONS (Items 1–15): Each of the numbered items or incomplete statements in this section is followed by answers or by completions of the statement. Select the ONE lettered answer or completion that is BEST in each case.

1. Primary-care physicians are often challenged to triage heart murmurs in children. To do so competently permits diagnosis of critical conditions while avoiding excessive utilization of technology and of consultation. You hear a low-frequency, crescendo-decrescendo murmur along the left sternal border in a 6-year-old boy. You suspect he has a Still's murmur. Which of the following would decrease the intensity of this type of murmur?

   (A) Fever of 102°F (38.8°C)
   (B) Hemoglobin of 8.0
   (C) Anxiety
   (D) Performing a Valsalva maneuver
   (E) Cutaneous vasodilatation

2. Which is true with respect to atrial septal defects?

   (A) They are the most common congenital heart defect.
   (B) They are usually recognized in infancy.
   (C) A loss of the change in the split of the second heart sound is present during inspiration.
   (D) The early systolic murmur at the left second intercostal space is pathognomonic.
   (E) The murmur is usually loud (grade IV-V/VI) in intensity.

3. Which is characteristic of a pulmonary flow murmur?

   (A) The inspiratory split in the second heart sound remains physiological.
   (B) It is frequently appreciated during the first trimester of pregnancy.
   (C) It is most often appreciated in the geriatric population.
   (D) It radiates to the neck.
   (E) It radiates to the back.

4. Which is characteristic of the murmur of a jugular venous hum?

   (A) It has only a diastolic component.
   (B) It has a coarse, harsh sound.
   (C) The murmur dissipates when the child lies supine.
   (D) It is produced by flow from the right subclavian vein hitting the right angle as it empties into the superior vena cava.
   (E) It is most often heard in teenagers and young adults.

5. During the well-baby visit of a 2-week-old male infant, you notice the baby has a harsh, pansystolic, loud murmur at the lower left sternal border. The infant has been eating normally, and the parent has not observed any episodes of cyanosis or dyspnea. In your earlier examinations of this baby at birth and before his discharge from the newborn nursery, you did not appreciate any murmurs. For which complication is the child at risk?

   (A) Heart failure
   (B) The Eisenmenger syndrome
   (C) Bacterial endocarditis
   (D) Failure of the defect to close spontaneously
   (E) All of the above

6. You are examining a 2-week-old infant with a ventricular septal defect. The infant has no symptoms, and has been eating and maintaining appropriate weight. Heart rate, respiratory rate, and pulses are normal. The murmur is of mild intensity (grade I/VI). The lung fields are clear. No cyanosis or edema is present. Which is true regarding this infant's condition?

   (A) The lack of symptoms predicts a favorable outcome without intervention.
   (B) Signs may develop over the following weeks as pulmonary vascular resistance drops.
   (C) The low intensity of the murmur speaks for a favorable prognosis without intervention.
   (D) This child should simply be observed during the next 1–2 years for spontaneous closure of this defect.
   (E) Further evaluation is necessary only if the child develops symptoms.

7. Which is characteristic of pulmonary stenosis?

   (A) The severity can be estimated by assessment of the degree of right ventricular hypertrophy on EKG.
   (B) A palpable lift is present at the fifth intercostal space, 1 centimeter lateral to the mid-clavicular line.
   (C) The gradient usually increases as the child grows.
   (D) Most cases require valve replacement.
   (E) The murmur usually radiates to the neck.

8. You detect a grade III/VI harsh murmur over the left sternal border and second right intercostal space in a 13-year-old boy. He has no dyspnea, orthopnea, syncope, or chest pains. You suspect he has congenital aortic stenosis. On physical examination, which finding correlates BEST with a significant gradient across the valve?

(A) The murmur radiates to the neck.
(B) An ejection click is present.
(C) The murmur is loud and harsh, both at the base and left sternal border.
(D) The murmur radiates to the back.
(E) A palpable thrill is present in the suprasternal notch.

9. You are evaluating a child for suspected coarctation of the aorta. Which physical finding correlates best with its presence?

(A) An ejection click at the second left intercostal space
(B) Diminished blood-pressure readings in the legs as compared with the arms
(C) A delay in the femoral pulse
(D) A continuous murmur over the back
(E) A systolic murmur over the left sternal border

10. What is the treatment of choice for a hemodynamically significant patent ductus arteriosus in a premature infant of 4 lbs and 5oz (1650 g) that persists for longer than 48 hours?

(A) Observation for clinical deterioration
(B) Thrombosing the patent ductus via cardiac catheterization
(C) Indomethacin
(D) Surgical ligation
(E) Vasodilators

11. You are examining a 2-day-old male infant in the nursery. The baby was born at term, via a normal, spontaneous vaginal delivery. No prenatal or perinatal complications occurred. The infant has been eating well. His color is good, and no tachypnea or cyanosis is present. His pulse rate is normal; his lungs are clear. You hear a mild, continuous murmur in the second left intercostal space. Which would you recommend?

(A) Observation only, with no testing or treatment if the murmur disappears in the next 1 or 2 days
(B) Chest x-ray and EKG
(C) 2-D echocardiogram with Doppler study
(D) Cardiac catheterization
(E) Indomethacin

12. You hear a carotid bruit in a 3-year-old who has been otherwise healthy and has been growing and developing appropriately for her age. She is on no medications. Which would you recommend?

(A) Aspirin 325 mg by mouth each day
(B) Dipyridamole by mouth, 3 times each day
(C) A carotid Doppler study
(D) A cerebral angiogram
(E) Nothing but observation

13. Which congenital heart lesion could present with cyanosis within the first 3 days of birth?

(A) Patent ductus arteriosus
(B) Transposition of the great vessels
(C) Coarctation of the aorta
(D) Atrial septal defect
(E) Hypoplastic left-heart syndrome

14. Which cardiac rhythm is cause for concern in an otherwise healthy, asymptomatic child?

(A) Premature atrial contractions
(B) Respiratory sinus arrhythmia
(C) Couplets of premature ventricular contractions
(D) All of the above
(E) None of the above

15. A 6-week-old boy was born via a normal, spontaneous vaginal delivery and required no resuscitation. Since birth, he had a mild systolic murmur over the second left intercostal space, but normal brachial pulses and clear lung fields. He had been doing well, but 1 week ago he developed episodes, lasting 10–15 seconds, of cyanosis and lethargy. These episodes were noted when he was irritated and crying. These findings best describe which of the following congenital heart lesions?

(A) Tetralogy of Fallot
(B) Transposition of the great arteries
(C) Patent ductus arteriosus
(D) Atrial septal defect
(E) Ventricular septal defect

DIRECTIONS (Item 16): The incomplete statement in this section is negatively phrased, as indicated by the capitalized word, EXCEPT. Select the ONE lettered answer or completion that is BEST.

16. Assume you are in a small community hospital. All of the following would be appropriate in the management of an infant with suspected cyanotic congenital heart disease EXCEPT

- (A) Obtaining a chest x-ray to evaluate for evidence of pulmonary disease
- (B) Obtaining a complete blood cell count (CBC) and arterial oxygen tension (PO_2)
- (C) Assessing the infant's response to the administration of 100% oxygen
- (D) Starting an IV infusion of prostaglandin E_1 and urgently transporting the infant to a tertiary center with expertise in pediatric cardiovascular surgery.
- (E) Holding the patient in your hospital until the following day, at which time a 2-D echocardiogram can be performed.

ANSWERS AND EXPLANATIONS

1. The answer is D. Performing a Valsalva maneuver usually decreases the intensity of a functional murmur. During the Valsalva maneuver, the patient is bearing down to exhale, but the glottis remains closed, which has the effect of transiently (for approximately 10 seconds) raising the intrathoracic pressure. The Valsalva maneuver diminishes end diastolic left-ventricular volumes and diminishes cardiac output; this either diminishes the murmur or produces no change in the murmur. Functional murmurs, such as Still's, increase in intensity in situations that increase cardiac output, such as with fever, anemia, anxiety, or cutaneous vasodilatation.

2. The answer is C. With respect to atrial septal defects, a loss of the change in the split of the second heart sound is present during inspiration. The murmur of atrial septal defect is systolic and of low intensity at the second or third left intercostal space, where it is easily confused with a pulmonary flow murmur. The murmur of atrial septal defect is associated with a fixed split of the second heart sound, whereas the split of S_2 only during inspiration is preserved in pulmonic flow murmurs. The murmur is frequently not appreciated in childhood. Ventricular septal defect, not atrial septic defect, is the most common congenital heart defect.

3. The answer is A. It is characteristic of pulmonary flow murmurs that the inspiratory split in the second heart sound remains physiological. The murmur of pulmonary flow is systolic and usually heard at the left second or third intercostal space. It does not radiate to the neck or back. It is frequently heard in adolescents and in women in the third trimester of pregnancy. In contrast to atrial septal defects, it is not associated with a fixed split in the second heart sound.

4. The answer is C. The murmur of a jugular venous hum dissipates when the child lies supine. A jugular venous hum, which is a buzz-like noise heard throughout the cardiac cycle in some children (especially toddlers), is produced by cerebral blood flow hitting the right angle at the innominate vein. It is heard best in infraclavicular regions, and it is not heard when the jugular vein is compressed or when the child lies supine. It has no clinical significance except that the sound must not be confused with cardiac murmurs.

5. The answer is E. The infant is at risk for all of the complications listed in the answer choices. Patients with ventricular septal defect (VSD) may develop several complications, most of which relate to the increased pulmonary blood flow which can lead to pulmonary hypertension and, eventually, right heart failure. Sometimes the pulmonary hypertension develops to the degree that a right-to-left shunt of blood occurs across the defect (the Eisenmenger syndrome), replacing the previous left-to-right shunt. Smaller VSDs often close spontaneously in the first few years of life, but larger defects and defects in older children are less likely to close spontaneously. Patients with VSD are prone to bacterial endocarditis; prophylaxis is recommended.

6. The answer is B. Signs may develop in this child in the following weeks as pulmonary vascular resistance drops. Symptoms may not be present in a child such as this with ventricular septal defects (VSDs), even large VSDs, until irreversible pulmonary hypertension and its sequelae develop. In infants, fetal pulmonary vascular resistance may persist to some degree, diminishing any left-to-right shunting, the intensity of the murmur, and symptoms. Smaller VSDs produce more turbulence and vibration (louder murmurs) with the passage of blood; thus, louder murmurs are usually appreciated in children with smaller VSDs, which have a better prognosis without intervention.

7. The answer is A. The severity of the gradient in pulmonary stenosis can usually be well estimated by assessing the degree of right ventricular hypertrophy on EKG. The gradient does not usually progress in the congenital variety. Pulmonary stenosis is associated with a harsh murmur at the second left intercostal space that radiates to the back. Antibiotic prophylaxis is recommended, and valvuloplasty is the common treatment if the gradient is severe.

8. The answer is E. On physical exam, a palpable thrill in the suprasternal notch is the best correlate for a significant aortic stenosis. (If a significant stenosis exists, a strong vibration is produced as the blood passes through, which is palpable in the suprasternal notch.) A murmur that radiates to the neck or back, a murmur that is loud and harsh both at the base and left sternal border, and an ejection click can all be seen with aortic stenosis, but they do not predict the gradient as well.

9. The answer is B. The physical finding that correlates best with the presence of coarctation of the aorta is diminished blood pressure readings in the legs compared to those in the arms, especially in a child. Other changes (e.g., changes of possibly associated bicuspid aortic valve, such as ejection clicks or systolic murmurs) are not always present. The femoral pulse delay and collateral formation (which produces a continuous murmur over the back) are usually not evident in children.

10. The answer is C. In most cases, a hemodynamically significant patent ductus arteriosus in a premature infant will close with the use of IV indomethacin if it does not close spontaneously within the first 2 days with supportive care. A patent ductus arteriosus permits a left-to-right shunt to occur, which eventually leads to left (and, later, right) ventricular hypertrophy; observation is appropriate only for the first 48 hours. Surgical ligation or thrombosis is considered only when the less invasive indomethacin treatment is not effective. Vasodilators can decrease the left-to-right shunt, but they only have a temporary effect.

11. The answer is A. For this infant, observation with no testing or treatment is recommended if the murmur disappears in the next 1 or 2 days. This is probably the common murmur of a transient ductus arteriosus. Other studies (listed in the other answer choices) would not be necessary. In newborns, evidence of cyanosis, tachypnea, increasing supplemental oxygen needs, poor pulses, and hypotension are more indicative of hemodynamically significant congenital heart disease than the presence or absence of a murmur.

12. The answer is E. In this child, one should recommend nothing but observation. Carotid bruits are a common physiologic murmur in children and can be heard in conjunction with a Still's murmur, a lower frequency, systolic, innocent murmur that can be heard along the left sternal border in many children.

13. The answer is B. Transposition of the great vessels is a congenital heart lesion that presents with cyanosis early in life, and could present within the first 3 days of birth. A patent ductus is necessary along with the transposition to allow any oxygenated blood to reach the systemic circulation. Atrial septal defect (ASD) could be associated with cyanosis, but not in infancy. ASD produces a left-to-right shunt which leads to pulmonary volume overwork. In adulthood, rare development of pulmonary hypertension can change the shunt to a right-to-left shunt and produce cyanosis, but this is much less likely to be seen in ASD than in ventricular septal defect or in cases where a patent ductus persists. Hypoplastic left heart is not characterized by a shunt; therefore, it is not associated with cyanosis. Coarctation of the aorta can produce disparity in blood pressure and pulse intensities between the two arms and between the arms and legs, but will not produce cyanosis.

14. The answer is C. A cardiac rhythm characterized by couplets of premature ventricular contractions (PVCs) is cause for concern, even in an otherwise healthy, asymptomatic child. Premature atrial contractions and most premature ventricular contractions are benign in childhood; however, PVCs that are multifocal, or are associated with known cardiac abnormalities, or are present in couplets or triplets, are of more concern because they are more likely to develop into ventricular tachycardia and because these rhythms are more likely to be seen when heart disease is present. Respiratory sinus arrhythmia is an altered rate of sinus discharge, depending on whether the patient is in inspiration or expiration; this is a normal physiologic variation which is more pronounced in children.

15. The answer is A. The tetralogy of Fallot would best explain the findings in this 6-week-old baby. Only the tetralogy of Fallot and transposition of the great arteries are associated with cyanosis in infancy, but the cyanosis that is secondary to the tetralogy is more likely to develop after 2 weeks of age, while the cyanosis in transposition is usually noted at birth or within the first few days, as the ductus arteriosus closes. A patent ductus is not associated with cyanosis. Atrial septal defect and ventricular septal defect can be associated with cyanosis only if a right-to-left shunt has developed secondary to pulmonary hypertension that results from pulmonary vascular overload (Eisenmenger syndrome). This shunt would take years to develop, even across large defects.

16. The answer is E. Obtaining a 2-D echocardiogram, an expensive use of time and money, is not appropriate in the management of an infant with suspected cyanotic congenital heart disease. Infants with cyanosis can and should be quickly evaluated for potential respiratory disorders via a chest x-ray and a check of the response in the PO_2 to supplemental oxygen. Echocardiography can have poor sensitivity for congenital heart disease in inexperienced centers, and a precise anatomical diagnosis could and should wait until the child is at a pediatric cardiovascular center. A prostaglandin E_1 infusion would help keep the ductus patent if cyanotic heart disease is present until a definitive work-up and treatment can be initiated.

BIBLIOGRAPHY

Bricker JT, Anderson JC: Cardiovascular problems in children. In *Family Medicine* (House Officer Series). Edited by Rudy DR, Kurowski K. Baltimore, Williams & Wilkins, 1997, pp. 133–144.

Test 9

Hypertension

1. A middle-aged, male patient, upon learning that his blood pressure is elevated, suggests that his cigarette smoking and stressful job may be responsible. Which of the following is the strongest risk factor for his primary (essential) hypertension?

   (A) Family history of type II diabetes mellitus
   (B) High-stress occupation
   (C) Obesity, with distribution in hips and thighs
   (D) History of smoking
   (E) Primary aldosteronism

2. A 45-year-old male patient, with a multiple family history of hypertension, weighs 180 lb. (81.8 kg) at a height of 5′10″ (1.78 m), and presents with a blood pressure (BP) of 145/95. You place the patient on a no-salt-added diet, which results in a consistent BP of 130/85 for the next 6 months. Then, as the patient's weight rises to 195 lb and the patient lapses on the low-salt diet, the BP rises again. Which of the following medications is most likely to be effective in controlling the BP in this patient?

   (A) Lisinopril
   (B) Propranolol
   (C) Atenolol
   (D) Triamterene/hydrochlorothiazide
   (E) Diazepam

3. A 47-year-old, male, African-American patient presents with a blood pressure (BP) of 150/105, confirmed over three visits. You consider the fact that the choice of first-line drug therapy may be influenced by the patient's race. Which of the following pathophysiologic mechanisms is likely to be at work in this case?

   (A) Less reduction of renal function for given average BP maintenance
   (B) Low risk for stroke for given BP level
   (C) A higher allowable therapeutic target BP
   (D) High renin state
   (E) A statistically more favorable response to diuretics

4. Before embarking on any treatment for the first time in a patient, you realize you should consider the possibilities of secondary forms of hypertension. The approximate proportion of hypertension that falls into the category of secondary hypertension is

   (A) 5%–10%
   (B) 1%–15%
   (C) 15%–20%
   (D) 25%
   (E) 35%

5. Which statement is true with respect to primary aldosteronism?

   (A) It comprises 5%–10% of all cases of hypertension.
   (B) It should be considered in the face of hypertension accompanied by hypokalemia.
   (C) It is caused, in 70%–90% of cases, by idiopathic hyperaldosteronism, which results from bilateral hyperplasia.
   (D) Idiopathic hyperaldosteronism, caused by bilateral hyperplasia, can be treated by angiotensin-converting enzyme inhibitors.
   (E) Adenomas causing this disease can be palpated transabdominally in the majority of cases.

6. Which statement is relevant with regard to pheochromocytoma?

   (A) The majority of cases of paroxysms of anxiety presenting to the primary-care physician result from pheochromocytoma.
   (B) Removal of the tumor guarantees cure.
   (C) Familial cases tend to occur in association with primary aldosteronism.
   (D) Sensitivity and specificity for 24-hour urine metanephrines are sufficient to diagnose pheochromocytoma.
   (E) Labetalol is useful in stabilizing the patient prior to definitive therapy because it blocks both alpha and reflex beta discharge.

7. Which of the following represents the "normal" deterioration of renal function with the passage of time in a nonhypertensive adult?

(A) BUN rising by 1 mg/dl per year
(B) Creatinine rising by 0.1 mg/dl per year
(C) Proteinuria increasing by 1 g/24 hr per year
(D) Uremic frost appearing by age 80
(E) Creatinine clearance falling by 1 ml/min/1.73 m^2 per year

8. Which is an acceptable definition of microalbuminuria in hypertension?

(A) 30–300 mg/24 hours
(B) 200–500 mg/24 hours
(C) 500–1000 mg/24 hours
(D) 2000–3000 mg/24 hours
(E) > 3000 mg/24 hours

9. Which statement describes the circumstances of polycystic kidney disease?

(A) It is always inherited by autosomal dominant mechanism.
(B) Associated hypertension is routinely treated with diuretics until late in the course.
(C) A generally lower-than-normal hemoglobin is associated with it.
(D) When renal function begins to deteriorate, creatinine clearance falls by one half every 36 months.
(E) It is characterized by hypokalemia.

10. For hypertensive patients whose race is not a factor, who are not diabetic, and who manifest no renal failure, the blood pressure target for therapy and follow-up of essential hypertension is

(A) ≤ 120/80
(B) ≤ 130/85
(C) 130–140/≤ 89
(D) 140–159/90–99
(E) ≤ 210/≤ 120

11. Which is true of hypertension in the elderly?

(A) Normal systolic pressure may be defined as 100 mm Hg plus the age of the patient.
(B) Therapeutic responses are suggestive of renin-driven physiology in the majority of cases.
(C) Hypertension responds readily to beta-blocking agents.
(D) The onset of diastolic hypertension suggests changing physiology, such as renovascular processes and high renin states.
(E) Systolic hypertension is not as significant a risk factor as diastolic hypertension for stroke and coronary heart disease.

12. Which statement is accurate with respect to thiazide diuretics in the treatment of hypertension?

(A) They are effective antihypertensive agents in a majority of Caucasian hypertensive patients.
(B) They are contraindicated in diabetes mellitus.
(C) Dosages (of hydrochlorothiazide) greater than 25 mg require potassium to be repleted or a potassium-saving agent employed.
(D) They are very effective in young, hyperreactive hypertensive patients.
(E) They are most effective in high-renin type hypertension.

13. As first-line drugs for therapy in essential hypertension, thiazide diuretics are effective in approximately what percentage of cases of hypertension?

(A) 10%–20%
(B) 20%–30%
(C) 30%–40%
(D) 40%–50%
(E) 60%–70%

DIRECTIONS (Items 14–16): Each of the numbered items or incomplete statements in this section is negatively phrased, as indicated by a capitalized word, such as NOT, LEAST, or EXCEPT. Select the ONE lettered answer or completion that is BEST in each case.

14. You are reviewing the multiple chemical profile of an obese, 55-year-old man who has a blood pressure (BP) of 160/100 and who has been under treatment for 25 years. His present BP treatment is triamterene/hydrochlorothiazide and a sustained-release diltiazem preparation. His creatinine is 2.8 mg/dL, and his blood urea nitrogen 35 mg/dL. He has a brother with diabetes mellitus type II, but his own random blood sugar is 90 mg/dL. You review the differential diagnosis of renal failure in preparation for instituting a correct diet and possible change in medication for his hypertension. Which is the LEAST likely of causes of this renal condition?

    (A) Diabetic nephropathy
    (B) Chronic pyelonephritis
    (C) Hypertensive nephropathy
    (D) Chronic glomerulonephritis
    (E) Polycystic kidney disease

15. Collection of 24-hour urine specimens, at least occasionally, is useful in assessing hypertensive patients. In primary care, relative reasons for doing such studies in hypertensive patients include all EXCEPT

    (A) Creatinine excretion for measurement of creatinine clearance
    (B) Evaluation of severity of pyelonephritis
    (C) Measurement of protein excretion to diagnose microalbuminuria
    (D) Urinary excretion of salt for estimation of salt intake
    (E) Measurement of urinary urea for estimation of dietary protein intake

16. All of the following apply to accelerated hypertension EXCEPT

    (A) Blood pressure of $\geq 180/110$
    (B) Papilledema
    (C) Association with 2-year survival of less than 50%, if untreated
    (D) Association with renal failure
    (E) Ready responsiveness to single drug therapy

ANSWERS AND EXPLANATIONS

1. The answer is A. Among the answer choices, type II diabetes is the ranking risk factor for primary (essential) hypertension. Because, most often, type II diabetes is associated with insulin resistance, a fundament of syndrome X, a family history of type II diabetes is tantamount to a family history of hypertension. (Type II diabetes is characterized by insulin resistance and hyperinsulinemia. Hyperinsulinemia is associated with, and probably causes, hypertension and dyslipidemia. This trio forms the basis of syndrome X.) A history of smoking is not in itself a risk factor for hypertension, although smoking and hypertension are independent risk factors for atherosclerotic vascular disease. Stress may result in elevated blood pressure, but only when other factors, particularly sympathetic hyperreactivity, are present. Obesity, with hips and thighs distribution, is a protective (not a risk) factor for syndrome X and hypertension. Primary aldosteronism causes secondary hypertension but not primary (essential) hypertension.

2. The answer is D. Triamterene/hydrochlorothiazide is most likely to be effective in controlling this patient's hypertension, which has demonstrated salt sensitivity (it has responded to dietary salt restriction). Such patients (typically two-thirds of hypertensive African Americans, two-thirds of elderly hypertensives, and 35% of Caucasian hypertensives) respond well to single-drug therapy consisting of thiazide diuretics. In the correct answer choice, hydrochlorothiazide is compounded with the potassium-saving, weak diuretic, triamterene. Angiotensin-converting enzyme inhibitors (e.g., lisinopril), beta-blockers (e.g., propranolol and atenolol), and sedatives (e.g., diazepam) are more effective in hypertension characterized by increased peripheral resistance.

3. The answer is E. Diuretic responsiveness occurs in approximately 65% of cases of primary hypertension in African-Americans. A high-renin state is not a particularly common characteristic of primary hypertension in African-Americans. In fact, approximately 66% of black American hypertensive patients exhibit low-renin states (hence with likely responsiveness to diuretic therapy). In contrast, only approximately 35% of Caucasian hypertensive patients feature low-renin states. None of the other answer choices apply to black Americans with hypertension. African-Americans with hypertension suffer more accelerated loss of renal function and higher risk of stroke.

4. The answer is A. Approximately 5%–10% of hypertension is secondary in origin. The causes are mainly re-

nal parenchymal hypertension (5% of cases of hypertension), renovascular hypertension (0.5%–5% of cases), primary aldosteronism (0.1%–1% of cases), polycystic kidney disease (0.5% of cases), and pheochromocytoma (0.1%–0.4%). Primary aldosteronism is ruled out by a potassium determination with an abnormally low finding before institution of drug therapy. The other causes should be considered, but need not be ruled out, in the absence of typical clinical presentation or failure to respond as essential hypertension.

5. The answer is B. In the absence of another cause for potassium wasting, primary aldosteronism should be considered whenever hypertension is accompanied by hypokalemia. Primary aldosteronism comprises 0.5%–1.0% of all cases of hypertension, probably much fewer in primary-care situations. Solitary adenomas, rather than idiopathic hyperplasia, cause 70%–90% of primary aldosteronism cases. Idiopathic hyperplasia, which causes the remaining 10%–30% of primary aldosteronism, can be managed for extended periods by the use of aldosterone antagonists, such as spironolactone. Adenomas that cause primary aldosteronism cannot be palpated transabdominally.

6. The answer is E. With respect to pheochromocytoma, labetalol is useful in stabilizing the patient prior to definitive therapy because it blocks both alpha and reflex beta discharge, thus preventing reflex peripheral vasospasm. The majority of patients presenting to the primary-care physician with paroxysms of anxiety are suffering from phobic reactions, anxiety neuroses, or panic disorder. Removal of the tumor results in only a 75% cure rate. Familial cases tend to occur in association with multiple endocrine neoplasms (MEN II A II B). Sensitivity and specificity for 24-hour urine metanephrines are insufficient to diagnose pheochromocytoma. However, if the specimen is also tested for free catecholamines and vanillylmandelic acid, the three results are sufficient to diagnose the disease, provided that the symptoms are not paroxysmal and that the collection does not coincide with the day of an attack.

7. The answer is E. Creatinine clearance falls by 1 ml/min/1.73 m^2/year from an average of 85–125 for the range of normal (nonhypertensive) adults whose average surface area is 1.73 m^2, starting from about the age of 30–35 years. Thus, the average 70-year-old person with normal kidneys has a creatinine clearance of 70 ml/min. The other answer choices do not represent the normal deterioration of renal function in adulthood with the passage of time. Creatinine clearance is calculated as follows:

$$\frac{\text{Urine creatinine (mg/dL)} \times \text{urine volume (ml/24 hr)}}{\text{Serum creatine} \times 1440 \text{ min}}$$

8. The answer is B. Microalbuminuria (microproteinuria) as a "red flag" for declining renal function in hypertension is defined as 200–500 mg/24 hours albumin. The accepted definition of microalbuminuria in diabetes is 30–300 mg/24 hours. The range defining nephrotic syndrome is approximately > 3000 mg/24 hours (in some sources, > 3.5 g/24 hours).

9. The answer is D. With respect to polycystic disease, once renal function begins to deteriorate, creatinine clearance falls by one half every 36 months. Polycystic kidney disease is inherited by autosomal dominant as well as autosomal recessive mechanism, and occurs sporadically. The hypertension associated with polycystic disease is renin driven until renal insufficiency sets in; until that point, it is treated effectively by angiotensin-converting enzyme inhibitors (ACEIs). As renal insufficiency supervenes, the hypertension becomes salt sensitive, thus diuretic responsive. Hemoglobin is often higher than normal in polycystic kidney disease, despite frequent presence of hematuria, as a result of the production of erythropoietin. Polycystic disease is not characterized by hypokalemia.

10. The answer is B. In nondiabetics and non-African-Americans, the blood pressure target for therapy and follow-up of essential hypertension is ≤ 130/80. For diabetics and African-Americans, because of the greater propensity for renal damage at given blood pressure levels, the target pressure is 125/75 or other combinations to produce the same mean arterial pressure. The upper limit of normal systolic blood pressure is 139. The pressure definition of stage-4 hypertension is ≥210/≥120 mm Hg, according to the Joint National Committee on Detection, Evaluation and Treatment of High Blood Pressure (*Arch Intern Med* 1993; 153:161).

11. The answer is D. With respect to hypertension in the elderly, the onset of diastolic hypertension suggests changing physiology, such as renovascular processes (e.g., renal artery obstruction, chronic glomerulonephritis, or nephrosclerosis) and high renin states. Hypertension in the elderly responds less well to beta blocking agents than does hypertension in younger patients; the elderly require larger dosages of beta blockers. This response may be related to the tendency for hypertension in the elderly to respond to diuretics (as low-renin hypertension would respond). Systolic hypertension is a significant risk factor for stroke, and the Systolic Hypertension in the Elderly Program (SHEP study) showed

that control of systolic hypertension to ≤ 143 mm Hg resulted in a 33% reduction in the incidence of stroke (*JAMA* 1991;265:3255–3264). Thus, normal systolic blood pressure, once accepted as "100 plus the age," is now defined for all ages as <140 mm Hg.

12. The answer is C. With regard to the use of thiazide diuretics in hypertension, if hydrochlorothiazide is used in dosages greater than 25 mg over long periods of time, potassium must be repleted or a potassium-saving agent must be employed. Thiazide diuretics are not very effective in young, hyperreactive hypertensives. The latter hypertension tends to be driven by catecholamines and by the renin-angiotensin system. Thiazide diuretics are effective antihypertensive agents in a clear majority of African-Americans and the elderly, but only in 30%–40% of Caucasian hypertensive patients. Thiazides are not contraindicated in diabetes mellitus, but may precipitate (reversible) diabetes on an idiosyncratic basis in a significant minority of potential diabetics or prediabetics (those with hyperinsulinemia resulting from incipient syndrome X) [see *Family Medicine* (House Officer Series), chapter 31]. Thus, thiazide diuretics are most effective in *low*-renin type hypertension.

13. The answer is C. As first-line drugs for therapy in essential hypertension, thiazide diuretics are effective in approximately 30%–40% of cases. This percentage corresponds to the proportion of cases that are generated by endogenous mineralocorticoids, salt-craving tendencies, and lower-than-normal renin activity for a given salt intake. With respect to the remaining 65% of hypertensive patients, 10% of total hypertensive patients are high renin. This 10% comprise the so-called "hot reactors," and they respond well to beta-adrenergic-blocking agents and to angiotensin-converting enzyme (ACE) inhibitors. The "normal renin" hypertension patients (approximately 55% of all hypertensives) respond to both families of drugs to varying degrees, but often best when diuretics are combined. Calcium channel-blocking agents are equally effective (significantly effective, often as single drug therapy) across the renin spectrum, but particularly in normal-renin and low-renin patients.

14. The answer is B. Chronic pyelonephritis is the LEAST likely cause of this man's renal failure. The four leading causes of endstage renal disease are diabetic nephropathy, hypertensive nephropathy, chronic glomerulonephritis, and polycystic kidney disease.

15. The answer is B. Pyelonephritis is NOT evaluated by a 24-hour urine study, but by the concentration of white blood cells (WBCs), WBC casts, and bacteria in a spot urinalysis. The other answer choices constitute relative indications for 24-hour urine studies. Creatinine excretion must be known for measurement of creatinine clearance and for validation of the adequate length of time of collection. Measurement of protein excretion is needed to diagnose microalbuminuria. If the latter is present, drugs should be changed (e.g., to angiotensin-converting enzyme inhibitors) to preserve renal function, and a diet should be prescribed to reduce intake of protein from the average of 1.25 g/Kg to 0.75 g/Kg. Measurement of urinary urea for estimation of dietary protein intake allows a check on baseline, as well as follow-up, protein intake. Urinary excretion of salt facilitates an estimation of salt intake.

16. The answer is E. Accelerated or malignant hypertension is not characterized by ready responsiveness to single-drug therapy. It is characterized by a blood pressure $\geq$ 180/110, papilledema, an untreated survival rate of $<$ 50%, and association with renal failure. The mainstays of management of accelerated and malignant hypertension are sodium nitroprusside, labetalol, hydralazine, trimethaphan, phentolamine, nitroglycerine, nifedipine, clonidine, and enalaprilat.

BIBLIOGRAPHY

Rudy DR: Hypertension. In *Family Medicine* (House Officer Series). Edited by Rudy DR, Kurowski K. Baltimore, Williams & Wilkins, 1997, pp 145–168.

SECTION III

Neurology

Test 10

Neurology in Primary Care

DIRECTIONS (Items 1–13): Each of the numbered items or incomplete statements in this section is followed by answers or by completions of the statement. Select the ONE lettered answer or completion that is BEST in each case.

1. Which is characteristic of lower motor neuron lesions?

    (A) Muscle weakness ipsilateral to the lesion
    (B) Hyperactive deep tendon reflexes for the involved muscle group
    (C) Spasticity in the involved muscle groups
    (D) An extensor plantar response
    (E) Hypertrophy of the involved muscles

2. Which feature is characteristic of Wernicke's aphasia?

    (A) The patient seems to struggle visibly to speak and express himself or herself.
    (B) The information in speech is incorrect.
    (C) Some words are mispronounced.
    (D) The patient seems to avoid speaking and says as little as possible.
    (E) Agrammatism is evident in the patient's speech.

3. Which feature is best associated with the clinical definition of multiple sclerosis?

    (A) A fluctuating course with multiple areas of demyelination in the central nervous system
    (B) An elevated immunoglobulin level in the cerebrospinal fluid
    (C) Transient visual loss in the right eye with scotomas noted frequently in the same eye
    (D) Plaque in the cerebral white matter visible on MRI of the cervical spine
    (E) Transverse myelitis associated with bilateral symmetrical spastic paresis of the legs

4. A 30-year-old woman has had episodes of complete visual loss in her left eye, bilateral pains in her upper abdomen and chest, and a spastic paresis, principally of her right leg. All of these symptoms have fluctuated since they began 3 years ago. An MRI of her brain and spinal cord reveals multiple areas of demyelination of the white matter within her central nervous system. You decide to treat her with an agent that has the best demonstrated efficacy in reducing exacerbations. During her treatment with this agent, particular monitoring will be needed for which of the following?

    (A) Increased BUN and creatinine
    (B) Hypercalcemia
    (C) Hyperlipidemia
    (D) Depression and suicidal ideation
    (E) Q-T wave prolongation on EKG

5. A 69-year-old woman has had progressive, short-term memory loss for 3 years. In the last year, she also had episodes of aphasia and two episodes of inability to find her way home. Assuming the most common diagnosis for these symptoms, which of the following would be most likely to exacerbate her condition?

    (A) Congestive heart failure, controlled by diuretics and angiotensin-converting enzyme inhibitors
    (B) Mild distal sensory neuropathy affecting the feet, secondary to type II diabetes mellitus
    (C) Cigarette smoking
    (D) Ibuprofen, 400 mg, three times a day, for osteoarthritis
    (E) Very poor visual acuity as a result of bilateral cataracts

6. You are considering tacrine therapy for a 72-year-old patient with Alzheimer's dementia. One of the major side effects of this therapy is

    (A) Renal failure
    (B) Thrombocytosis
    (C) Elevation of serum transaminases
    (D) Formation of cataracts
    (E) Development of deep venous thrombosis

7. Which feature is commonly seen in untreated patients with Parkinson's disease?

    (A) Choreiform movements
    (B) A bilateral, symmetrical, resting tremor at onset of Parkinson's
    (C) Loud speech of widely variable tone
    (D) Orthostatic hypotension
    (E) Delirium

8. You are examining a 65-year-old patient with Parkinson's disease. She is on no medication. Although she has some features of bradykinesia and demonstrates some cogwheel rigidity, she says that only her tremor interferes with her functioning. Which of the medications listed below would be most appropriate for her?

    (A) Amantadine
    (B) Carbidopa/levodopa
    (C) Benztropine
    (D) Deprenyl (selegiline)
    (E) Pergolide

9. A parent reports that, during the past 2 months, her 4-year-old son has been having multiple episodes each day in which he stares ahead, sometimes nods his head, but does not respond to his parents or others. Each episode lasts about 10 seconds. The boy, who has been otherwise healthy and taking no medication, is fully awake after the attacks have ended. He is afebrile, with a pulse of 80, and a blood pressure of 97/65. No trauma is reported. No skin lesions are present. The boy's sensation to light touch is intact to his face and all extremities. His gait is normal, and his motor strength is 5/5 in all proximal and distal extremities. His cranial nerves I-XII and all deep tendon reflexes test normal. Which medication is the preferred initial agent in the treatment of this child's seizures?

(A) Phenytoin
(B) Diazepam
(C) Valproic acid
(D) Primidone
(E) Phenobarbital

10. You are examining a 38-year-old woman who complains of bilateral leg weakness which started in her feet 3 days ago, and is now progressively affecting her ability to walk. She reports she had cold symptoms 2 weeks earlier. She denies any trauma or falls and reports being otherwise in good health and taking no medications. She is experiencing some numbness in her feet, and you cannot elicit a deep tendon reflex at her ankles or knees. No atrophy is present. The woman now demonstrates a significantly reduced ventilatory peak flow. The diagnosis most consistent with this presentation is

(A) A herniated lumbar disc
(B) Lateral femoral cutaneous-nerve syndrome
(C) Diabetic neuropathy
(D) Cerebrovascular accident
(E) Guillain-Barré syndrome

11. A patient has his blood pressure and pulse checked after he has been lying supine for 5 minutes and again after sitting up. The accepted cutoff change for orthostatic hypotension is a decrease of

(A) 40 mmHg in the systolic reading and 20 mmHg in the diastolic
(B) 30 mmHg in the systolic or 20 mmHg in the diastolic
(C) 20 mmHg in the systolic and 5 mmHg in the diastolic
(D) 20 mmHg in the systolic or 10 mmHg in the diastolic
(E) 10 mmHg in the systolic or 5 mmHg in the diastolic

12. A 41-year-old woman, walking through a grocery store, senses that the walls of the store are circling around her. She feels uncertain on her feet but cannot get to a chair to sit down. She remains conscious throughout the episode. She has otherwise been in good health, takes no medication, and drinks no alcohol. Her episode is best described as

(A) Syncope
(B) Presyncope
(C) Vertigo
(D) A drop attack
(E) Subclavian steal

13. A 32-year-old woman with a history of generalized tonic-clonic seizures complains of a 2-week history of dysequilibrium without vertigo, accompanied by some nausea. She denies alcohol use or head trauma. She is taking phenytoin, 400 mg per day, and has not had a seizure in 5 years. She started taking isoniazid for TB skin test conversion 1 month ago. On physical examination, she is afebrile, with a blood pressure of 120/80. She has some nystagmus on lateral gaze. Her speech is understandable, but somewhat slurred. Her motor and sensory strength is intact in all extremities and in her face. Which of the following is the most likely cause of her symptoms?

(A) Phenytoin toxicity
(B) Isoniazid toxicity
(C) Labyrinthitis
(D) Cerebellar neoplasm
(E) Orthostatic hypotension

DIRECTIONS (Items 14–15): Each of the numbered items or incomplete statements in this section is negatively phrased, as indicated by a capitalized word, such as NOT, LEAST, or EXCEPT. Select the ONE lettered answer or completion that is BEST in each case.

14. You are examining a 70-year-old woman with a slowly progressing, chronic dementia not previously evaluated in her. Your evaluation for treatable causes would typically include all of the following tests EXCEPT

   (A) A thyroid-stimulating hormone level
   (B) A CT scan of the brain
   (C) A rapid plasma reagin test
   (D) Serum B_{12} and folate levels
   (E) A serum iron level

15. Family physicians regularly encounter and diagnose vasovagal syncope. However, this syndrome is a non-specific response to various dysfunctions, which must be diagnosed in turn. Which is NOT known to precipitate a vasovagal response?

   (A) Coughing
   (B) Swallowing
   (C) Urinating
   (D) Taking a deep breath
   (E) Defecating

ANSWERS AND EXPLANATIONS

1. The answer is A. Lower motor neuron injury produces a flaccid, ipsilateral muscle weakness with atrophy, fasciculation, and loss of deep tendon reflexes. Upper motor neuron disease usually produces contralateral weakness associated with spasticity and extensor plantar reflexes (positive Babinski reflex).

2. The answer is B. Incorrect information in speech is characteristic of Wernicke's aphasia. In contrast to global or Wernicke's aphasia, information content is preserved in Broca's aphasia, but patients with this aphasia may avoid grammatical construction in order to use fewer words in speaking. Broca's aphasia is characterized by good comprehension, but a nonfluent, effortful speech, often with an associated right hemiparesis. The lesion is in the lower posterior frontal lobe. Wernicke's aphasia is characterized by poor comprehension and an abundant, fluid, well-articulated speech that makes no sense. The lesion is in the posterior and superior temporal lobe.

3. The answer is A. The clinical definition of multiple sclerosis is best associated with clinical evidence, which has changed over time, of lesions affecting more than one area of the central nervous system, for which no other explanation can be found. Multiple sclerosis involves multiple plaques in the central nervous system (including the optic nerve), which changes over time. Elevated immunoglobulin level in the cerebrospinal fluid, transient visual loss and scotomas in the right eye, and transverse myelitis associated with bilateral symmetrical spastic paresis of the legs may or may not be seen in multiple sclerosis patients and do not clinically define the disease.

4. The answer is D. Particular monitoring for depression and suicidal ideation is needed with beta-1b interferon treatment, the agent with the best proven efficacy in reducing exacerbations of multiple sclerosis. The patient presents with the clinical and MRI features of this disease. Monitoring is also necessary for marked increase in liver enzyme. The most commonly reported side effects are injection-site reactions and flu-like symptoms, but these effects are not usually serious enough to force termination of treatment. Interferon can also produce a neutropenia, but does not tend to effect renal function, calcium levels, lipid levels, or the Q-T waves on EKGs.

5. The answer is E. Significant sensory deficits, especially visual ones (e.g., poor visual acuity, secondary to bilateral cataracts), can exacerbate the patient's symptoms of Alzheimer's dementia and should be corrected if possible. The other answer choices—congestive heart failure controlled by diuretics and ACE inhibitors, mild distal sensory neuropathy affecting the feet as a result of type II diabetes mellitus, cigarette smoking, and ibuprofen three times a day—are not associated with significant exacerbation of Alzheimer's symptoms.

6. The answer is C. Elevation of serum transaminases is one of the major side effects of tacrine therapy. Approximately 50% of patients treated with this drug develop at least one transaminase elevation above normal limits. Tacrine is usually withdrawn if the elevation is greater than three times the upper limit of normal. With respect to other side effects, neutropenia has also been reported (rarely), but thrombocytosis, renal failure, cataracts, and deep venous thrombosis have not.

7. The answer is D. Orthostatic hypotension is one of a number of autonomic features commonly seen in patients with Parkinson's disease (PD). Constipation and impotence can also be seen. Although the striatonigral tract is the most affected in PD, other dopaminergic pathways and other neurotransmitters are also affected. The resting tremor common in PD is initially unilateral. The gait is shuffling with little arm swing. The speech is very soft and monotonal. Swallowing some foods may be difficult. The most common symptoms in PD include rigidity, difficulty in initiating movement, slow movement, a resting tremor, an expressionless face ("Parkinson's mask"), and depression. Only about 20% of PD patients eventually develop dementia. (Some patients develop medication-induced hallucinations.) Choreiform movements, which are rapid, purposeless, and jerky, occur in Huntington's and Sydenham's chorea, but not in untreated PD (although these movements are often seen as a side effect of some Parkinson's medications).

8. The answer is C. Benztropine mesylate (or other anticholinergic medication) is most likely to relieve the tremor of Parkinson's disease (PD). Although other types of medications (especially levodopa preparations) are superior in improving the rigidity and bradykinesia of PD, the anticholinergics are more effective in diminishing the tremor. Amantadine, originally a flu medication (and relatively inexpensive), can be used for bradykinesia and rigidity in early, mild disease. Deprenyl (also called selegiline), an MAO-B inhibitor, is used mostly in combination with levodopa preparations to diminish the required amount of levodopa. Pergolide, a dopamine agonist, is also used mostly in combination with levodopa preparations.

9. The answer is C. Valproic acid and ethosuximide are the preferred agents for treatment of absence seizures. Absence seizures do not result in status epilepticus and are not treated with phenytoin or diazepam. The seizures last for less than 30 seconds and are not preceded by auras or followed by post-ictal states. An EEG shows a 3-per-second spike and wave abnormality. Absence seizures will stop occurring in most children after the beginning of adolescence. Phenytoin and phenobarbital are first-line agents for generalized and focal seizures. Primidone is one of the first-line agents for focal seizures or partial complex seizures. Diazepam can be used in status epilepticus.

10. The answer is E. A diagnosis of Guillain-Barré syndrome would be most consistent with the presentation in this woman's case. Guillain-Barré usually presents as a distal, ascending paralysis, sometimes accompanied by less-pronounced sensory deficits, after a viral illness. Absence of reflexes is common. This syndrome can lead to respiratory arrest. Patients need frequent monitoring of their vital capacity, with endotracheal intubation and respiratory support, if it falls to 30% of normal. Plasma exchange (3–5 exchanges per day) is useful in the first week. If this fails, intravenous immunoglobulin is used. The differential diagnosis should include AIDs, botulism, arsenic exposure, and collagen vascular disease. A centrally herniated disc can produce bilateral leg weakness, but does not affect the muscles of respiration. Diabetic neuropathy can produce muscle weakness and loss of deep-tendon reflexes, but not as rapidly as in this situation. Cerebrovascular accidents are characterized by unilateral (rather than bilateral) spastic weakness with hyperactive reflexes.

11. The answer is D. A decrease of 20 mmHg in the systolic or a decrease of 10 mmHg in the diastolic is the accepted cutoff change for orthostatic hypotension. These decreases are considered significant, especially if associated with an elevation in pulse rate of 10 bpm or greater.

12. The answer is C. Vertigo, a sense that either the environment or one's own body is rotating, best describes this woman's episode. Syncope is a loss of consciousness from a temporary reduction in cerebral blood flow. Presyncope is a sensation that one is going to faint, not followed by fainting. A drop attack involves loss of postural tone only. In subclavian steal, the patient may experience syncope or near syncope with left (or right) arm exertion. A partial obstruction in the left subclavian

and anomalies of the vertebral arteries cause reversal of vertebral artery flow and, thus, brain stem ischemia. With ataxia (muscular incoordination), a patient may fall because of the poor coordination in their extremities and gait but will not lose consciousness.

13. The answer is A. Phenytoin toxicity is the most likely cause of this woman's symptoms. Phenytoin toxicity is most commonly manifested by nystagmus, ataxia, slurred speech, poor coordination, and confusion, and is sometimes accompanied by nausea and emesis. Rashes and granulocytopenia may also occur, but are not as dose related. Several medications, including alcohol, amiodarone, benzodiazepines, H-2 antagonists, and isoniazid, can raise phenytoin levels. Isoniazid toxicity and orthostatic hypotension do not produce ataxia nor nystagmus. Labyrinthitis and cerebellar lesions do not produce slurred speech.

14. The answer is E. A serum iron level test would NOT be included in your evaluation of treatable causes of this woman's dementia. Abnormalities of the serum iron level would not typically present as an isolated dementia in the elderly. A thyroid-stimulating-hormone level is ordered to exclude hypothyroidism, which, particularly in the elderly, can present with decreased memory, loss of calculation abilities, and social withdrawal that can be confused with senile dementia. A rapid plasma reagin test (although only approximately 80% sensitive) is ordered to detect neurosyphilis, in which the general paresis can produce impaired memory and judgment, paranoia, and depression or euphoria. The level of serum B_{12} is checked to exclude the dementia that can be produced by a deficiency of this vitamin. A CT scan of the brain is performed to exclude a brain tumor (especially in the frontal lobe), multi-infarcts, and hydrocephalus. (Cerebral atrophy in both Alzheimer's and nondemented elderly patients can frequently be seen in these scans.)

15. The answer is D. Taking a deep breath is NOT known to precipitate a vasovagal response. The underlying mechanism of a vasovagal response, believed to be second to production of a Valsalva maneuver, does not occur with deep breathing. Coughing, swallowing, urinating, and defecating can precipitate vasovagal syncope.

BIBLIOGRAPHY

Olsen CG, Clasen ME: Neurology in primary care. In *Family Medicine* (House Officer Series). Edited by Rudy DR, Kurowski K. Baltimore, Williams & Wilkins, 1997, pp 169–184.

SECTION IV

Diseases of the Respiratory Tract

Test 11

Pneumonias, Bronchitides, and Chronic Lung Disease

DIRECTIONS. (Items 1–12): Each of the numbered items or incomplete statements in this section is followed by answers or by completions of the statement. Select the ONE lettered answer or completion that is BEST in each case.

1. A 32-year-old woman complains of a 2-day cough with chills and fever, pain in her right lower chest, but no shortness of breath. Otherwise, she has been in good health, does not smoke, has no allergies, and denies any activities that would put her at high risk for acquiring HIV. She is menstruating at this time. Her temperature is 101°F (38.3°C), pulse is 96, and blood pressure is 124/82. She docs not appear in distress, but looks ill. Lung examination reveals bronchophony, egophony, and dullness to percussion in the right posterior chest, below an approximate T5 level. Some rales are also present in this area. No accessory muscle use, clubbing, nor cyanosis is found. Sputum Gram's stain reveals lancet-shaped, gram-positive diplococci. Chest x-rays reveal a right lower-lobe infiltrate. Which therapeutic intervention is most likely to benefit this patient?

    (A) Penicillin
    (B) Trimethoprim/sulfamethoxazole
    (C) Chest percussion treatment on the right lower lobe
    (D) Tetracycline
    (E) Furosemide

2. Which characteristic is typically seen with *Mycoplasma pneumoniae* infections?

    (A) A cough productive of copious amounts of yellow sputum
    (B) A lobar infiltrate on chest x-ray
    (C) Associated headaches
    (D) Associated severe myalgias
    (E) Clinical improvement on oral cephalosporin antibiotics

3. Which clinical characteristic is typical of legionella pneumonia?

    (A) A relative bradycardia
    (B) An associated sore throat
    (C) An associated rash
    (D) Associated ear pain
    (E) An occurrence in teenagers more than in other age groups

4. Which of the following is a correct way of confirming *Legionella pneumofila* infection?

    (A) A positive direct fluorescent antibody smear of a sputum sample
    (B) Detection of legionella antigen in the patient's serum
    (C) A standard sputum culture
    (D) A doubling of legionella antibody titers from acute to convalescent samples
    (E) A legionella titer of greater than 1:16

5. You are examining a 50-year-old woman who had viral influenza 1 week ago. Her other symptoms have resolved, but she has noted a progressive cough and fever in the last 3 days. She has no smoking history, no immune deficiency, no chronic respiratory disease, and has had no recent stays at hospitals or nursing homes. Her temperature is 101°F (38.3°C), pulse is 96 and regular, blood pressure is 130/70, and respiratory rate is 16. Her tympanic membranes are gray and translucent, with good light reflexes. Her lung examination shows increased tactile fremitus in the left lung base, with crackles and egophony appreciated in the same area on auscultation. Which of the organisms listed below is most likely responsible for her symptoms?

    (A) *Moraxella catarrhalis*
    (B) *Klebsiella pneumoniae*
    (C) *Streptococcus pneumoniae*
    (D) Mixed anaerobes
    (E) *Escherichia coli*

6. In which clinical situation are you most likely to see an anaerobic bacterial pneumonia?

    (A) A 49-year-old patient who has smoked two packs of cigarettes per day for 30 years and has a history of chronic bronchitis
    (B) A stroke patient who has recently aspirated
    (C) A 30-year-old patient who had an influenza infection 1 week earlier
    (D) A 55-year-old nonsmoker who recently traveled to Arizona.
    (E) A 34-year-old nonsmoker with AIDS

7. Which is the most common causative agent for viral pneumonia in an adult?

    (A) Influenza virus
    (B) Adenovirus
    (C) Parainfluenza virus
    (D) Respiratory syncytial virus
    (E) Varicella

8. A 70-year-old woman complains of increasing dyspnea for the past 2 weeks, but she denies any chest pain. She has been smoking half a pack of cigarettes each day for 40 years. She denies any history of alcohol consumption. Examination of her lungs shows dullness to percussion and diminished breath sounds over the right base. A chest x-ray shows a moderate, right pleural effusion. A thoracentesis yields clear fluid with a protein of 1.5 grams/dL (her serum protein is 3.2 grams/dL) and a lactate dehydrogenase (LDH) of 100 IU/liter (her serum LDH is 190 IU/liter). The most likely diagnosis for her effusion is

    (A) Metastatic breast carcinoma
    (B) Pulmonary neoplasm
    (C) Rheumatoid lung
    (D) Congestive heart failure
    (E) Pneumonia

9. For which patient would a test for $alpha_1$-antitrypsin level be most appropriate in evaluating chronic obstructive pulmonary disease (COPD)?

    (A) A 75-year-old patient with severe emphysema and cor pulmonale who is now homebound, on continuous oxygen, with a forced expiratory volume in 1 second (FEV_1) of 0.9 liters, marked hypoxemia, mild CO_2 retention, and a smoking history of only 15 packs per year
    (B) A 70-year-old male patient with a 10-year history of increasing shortness of breath and a smoking history of 30 packs per year
    (C) A 52-year-old patient with a 1-year history of mild shortness of breath brought on by heavy exertion, who has a smoking history of only 1 pack per year
    (D) A 48-year-old male patient with a 1-year history of mild shortness of breath brought on by exertion and with a smoking history of 40 packs per year
    (E) A 55-year-old patient with a 5-year history of shortness of breath, a smoking history of 20 packs per year, which she stopped 5 years ago, and a husband who smokes 2 packs per day in their home

10. Which is a chest x-ray feature of moderate to severe COPD?

    (A) Diffuse bilateral infiltrates
    (B) Raised diaphragms bilaterally
    (C) Cardiomegaly
    (D) Increased retrosternal air space
    (E) Hypoinflation

11. Which value of forced expiratory volume in 1 second (FEV_1) correlates with the START of CO_2 retention in a patient with COPD?

    (A) $FEV_1 = 3.0$ liters
    (B) $FEV_1 = 2.0$ liters
    (C) $FEV_1 = 1.0$ liter
    (D) $FEV_1 = 0.5$ liter
    (E) Normal FEV_1, but diminished forced expiratory flow (FEF) 25–75

12. Assuming no contraindications, which medication is the first-line agent of choice in treating mild to moderate COPD?

    (A) Inhaled corticosteroids
    (B) Oral corticosteroids
    (C) Inhaled beta-agonist
    (D) Oral theophylline
    (E) Inhaled ipratropium bromide

DIRECTIONS (Items 13–14): Each of the numbered items or incomplete statements in this section is negatively phrased, as indicated by a capitalized word, such as NOT, LEAST, or EXCEPT. Select the ONE lettered answer or completion that is BEST in each case.

13. You are managing a patient with severe COPD. Which one of the following does NOT indicate the need for an arterial blood gas measurement?

    (A) The patient has continued to smoke.
    (B) The patient has developed cor pulmonale.
    (C) The patient is about to undergo a laparoscopic cholecystectomy.
    (D) The patient has recently become confused.
    (E) The patient has developed brief (3-beat) runs of ventricular tachycardia.

14. You have a homebound patient who has severe COPD. His partial pressure of oxygen in arterial blood (PaO_2) is 62 mmHg at rest and 54 mmHg with ambulation in the house. Many interventions that tend to improve prognosis are available. Which of the following has NOT been shown to decrease mortality and morbidity in patients with this condition?

    (A) Smoking cessation
    (B) Annual, autumnal influenza vaccination
    (C) Pneumonococcal vaccine every 5–10 years
    (D) Supplemental oxygen
    (E) Chest physiotherapy every 2 months

DIRECTIONS (Items 15–17): For each numbered alteration on pulmonary function testing, select the letter of the lung disease that is most likely to be associated with it. Each lettered option may be selected once, more than once, or not at all. (FEV_1 is forced expiratory volume in 1 second. FVC is forced vital capacity. VC is vital capacity. RV is residual volume.)

    (A) Emphysema
    (B) Asthma
    (C) Pulmonary fibrosis
    (D) Pulmonary embolism
    (E) Solitary, 2-cm, peripheral lung nodule

15. FEV_1 and FVC are both reduced, but with normal ratio. VC and RV are increased. FEV_1 is unchanged after bronchodilator is used.

16. FEV_1 is reduced, but FVC is normal, resulting in FEV_1:FVC ratio of 64%. RV is increased. FEV_1 improves by 5% after bronchodilator is used.

17. FEV_1 is decreased, and FEV_1:FVC is reduced. RV is increased. FEV_1 increases by 60% after bronchodilator is used.

ANSWERS AND EXPLANATIONS

1. The answer is A. For this typical presentation of a *Streptococcus pneumoniae* pneumonia, penicillin is the treatment of choice (unless high rates of pneumococci resistant to penicillin exist in the community).

2. The answer is C. Associated headaches are typical with *Mycoplasma pneumoniae* infections. These infections, which most often affect young adults as well as adolescents and older children, typically present with a dry cough and fever. In contrast to viral pneumonia, severe myalgias are not typical, but extrapulmonary manifestations (e.g., headache, malaise, symptoms of upper respiratory infection, and diarrhea) are frequently experienced. Cephalosporin antibiotics and penicillin derivatives are not effective against this organism. Chest x-rays typically show diffuse infiltrates, rather than lobar patterns.

3. The answer is A. A relative bradycardia, mental confusion, abdominal pain, and diarrhea are frequent clinical characteristics typical of legionella pneumonia, which mostly affects elderly patients with co-morbid conditions. Not frequently seen are sore throat, ear pain, and rash. (Although many different strains and species of *Legionella* exist, approximately 95% of legionella pneumonia cases are caused by *Legionella pneumophila*.)

4. The answer is A. A positive direct fluorescent antibody smear of a sputum sample is a correct way of confirming *Legionella pneumophila* infection. A standard sputum culture cannot be used because, even if *Legionella pneumophila* is present in sputum, it will not grow on a standard culture. A random legionella titer would need to be ≥ 1:264 or at least a four-fold rise of legionella antibody titers between acute and convalescent titers to indicate legionella infection. Legionella antigen can be detected in the urine but not in the serum.

5. The answer is C. *Streptococcus pneumoniae* is the organism most likely responsible for the woman's symptoms. *Haemophilus influenzae* and *Staphylococcus aureus* are other bacterial pathogens that most commonly complicate an influenza infection. *Klebsiella pneumoniae* and *Escherichia coli* are often causes of pneumonia acquired during a hospitalization. *Moraxella pneumoniae* is usually seen only in smokers with chronic obstructive pulmonary disease. Anaerobe pneumonias result from aspiration.

6. The answer is B. A stroke patient who has recently aspirated is the one most likely to have an anaerobic bacterial pneumonia. Oral anaerobes that have been aspirated are the usual cause of aspiration pneumonia. A number of factors can cause aspiration: neurologic deficits that affect swallowing or concentration; seizures; drug overdose; alcoholism; and recent dental procedures. The middle-aged smoker with chronic bronchitis is at increased risk for nonencapsulated *Haemophilus influenzae,* and the Arizona traveler is at increased risk for coccidioidomycosis, but neither at increased risk for anaerobic bacterial pneumonia. The patient who had influenza a week ago is at increased risk for *Streptococcus pneumoniae.* AIDS patients are at increased risk for *Pneumocystis carinii* pneumonia, tuberculosis, and encapsulated organisms.

7. The answer is A. The influenza virus is the most common causative agent in viral pneumonia, although each of the organisms listed in the answer choices can cause viral pneumonia in an adult. Influenza symptoms in a young adult include chills, headache, sore throat, myalgias, cough, malaise, and anorexia. In elderly adults, symptoms frequently include only cough and fever.

8. The answer is D. Congestive heart failure (CHF) is the most likely cause of this woman's effusion. The clear thoracentesis fluid with relatively low levels of protein and lactate dehydrogenase (compared to her serum) is consistent with a transudate, produced only by CHF and by diseases not included among the answer choices (e.g., ascites secondary to liver cirrhosis). Metastatic carcinoma, primary pulmonary neoplasms, rheumatoid lung, and pneumonia (empyema), all produce exudates, defined as pleural fluid to serum protein greater than 0.5 and pleural fluid to serum LDH greater than 0.6.

9. The answer is C. An alpha$_1$-antitrypsin level would be most appropriate in evaluating chronic obstructive pulmonary disease (COPD) in the 52-year-old patient with a 1-year history of mild shortness of breath brought on by heavy exertion, who has a smoking history of only one pack per year. (Alpha$_1$-antitrypsin is a serum glycoprotein that inhibits a variety of proteolytic enzymes. Deficient alpha$_1$-antitrypsin is associated with progressive destruction of lung and liver.) The patients presented in answer choices A and C both seem to have developed COPD, despite a relatively small exposure to cigarette smoke, but the patient in situation A already has end-stage COPD with cor pulmonale. This carries a very poor prognosis and would not be reversible with alpha$_1$-antitrypsin at such an advanced stage. The patients in answer choices B and D have symptoms consistent with their smoking history and do not require a search for enzymatic causes.

10. The answer is D. Increased retrosternal air space is one of the chest x-ray features of moderate to severe, chronic obstructive pulmonary disease (COPD). Patients with COPD show evidence of *hyper*inflation, reflecting the increase in total lung capacity and functional residual volume. The overdistension results in visibly depressed diaphragms and increased retrosternal air space. Even if right ventricular hypertrophy develops, no cardiomegaly is seen on chest x-ray. Bi-basilar infiltrates can have many potential etiologies, including pneumonia and left-sided heart failure, but these infiltrates do not suggest COPD.

11. The answer is C. A forced expiratory volume in 1 second (FEV$_1$) of 1.0 liter correlates with the start of CO$_2$ retention in a patient with COPD. CO$_2$ retention is typically seen when the FEV$_1$ is smaller than, or equal to, 1.0 liter. The forced expiratory flow (FEF) 25–75 is used to detect early COPD that is primarily affecting the small airways, but CO$_2$ retention would not be present. Thus, though diminished FEF 25–75 is more sensitive for earlier phase disease, a finding of this abnormality is not indicative of incipient CO$_2$ retention.

12. The answer is E. Inhaled ipratropium bromide is the first-line agent of choice (in the absence of contraindications) in the treatment of mild to moderate COPD. Inhaled corticosteroids, oral corticosteroids, inhaled beta-agonist, and oral theophylline are sometimes used in COPD patients (although inhaled corticosteroids have been shown to have little effect), but inhaled ipratropium bromide is the preferred starting agent because of its better side-effect profile.

13. The answer is A. Continued smoking is NOT an indicator for an arterial blood-gas measurement in a patient with severe COPD. Even with continued smoking, the disease progression is not fast enough to show changes at every 3–6 month periodic examination, and treatment is unlikely to be affected. Nevertheless, continued smoking will accelerate the progression of the COPD. Confusion and ventricular tachycardia can be manifestations of hypoxia in COPD patients. Postoperative pain, especially from incisions made near the diaphragm, may inhibit ventilation, and preoperative blood gas measurement is indicated in COPD patients.

14. The answer is E. Periodic chest physiotherapy has NOT been shown to improve the morbidity and mortality of patients with COPD. Smoking cessation, annual autumnal influenza vaccination, pneumococcal vaccine every 5–10 years, and supplemental oxygen have been shown to be helpful, the latter only to maintain a PaO$_2$ of 60 mmHg or oxygen saturation of greater than 90%. Excessive oxygen can suppress carbon-dioxide-dependent respiratory drive and lead to hypercapnia.

15. The answer is C. Pulmonary fibrosis is the disease that is most likely to show the listed alterations. It is an example of a restrictive lung disease, a disorder in which lung compliance is reduced, so all lung volumes (e.g., VC and RV) are reduced. The FEV$_1$ and FVC are both reduced, but usually to the same degree (preserving a normal ratio). Asthma and COPD both lower the FEV$_1$:FVC ratio and increase the RV. Pulmonary embolism could produce hypoxemia through ventilation-perfusion mismatches but does not alter pulmonary function tests (PFTs). A small, peripheral nodule produces neither hypoxemia nor altered PFTs.

16. The answer is A. Emphysema is the most likely disease. A fairly pure pattern in an emphysema patient shows little reversibility with bronchodilators, whereas an asthmatic or chronic bronchitis patient improves. Emphysema is an obstructive disease producing a particular reduction in FEV$_1$, and, thus, the FEV$_1$:FVC ratio. The destroyed alveoli are replaced with dead air space, so RVs increase.

17. The answer is B. Asthma is the most likely condition. It is also an obstructive lung disease, and, thus, the PFT pattern is similar to that of emphysema. Dramatic reversibility with bronchodilators suggests asthma.

BIBLIOGRAPHY

Lipsky MS, Sternbach M: Pneumonias, bronchitides, and chronic lung disease. In *Family Medicine* (House Officer Series). Edited by Rudy DR, Kurowski K. Williams & Wilkins, 1997, pp 185–200.

Test 12

Respiratory Diseases in Infants and Children

DIRECTIONS (Items 1–12): Each of the numbered items or incomplete statements in this section is followed by answers or completions of the statement. Select the ONE lettered answer or completion that is BEST in each case.

1. In which age group do the most cases of bronchiolitis occur?

- (A) 0–2 years
- (B) 1–3 years
- (C) 3–4 years
- (D) 4–5 years
- (E) 5–10 years

2. Which organism accounts for the most cases of bronchiolitis?

- (A) Parainfluenza virus
- (B) Adenovirus
- (C) Influenza virus
- (D) *Mycoplasma pneumoniae*
- (E) Respiratory syncytial virus

3. Which of the following pairs of organisms are typically involved in respiratory infections in infants from birth through 3 months of age?

- (A) *Chlamydia pneumoniae* and *Staphylococcus albus*
- (B) *Mycoplasma pneumoniae* and *Haemophilus influenzae*
- (C) *Chlamydia pneumoniae* and group B streptococci
- (D) *Chlamydia trachomatis* and group B streptococci
- (E) *Haemophilus influenzae* and *Streptococcus pneumoniae*

4. A 4-year-old girl has a 3-day history of high fevers [to 103°F (39.4°C)]; deep alveolar cough (finely bubbly); chest x-ray findings of lobar infiltrates; and a painful left knee, manifesting effusion. The parents and patient deny the possibility of trauma. What is the best choice of antibiotic therapy for this patient?

- (A) Erythromycin 125 mg orally 4 times daily
- (B) Amoxicillin 40 mg/kg in 3 divided doses daily
- (C) Penicillin V potassium 250 mg 4 times daily
- (D) Ceftriaxone 50–100 mg/kg/day, intramuscularly
- (E) Dihydrostreptomycin 150 mg twice daily

5. When upper respiratory symptoms are present at onset and evidence of interstitial pulmonary infiltrates are evident on x-ray, what is the best empiric choice of antibiotic therapy in children 3 months to 5 years of age?

- (A) Penicillin
- (B) Amoxicillin
- (C) Erythromycin
- (D) Gentamicin
- (E) Methicillin

6. You are called at night because a 3-year-old boy has the onset of inspiratory stridor. He has had coryza, followed by a tracheal cough, for 4 days. Which organism is the most likely cause of this condition?

- (A) Parainfluenza virus, types 1, 2, or 3
- (B) Influenza virus A or B
- (C) *Haemophilus influenzae*
- (D) Adenovirus
- (E) Respiratory syncytial virus

7. What is the chance that the 3-year old patient with inspiratory stridor caused by croup, in question 6, will require hospitalization?

- (A) < 10%
- (B) 10%–15%
- (C) 15%–25%
- (D) 25%–40%
- (E) ≥ 50%

8. The peak age range for croup is

- (A) 0–1 month
- (B) 1–6 months
- (C) 6 months–3 years
- (D) 2–6 years
- (E) 6–12 years

9. You are called by an alarmed father whose 5-year-old son has manifested a sudden onset of inspiratory stridor after complaining of chills and showing a fever of 102°F (38.8°C). No coryza, cough, nor other prior symptoms had been seen. This condition is caused by

- (A) Parainfluenza virus, type 1, 2, or 3
- (B) Influenza virus A or B
- (C) *Haemophilus influenzae*
- (D) Adenovirus
- (E) Respiratory syncytial virus

10. Which statement is true with respect to epiglottitis?

   (A) The incidence has increased over the past 10 years.
   (B) Characteristic symptoms are stridor, drooling, muffled speech, and agitation.
   (C) Penicillin dosages should be at least 1 million units every 6 hours.
   (D) A chest X-ray may be diagnostic.
   (E) The child prefers the supine position, in which the abdominal viscera provide increased expiratory assistance.

11. In the first 6 years of life, children are exposed to, and infected by, a variety of viral and bacterial agents, some of which have long-term effects. For example, repeated infection with which organism may result in subsequent asthma?

   (A) Influenza A virus
   (B) Respiratory syncytial virus
   (C) *Staphylococcus aureus*
   (D) *Klebsiella pneumoniae*
   (E) *Moraxella (Branhamella) catarrhalis*

12. In the treatment of childhood asthma, which of the following is a valid indication for the addition of an anti-inflammatory agent, such as inhaled glucocorticoid or a basophile-stabilizing drug?

   (A) Any variance in twice-daily peak-flow measurements at home
   (B) A normal peak-flow measurement that is less than predicted
   (C) A peak-flow performance that is less than the patient's historical best
   (D) A need for beta-agonist medication more than 3 times per week
   (E) A positive skin or serum allergy test

DIRECTIONS (Items 13–14): Each of the numbered items or incomplete statements in this section is negatively phrased, as indicated by a capitalized word, such as NOT, LEAST, or EXCEPT. Select the ONE lettered answer or completion that is BEST in each case.

13. If the patient in question 6 (3-year-old boy with onset of inspiratory stridor caused by croup) requires hospitalization, any of the following treatment modalities are useful EXCEPT

   (A) Racemic epinephrine
   (B) Glucocorticoids
   (C) An oxygen-mist tent
   (D) Endotracheal intubation
   (E) Ceftriaxone

14. An adolescent boy complains of bouts of shortness of breath. However, each time you examine him, his lung fields are clear to percussion and auscultation. With further questioning, you learn that his shortness of breath is likely to be greater when he is resting than when he is exercising. He denies orthopnea and paroxysmal nocturnal dyspnea. In preparing to order ancillary tests, you consider that each of the following is characteristic of this condition EXCEPT

   (A) A prolonged expiratory phase
   (B) An increased forced expiratory volume in 1 second (FEV_1) on pulmonary-function testing
   (C) Increased dyspnea at rest, decreased dyspnea with exercise
   (D) A lowered PO_2 and PCO_2 in arterial blood gases
   (E) A lowered PO_2 and increased PCO_2 in arterial blood gases

ANSWERS AND EXPLANATIONS

1. The answer is A. Most cases of bronchiolitis (inflammation of the bronchioles as a result of a virus infection) occur in children younger than 2 years, and the clinically most significant cases occur in children younger than 1 year of age, in whom it may cause respiratory failure. The disease is characterized by wheezing, coughing, and dyspnea, and it is most serious in infants under 3 months of age. Many affected children are likely to have recurrent wheezing during future respiratory virus infections, or even to develop asthma later in life.

2. The answer is E. Respiratory syncytial viruses (RSV) cause the majority of bronchiolitis cases. Other viral causes are parainfluenza virus, adenovirus, influenza virus, and other viruses, as well as *Mycoplasma pneumoniae.*

3. The answer is D. *Chlamydia trachomatis* and group B streptococci are a pair of organisms typically involved in respiratory infections (pneumonitides) in infants from birth to 3 months of age. [See Table 12.1, pages 204–205, in *Family Medicine* (House Officer Series), for a listing of the most common organisms, symptoms, and treatments, in the various pediatric age groups.]

4. The answer is D. Ceftriaxone 50–100 mg/kg per day is the best choice of antibiotic therapy for this patient, who has a community-acquired lobar pneumonia, for which the most likely etiology in a 4-year-old is *Streptococcus pneumoniae* or *Haemophilus influenzae.* The patient also has a probable case of septic arthritis of the left knee, which suggests *H. influenzae B,* the most common cause of septic arthritis in children. Ceftriaxone is the treatment of choice for a moderately severe form of this infection, and it is also effective against *S. pneumoniae.* While amoxicillin is theoretically effective against *H. influenzae,* it is not effective against the lactamase-producing 15% of this organism that are resistant to it. Neither penicillin nor erythromycin is effective against *H. influenzae,* but both are effective against the majority of *S. pneumoniae* organisms. Dihydrostreptomycin, which is ineffective against gram-positive organisms (i.e., *S. pneumoniae*), is no longer used because of its toxicity.

5. The answer is C. Erythromycin or another macrolide antibiotic is the best empiric choice for children of 3 months to 5 years of age when upper respiratory symptoms are present at onset and evidence of interstitial pulmonary infiltrates are evident on x-ray. Erythromycin is effective against *Streptococcus pneumoniae* as well as *Chlamydia pneumoniae* and *Mycoplasma pneumoniae.* The newer macrolides, azithromycin and clarithromycin, are effective against *Haemophilus influenzae* as well. (When *H. influenzae* is suspected, ceftriaxone is an even more potent choice.)

6. The answer is A. Parainfluenza virus, type 1, 2, or 3, is the organism that usually causes laryngotracheobronchitis (LTB), commonly known as "the croup," to which this child's symptoms point. LTB results in 90% of cases of stridor, a high-pitched, harsh inspiratory sound that indicates narrowing of the larger airways. Other organisms (e.g., influenza virus, adenovirus, respiratory syncytial virus) may also be involved.

7. The answer is A. Less than 10% of cases of laryngotracheobronchitis (LTB) require hospitalization. Hospitalization is necessary when obstruction causes respiratory failure, unusual because obstruction generally responds to humidified air, especially cool mist. Hospitalization is indicated when the respiratory rate rises persistently above 40 per minute or when the patient exhibits persistent stridor at rest.

8. The answer is C. The peak age range for croup is from 6 months to 3 years. The further the child is beyond the age of 3 years when an attack of the croup is experienced, the more benign is the course of the disease. Antibiotics are irrelevant, except as empiric coverage of possible epiglottitis.

9. The answer is C. *Haemophilus influenzae* is the cause of epiglottitis, to which this boy's symptoms point. *H. influenzae* differentiates epiglottitis from croup, the latter caused by viruses and occasionally by mycoplasma. In contrast to the viral laryngotracheobronchitis (croup), epiglottitis has an acute onset that is not preceded by coryza, and it manifests more severe respiratory obstruction. It is a genuine emergency, and when suspected, is cause for hospitalization and close observation for tracheal intubation or emergency tracheotomy.

10. The answer is B. Characteristic symptoms of epiglottitis are stridor, drooling, muffled speech, and agitation. The child's head is held guardedly forward in the "sniffing position." The incidence has *decreased* since the introduction of *Haemophilus influenzae* vaccine approximately 9 years ago. Penicillin dosages are irrelevant because, for *H. influenzae,* the antibiotics of choice are ceftriaxone and ampicillin (the vast majority of cases are bacteremic at the time of presentation). Chest X-rays are not diagnostic, but a lateral X-ray of the neck may show the thumb sign, pathognomonic of epiglottitis. The child with this illness *abhors* the supine position. Although a classic sign of this disease is a cherry-red epiglottis, which may be seen accidentally, the sign should not be sought because stimulation of the epiglottal region may precipitate laryngospasm, an emergency requiring intubation, tracheotomy, or cricothyrotomy.

11. The answer is B. Repeated infection with respiratory syncytial virus (RSV) in children under the age of 5 years may result in subsequent asthma.

12. The answer is D. The need for beta-agonist medication more than 3 times per week is the most common indication for adding an anti-inflammatory agent, such as inhaled glucocorticoids, in the management of asthma. Other indications are: greater than 20% variance in twice-daily peak flow measurements; less than 80% of the predicted normal peak flow measurement; less than 80% of the patient's best peak flow performance historically. A positive test result for skin allergy or serum allergy is not in itself an indication for anti-inflammatory therapy. Such testing shows the association of asthmatic symptoms with atopic disease, which may lend support to a diagnosis of asthma. It has no implications for the severity or refractoriness of asthma, the true indicators for the need of therapy beyond bronchodilation.

13. The answer is E. Laryngotracheobronchitis (croup) is NOT treated by ceftriaxone or other antibiotics. It is a viral infection, except for the occasional case of mycoplasma infection, which causes croup, and which does not respond to ceftriaxone. Racemic epinephrine (empiric use), glucocorticoids (to reduce edema), an oxygen mist tent (to maintain oxygenation while reducing accumulated secretions), and endotracheal intubation are used in hospitals.

14. The answer is C. Increased dyspnea with rest and decreased dyspnea with exercise are not characteristics of asthma, of which this case is a common early presentation. Virtually all asthmatics exhibit a degree of exercise-induced, reactive airway disease (i.e., bronchospasm, wheezing): With exercise, they would either experience no change in symptoms or a worsening of symptoms. Characteristics of asthma include: a prolonged expiratory phase; an increased FEV_1 on pulmonary functioning testing; a lowered PO_2 and lowered PCO_2 in arterial blood as a result of hyperventilation; and, when asthma enters a severe phase, a lowered PO_2 with a rise in PCO_2 in arterial blood, as a result of retention. Circumstantial evidence includes seasonality of symptoms (dyspnea or hay fever), family history of atopic (allergic) diseases, and precipitation of symptoms in certain environments, such as in the presence of animals.

BIBLIOGRAPHY

King MS: Respiratory diseases in infants and children. In *Family Medicine* (House Officer Series). Edited by Rudy DR, Kurowski K. Baltimore, Williams & Wilkins, 1997, pp 201–216.

SECTION V

Problems of the Gastrointestinal Tract

Test 13

Medical Problems of the Gastrointestinal Tract

DIRECTIONS (Items 1–10): Each of the numbered items or incomplete statements in this section is followed by answers or by completions of the statement. Select the ONE lettered answer or completion that is BEST in each case.

1. Dysphagia that results from an esophageal motor disorder is characterized by which of the following patterns of symptoms?

    (A) Rapidly progressing dysphagia with weight loss

    (B) Slowly progressing dysphagia, over months or years

    (C) Intermittent acute symptoms, or even acute obstruction

    (D) Dysphagia for both solids and liquids

    (E) Odynophagia

2. In treatment of GERD, which of the following modalities is the most reliably successful?

    (A) Omeprazole

    (B) H-2 blocking agents

    (C) Antacids

    (D) Elevation of the head of the bed during sleep

    (E) Prokinetic agents metoclopramide, cisapride, or both

3. Which of the following is a risk factor for squamous cell carcinoma of the esophagus?

    (A) Female sex

    (B) Asian-American race

    (C) Long-standing use of caffeine

    (D) Nasopharyngeal carcinoma

    (E) Duodenal ulcer disease

4. A 54-year-old female patient experiences substernal chest pain, which often occurs when she exercises immediately after a meal, and which is relieved by cessation of exercise. Her exercise includes leg lifts among other activities. She has a family history of coronary artery disease (CAD) and diabetes type II. She weighs 180 pounds (81.82 kilograms) at a height of 5 feet 4 inches (1.63 meters). Her symptoms abated significantly after she began following your suggestions that she elevate the head of her bed by 6 inches and avoid meals within 3 hours of retiring and within 1 hour of exercise. Examination of the abdomen is negative for masses or tenderness. Which of the following laboratory or ancillary findings is most likely in this patient?

    (A) ST elevation in the precordial leads during treadmill exercise test

    (B) Elevation of creatine phosphokinase (CPK) within 12 hours after a bout of chest pain

    (C) Elevation of lactic dehydrogenase (LDH) within 3 days of a bout of chest pain

    (D) A crater in the duodenum on upper gastrointestinal x-rays (UGI)

    (E) Erosion of the lower end of the esophagus on upper endoscopy

5. What is the approximate proportion of recurrent chest pain accounted for by gastrointestinal causes?

    (A) 10%

    (B) 20%

    (C) 30%

    (D) 40%

    (E) 50%

6. You are instructing a 25-year-old male patient about avoiding gastritis while treating his tension headaches. In addition to advising the use of antacids, you inform him that the most ulcerogenic of the nonsteroidal anti-inflammatory drugs (NSAIDs) is

    (A) Aspirin

    (B) Ibuprofen

    (C) Naproxen

    (D) Indomethacin

    (E) Acetaminophen

7. Early referral of Crohn's disease for surgery is inadvisable because the average 5-year recurrence rate of Crohn's disease after surgical treatment is

(A) 10%
(B) 25%
(C) 50%
(D) 75%
(E) 100%

8. A male patient complains of postprandial cramps and occasional colicky pain that is unrelated to meals. The most compelling reason to completely "work up" the lower bowel of a patient in whom you suspect irritable bowel syndrome would be the presence of which of the following?

(A) Heartburn among the symptoms
(B) A family history of colon cancer
(C) Age younger than 40 years
(D) Alternating constipation and diarrhea
(E) Specific and predictable intolerances of secretagogues in the diet

9. The odds that people with diverticulosis will develop diverticulitis are

(A) 10%
(B) 15%
(C) 20%
(D) 30%
(E) 50%

10. A 75-year-old male patient complains of fatigue. Thyroid studies are normal, but the hemoglobin is 8 g/dl. Mean cell corpuscular volume (MCV) is 106 μm^2 (80–96). A gastrin level is drawn and found to be 1000 pg/ml (0–110). Which of the following should you choose as the correct next step?

(A) Prescribe ferrous sulfate ($FeSO_4$) 325 mg twice daily.
(B) Order or perform a bone marrow aspiration.
(C) Check for elevated urine urobilinogen.
(D) Require upper endoscopy on a repeated schedule.
(E) Check for elevated blood urea nitrogen (BUN) and serum creatinine.

DIRECTIONS (Items 11–13): Each of the numbered items or incomplete statements in this section is negatively phrased, as indicated by a capitalized word such as NOT, LEAST, or EXCEPT. Select the ONE lettered answer or completion that is BEST in each case.

---

11. A 48-year-old female patient complains of substernal chest pain of a burning nature, which is aggravated by reclining supine within 2 hours after a substantial meal, and is relieved by antacids to varying degrees. The pain is often precipitated by coffee or alcoholic beverages. All of the following are known complications of this condition EXCEPT

(A) Barrett's esophagus
(B) Coronary artery disease
(C) Dental caries
(D) Pharyngitis
(E) Dyspareunia

12. For several months, a 28-year-old female patient has had chronic diarrhea, with 3–10 stool movements daily. Lately her soft-to-liquid stools have also begun to manifest pyosanguineous discharge. Flexible sigmoidoscopy reveals large areas of raw denudation interspersed with islands of intact mucosa. The extraintestinal processes include all of the following EXCEPT

(A) Uveitis
(B) Sclerosing cholangitis
(C) Arthropathies
(D) Pyoderma gangrenosum
(E) Erythema nodosum

13. A 45-year-old Caucasian woman presents with the third bout of peptic ulcer disease symptoms in 2 years, the eighth in 8 years. Ten years ago, she was diagnosed (by upper gastrointestinal series) with a visible ulcer in the gastric mucosa and was treated successfully with histamine-2 blockers for 3 weeks. Since then, she has been treated with varying success. The patient denies depression and alcoholism, and manifests no depression on interview. All of the following statements are correct with respect to this patient's condition EXCEPT

(A) An infectious agent is very likely involved in this condition.
(B) The causative agent is confirmed by a color change on addition of ammonia to a pH-sensitive medium containing a biopsy specimen.
(C) The best test at present for diagnosis of this condition is 95% sensitive and 95% specific.
(D) Culture of the involved mucosa is the gold standard for diagnosis of the causative agent.
(E) Patients who have this condition have a risk six times the expected rate for carcinoma of the stomach.

DIRECTIONS (Items 14–18): For each numbered type of bacterial food poisoning in these matching questions, select the letter of the identifying characteristics. Each lettered option may be selected once, more than once, or not at all.

(A) Incubation period 8–24 hours; symptoms last < 24 hours

(B) Incubation period 6–48 hours; accounts for 33% of all bacterially caused food poisoning

(C) Causes watery diarrhea; is associated with seafood; causes 17% of non-typhoidal food-poisoning cases

(D) Causes diarrhea or vomiting; incubation period 9–18 hours; symptoms last 3 days

(E) Causes vomiting and diarrhea; incubation period 3–6 hours; symptoms last 24–48 hours

14. *Salmonella* (nontyphoidal)

15. *Staphylococcus aureus*

16. *Clostridium perfringens*

17. *Vibrio parahemolyticus*

18. *Bacillus cereus*

ANSWERS AND EXPLANATIONS

1. The answer is D. Dysphagia that results from an esophageal motor disorder characteristically involves difficulty swallowing both solids and liquids. Rapidly progressing dysphagia with weight loss is suggestive of esophageal cancer. Slowly progressing dysphagia, over months or years, is suggestive of benign stricture. Intermittent acute symptoms or spasmodic acute obstruction is characteristic of symptomatic esophageal ring (Schatzki's ring, at the lower end of the esophagus). Odynophagia of recent onset usually indicates ulcerative esophagitis caused by aphthous disease; odynophagia of longer duration could indicate ulcerative disease from a more serious underlying condition, such as immune compromise emanating from such diseases as cancer, blood dyscrasias, cancer chemotherapy, or AIDS.

2. The answer is A. Omeprazole is the most potent and reliably successful therapy in treating gastroesophageal reflux disease (GERD). It belongs to the relatively new category of drugs called proton (H+) pump inhibitors. H-2 blocking agents, antacids, elevation of the head of the bed, metoclopramide, and cisapride are also helpful in given patients; however, the H+ pump inhibitor has revolutionized medical treatment of GERD.

3. The answer is D. Nasopharyngeal carcinoma is a risk factor for carcinoma of the esophagus, as is long-standing achalasia, as well as tylosis (constitutional hyperkeratosis of the palms, soles, and esophagus). Duodenal ulcer disease is not a known risk factor for squamous carcinoma of the esophagus. Males have a 3-to-4 times greater chance of nasopharyngeal carcinoma than females. Blacks have 5 times the risk of the remaining population; Asian-Americans are not mentioned as having an increased risk. Alcohol use, but not caffeine, is a risk factor.

4. The answer is E. Erosion of the lower end of the esophagus on upper endoscopy is the most likely finding in this patient, who has symptoms typical of gastroesophageal reflux disease (GERD). Although she has two clear risk factors for ischemic heart disease (family history of CAD and diabetes type II), as well as obesity, the latter is also a risk factor for GERD. Patients with GERD may have symptoms during exercise after substantial meals, especially when exercises increase intraabdominal pressure. Elevation of creatine phosphokinase (CPK) occurs within hours of the onset of a myocardial infarction; lactic dehydrogenase (LDH) is el-

evated from about 2 days, for about 5 days. A myocardial infarction is not likely, not only because of the positive evidence for GERD, but because the patient's bouts of pain were short-lived and apparently related to exercise and supine position within a short time after meals. A duodenal crater on upper gastrointestinal x-rays represents a peptic ulcer. Active peptic ulcer is unusual in the absence of epigastric tenderness. ST elevation in the precordial leads is typical of exercise-induced angina. Such angina often occurs after a substantial meal, but not while the patient is reclining after a meal. This patient must still be evaluated for heart disease, with use of the exercise tolerance test, employing EKG during exercise, or EKG followed by a heart scan such as with the thallium stress test.

5. The answer is D. Approximately 40% of recurrent chest pain is accounted for by gastrointestinal causes. This fact is useful when chest pain is evaluated in a primary care office or emergency department.

6. The answer is A. Aspirin (acetylsalicylic acid) is the most ulcerogenic of the NSAIDs. Ibuprofen, naproxen, and indomethacin, as well as virtually all other NSAIDs, are potently ulcerogenic, but not to the same extent as aspirin. Acetaminophen is not an NSAID.

7. The answer is D. The average 5-year recurrence rate of Crohn's disease after surgical treatment is 75%. Thus, surgery is seldom the best approach; it is reserved for a complicating obstruction or an abscess, when manifestations are refractory to medical therapy.

8. The answer is B. A family history of colon cancer would be the most compelling reason to evaluate this patient definitively for colorectal cancer. Symptoms of heartburn suggest esophageal reflux. A patient under the age of 40 has *less* than the average risk of colon cancer. Alternating constipation and diarrhea, while sometimes signaling colon cancer, is caused, in the vast majority of cases, by irritable bowel syndrome, especially in younger individuals. Intolerances to secretagogues (e.g., caffeine, ethanol) suggests peptic ulcer, gastritis, or reflux.

9. The answer is C. The odds are 20% that people with diverticulosis (diverticula without inflammation) will develop diverticulitis (infection of individual diverticula, which causes pain, sometimes fever, and, occasionally, abscess formation or hemorrhage). An incidental finding of asymptomatic diverticulosis permits inexpensive preventive care, consisting of a high-fiber diet, preferably fortified with bulk additives (e.g., psyllium).

10. The answer is D. Referral for repeated upper endoscopy is indicated in this patient in order to be alert to the possibility of adenocarcinoma of the stomach. This patient has atrophic gastritis, as indicated by the elevated gastrin level and pernicious anemia. Atrophic gastritis is a risk factor for carcinoma of the stomach. Although elevated gastrin is a sign of atrophic gastritis, it cannot be said that elevated gastrin causes gastric carcinoma. The anemia is macrocytic and is based on malabsorption of vitamin B-12, caused by lack of intrinsic factor (normally contained in healthy gastric mucosa). Ferrous sulfate is the treatment for iron deficiency. Although you may test for transferrin saturation and serum ferritin to rule out iron deficiency, you would not treat with iron without such confirmation. A bone marrow aspiration is not indicated because the diagnosis is readily apparent. Although you should test for occult blood in the stool, the results will be negative because elevation of gastrin is not associated with iron deficiency, unless it is secondary to carcinoma of the stomach. Urine urobilinogen is elevated in hemolytic anemia. Elevated BUN and creatinine are indicative of renal failure, a cause of anemia; however, gastrin is not particularly elevated in renal failure.

11. The answer is B. Coronary artery disease is NOT particularly associated with gastroesophageal reflux (GERD), the condition to which the symptoms point. However, many people with GERD are admitted to hospitals because of the confounding nature of the "heartburn" symptom. Barrett's esophagus is the metamorphosis of esophageal mucosa into gastric mucosa in the region of the lower esophagus affected by reflux. Reflux must be present for extended periods for Barrett's esophagus to develop, but when it does, symptoms become much more difficult to control, and the risk of esophageal carcinoma is increased. Dental caries and pharyngitis, as well as chronic cough, result from nocturnal regurgitation and aspiration. Dyspareunia (in the form of genital discomfort) in female patients may be associated with GERD for unknown reasons; however, it is postulated that it may result from lack of lubrication or vaginismus secondary to diminished well-being during bouts of esophageal reflux and esophagitis.

12. The answer is A. Uveitis is NOT one of the extraintestinal processes involved in ulcerative colitis, the condition to which the symptoms point. (Although the two conditions may co-exist, they are not associated. In fact, if uveitis is present, the doctor should consider a different enteropathy, such as Reiter's syndrome.) Sclerosing cholangitis, arthropathies, and pyoderma gangrenosum are well known to be associated with ulcerative colitis, although the basis for the association is poorly understood. Erythema nodosum is also associated with ulcerative colitis, but less frequently than the other entities.

13. The answer is D. Culture of the involved mucosa is NOT the most sensitive nor specific test for this condition, upper gastrointestinal infection by *Helicobacter pylori*. (This infection accounts for the persistence and recurrence of gastric ulcer and chronic gastritis.) The best test is the probe for urease activity in which ammonia is added to a pH-sensitive medium which has been inoculated with a biopsy specimen from the affected area of the gastrointestinal mucosa. (Urease, produced by the organism, raises the pH and produces the color change.) Patients who have chronic gastritis and infection with *H. Pylori* have a sixfold increase in the risk of gastric carcinoma.

14. The answer is B. *Salmonella* poisoning (non-typhoidal) has an incubation period of 6–48 hours; and it accounts for 33% of all bacterially caused food poisoning. It tends to be acquired from contaminated eggs, meat, or poultry.

15. The answer is E. *Staphylococcus aureus* food poisoning causes vomiting and diarrhea after an incubation period of 3–6 hours, and its symptoms last 24–48 hours. Foods classically contaminated include ham, pork, canned beef, and (especially) cream-filled pastry that has been left for too long at room temperature.

16. The answer is A. *Clostridium perfringens* is the cause of 17% of nontyphoidal cases of food poisoning. It has an incubation period of 8–24 hours, lasts less than 24 hours, and may be acquired from contaminated beef, turkey, or chicken.

17. The answer is C. *Vibrio parahaemolyticus* produces watery diarrhea; it is associated with contaminated seafood.

18. The answer is D. *Bacillus cereus* produces either diarrhea or vomiting, has an incubation period of 9–18 hours, and lasts for 3 days.

BIBLIOGRAPHY

Nidiry JJ: Medical problems of the gastrointestinal tract. In *Family Medicine* (House Officer Series). Edited by Rudy DR, Kurowski K. Baltimore, Williams & Wilkins, 1997, pp 217–234.

Test 14

Surgical Problems of the Gastrointestinal Tract

DIRECTIONS (Items 1–9): Each of the numbered items or incomplete statements in this section is followed by answers or by completions of the statement. Select the ONE lettered answer or completion that is BEST in each case.

1. A patient complains of colicky abdominal pain. As you differentiate common duct obstruction from renal colic, which information would assist you most?

   (A) White blood cell count
   (B) Temperature curve
   (C) Location of the pain
   (D) Gender of the patient
   (E) Relation of pain to meals

2. A 28-year-old, white male has had abdominal pain for the past 36 hours. Examination of the anterior aspect of the abdomen is negative for rebound tenderness, but some guarding is evident in the right lower quadrant, close to the midline. The white blood count is elevated to 25,000, with 80% neutrophils, of which 30% are bands. You attempt to elicit the obturator sign. The obturator sign may denote which of the following conditions?

   (A) Cholecystitis
   (B) Retrocecal appendicitis
   (C) Femoral hernia
   (D) Irritable bowel syndrome
   (E) Bowel obstruction

3. A 6-week-old infant is presented by his parents with a history of increasingly frequent vomiting during the past 7 days. In the past 24 hours the vomiting has become projectile. On examination, the abdomen manifests a rippling visible through the skin, moving from the patient's left to right, preceding bouts of vomiting. A 2-centimeter nodule is palpable deep in the right epigastrium. Which of the following settings most typifies this condition?

   (A) Female infant, 2 weeks to 4 months of age
   (B) Newborn with Apgar score of 5–7
   (C) Male infant, 2 weeks to 4 months of age
   (D) Baby with birth weight of 9 lbs (4.08 kg), mother with diabetes
   (E) Infant who had benign tachypnea of the newborn

4. The most common cause of bowel obstruction (as opposed to pyloric obstruction) in the first 2 years of life is which of the following?

   (A) Meconium plug
   (B) Hirschsprung's disease
   (C) Ileal atresia
   (D) Colonic atresia
   (E) Intussusception

5. The differing presentation between small and large bowel obstruction is best exemplified by which of the following?

   (A) Vomiting versus distention
   (B) Presence versus absence of occult blood
   (C) Rapidity versus slowness of onset
   (D) Intermittency versus steadiness of symptoms
   (E) Presence versus absence of weight loss

6. The 67% decrease in the U.S. incidence of carcinoma of the stomach in the last 30 years is probably a result of

   (A) A decrease in the national per capita intake of caffeine
   (B) Changes in the prevalence of *Helicobacter pylori*
   (C) A decrease in overuse of hot spices in cooking
   (D) An increase in average life expectancy
   (E) A decrease in the rate of smoking

7. The lifetime risk of carcinoma of the colon is approximately 2.5% for the average American. For a person who has a first degree relative with either colon cancer or adenomatous polyp, what is the approximate risk?

   (A) 2.5%–3%
   (B) 7%–7.5%
   (C) 10%–10.5%
   (D) 18%–19%
   (E) 22%–23%

8. In patients whose colon cancer is in Duke's Stage A, what is the approximate percentage of patients that survive for 5 years?

(A) 90%
(B) 70%
(C) 60%
(D) 30%
(E) 5%

9. A 45-year-old female patient complains of "indigestion" that has occurred with increasing frequency during the past 2 months. Her symptoms consist of abdominal bloating, epigastric pain, and nausea. Sometimes the pain is felt in the right upper quadrant of the abdomen and simultaneously in the area of the right rib cage. The last attack started rapidly yesterday, within 20 minutes after a substantial evening meal. Throughout the night it caused pain, associated with fever and colicky waves of pain. Which of the following statements is correct with regard to this condition?

(A) Fair-complexioned people experience this condition more often than others do.
(B) Men have a higher risk than women of developing this disease.
(C) A history of pregnancy protects against this disease in women.
(D) A urinalysis is likely to show gross or microscopic hematuria.
(E) Abdominal examination will differentiate this condition from coronary insufficiency or myocardial infarction.

DIRECTIONS (Item 10): The incomplete statement in this section is negatively phrased, as indicated by the capitalized word EXCEPT. Select the ONE lettered completion that is BEST.

10. The many risk factors for carcinoma of the esophagus include all of the following EXCEPT

(A) Alcohol abuse
(B) Cigarette smoking
(C) Achalasia
(D) Reflux esophagitis
(E) Excessive coffee intake

DIRECTIONS (Items 11–15): For each numbered sign in these matching questions, select the letter of the correct description. Each lettered option may be selected once, more than once, or not at all.

(A) Tenderness at a point two thirds of the distance from the umbilicus to the anterior superior spine of the right iliac crest
(B) Pain upon hyperextension of the hip, denoting contact between the psoas muscle and an inflammatory process
(C) Pain over McBurney's point upon sudden release of deep pressure over the corresponding point in the left lower quadrant
(D) Cessation of inspiratory effort when the examiner's hand is deeply pressed into the right subcostal space
(E) Pain in the right subscapular area associated with anterior abdominal pain

11. Boas' sign

12. Murphy's sign

13. Rovsing's sign

14. McBurney's sign

15. Iliopsoas or psoas sign

ANSWERS AND EXPLANATIONS

1. The answer is C. Location of the pain would assist most in differentiating common duct obstruction from renal colic. Renal colic is the only colicky or cramping pain that is lateralized. It begins high in the ipsilateral flank and descends gradually to the scrotum (males) or labium majorum (females) with descension of the stone to the ureterovesical junction. All other colicky abdominal pains, invariably caused by a hollow organ partially or completely obstructed or hypersensitive to the contents in the lumen, are located in the midline (because their sources are midline derived organs). The white blood count, as well as the temperature, may be elevated or not in either condition. While cholelithiasis is more common in females, the gender factor is not sufficient to assist in making the diagnosis in a given case. Similarly, while gallbladder symptoms tend to be precipitated by meals, the relationship is not strong enough to determine the presence or absence of cholelithiasis or ureterolithiasis.

2. The answer is B. Retrocecal appendicitis is denoted by the obturator sign, defined as pain upon internal or external rotation of the thigh with the knee flexed. As with the psoas sign, this finding is most often present in appendicitis when the appendix is located (atypically) in a retrocecal position.

3. The answer is C. A male infant of 2 weeks to 4 months is the most likely infant to have pyloric stenosis, of which this patient's presentation is typical. Male infants are affected four times as frequently as female infants.

4. The answer is E. Intussusception is the most common cause of bowel obstruction (as opposed to pyloric obstruction) in the first 2 years of life, when approximately 80% of cases occur (peaking in the 5–9 months era). Males are affected three times more frequently than females; presentation includes colicky abdominal pain, "currant-jelly stools," reflex vomiting, leukocytosis, hemoconcentration, and a palpable mass. Hirschsprung's disease is congenital absence of ganglion cells in the colon walls, producing congenital megacolon. Meconium plug is a cause of obstruction in the newborn. Ilial and colonic atresias are congenital absences of lumina in the ilium and colon; both are causes of congenital bowel obstruction.

5. The answer is A. Vomiting in clinical obstruction signifies an upper gastrointestinal locale, especially at the pylorus, while a dominant symptom of distention signifies lower bowel obstruction. Intermittency (as opposed to steadiness) of symptoms is present in both small and large bowel obstruction. Constancy or steadiness of symptoms in an abdominal emergency is suggestive of peritoneal irritation (e.g., appendicitis, perforated viscus, or ischemic bowel disease). The higher or more proximal the location of the obstruction, the more rapid the onset, but rapidity of onset is not as reliable nor as precisely defined a sign as vomiting versus distention. Presence of occult blood in the stool, while more likely in upper GI obstruction, is not specific nor sensitive for either type. Weight loss is not a prominent characteristic of either type of obstruction.

6. The answer is B. A diminished prevalence of *Helicobacter pylori* is a likely reason for the 67% decrease in the U.S. incidence of carcinoma of the stomach during the last 30 years. *H. pylori*, a risk factor for stomach carcinoma, is close to being a proven cause. Along with the decrease in carcinoma is a decreased incidence of peptic ulcer, a disease that also appears to be caused by *H. pylori*. (Whether the decrease is a side effect of "indiscriminate" use of antibiotics during these years is not known.) Although caffeine is a secretagogue, its consumption in the US has not decreased during the past 30 years. No decreased use of hot spices in cooking nor decrease in the rate of smoking in the US is known. An increase in life expectancy should have the effect of increasing rather than decreasing the incidence of carcinoma of the stomach, because the disease is rare under the age of 40 years and more prevalent in later life.

7. The answer is B. The lifetime risk of carcinoma of the colon for a person who has a first-degree relative with either colon cancer or adenomatous polyp is approximately 7%–7.5%, or roughly triple the average American's lifetime risk of 2.5%. Because the incidence increases with each decade of life, the risks for both groups are greater among the elderly.

8. The answer is A. Duke's Stage A, carcinoma of the colon which is confined to the mucosa and submucosa, confers a 5-year cure rate of 90%. Stage B, confined to the muscularis or serosa, confers a 5 year cure rate of 60%-75%. Stage C, in which positive lymph nodes are present but without distant metastases, confers varying 5-year survival rates, depending on the number of positive lymph nodes (69% with one; 27% with six or more). Stage D, in which distant metastases (to liver, bone, lung) are present, regardless of the status of the site of origin and lymph nodes, confers a 5-year survival rate of only 5%. Cancers in the ascending and transverse colon are more likely to present in Stages C or D because early bleeding is not as likely to be noted by the patient. Carcinomas arise virtually always from adenomatous polyps that exist for a period of 10 years before becoming cancerous. More than half of all polyps found in the colon are of the hypertrophic variety and have no malignant potential. Adenomatous polyps occur in three histological types: tubular, with the least malignant potential; villous, with the greatest malignant potential; and tubulovillous, with malignant potential intermediate between the tubular and the villous.

9. The answer is E. Abdominal examination will differentiate this condition from coronary insufficiency or myocardial infarction on evidence of the tenderness in the right upper quadrant, aggravated by the patient's deep, inspiratory movement (the so-called "Murphy sign"). The patient's epigastric and right upper quadrant pain following meals that probably contain significant amounts of fat indicates that she has acute and chronic cholecystitis, and possibly cholelithiasis. ("Female, fertile, fat, and forty" is a medical students' mnemonic for remembering that middle-aged women who have had pregnancies and who are overweight fit the stereotype of susceptibility to gall bladder disease.) Shade of complexion is not associated with risk of gall bladder disease. (Formerly "the fair" was used in the mnemonic, for "the fair sex"; the term has sometimes been mistakenly interpreted as "fair complexion" by more recent trainees.) Heart pain, although often presenting as abdominal pain, especially in the case of insufficiency or occlusion in the right coronary circulation, is not characterized by abdominal tenderness. Colicky pain associated with gall bladder disease signifies impaction by a stone in the cystic duct or the common bile duct. The cramps are felt at the midline (unlike renal colic, in which the colicky pain is lateralized). Gall bladder colic, unlike renal colic, is not associated with hematuria.

10. The answer is E. Excessive coffee intake is NOT known to be a risk factor for carcinoma of the esophagus. Alcohol abuse, cigarette smoking, achalasia, and reflux esophagitis are among the known risks. Prolonged esophageal reflux leads to metaplasia of the lower esophageal mucosa into the gastric mucosa, a condition called Barrett's esophagus, itself a most powerful risk factor.

11. The answer is E. Boas' sign, actually a symptom rather than a sign, is pain in the right subscapular area associated with anterior abdominal pain. This is present in cholelithiasis and is a *forme fruste* (atypical or mild or incomplete expression of another, more recognized sign or symptom) of the right bandlike radiation of pain in this condition.

12. The answer is D. Murphy's sign is cessation of inspiratory effort when the examiner's hand is deeply pressed into the right subcostal space, a sign highly suggestive of cholelithiasis.

13. The answer is C. Rovsing's sign is pain over McBurney's point upon sudden release of deep pressure over the corresponding point in the left lower quadrant, a form of rebound tenderness, which is a sign of peritoneal irritation. It is highly suggestive of appendicitis.

14. The answer is A. McBurney's sign is tenderness at a point two thirds of the distance from the umbilicus to the anterior superior spine of the right iliac crest, a sign highly suggestive of appendicitis.

15. The answer is B. The psoas sign is pain upon hyperextension of the hip, denoting contact between the psoas muscle and an inflammatory process, most often present in appendicitis when the appendix is located (atypically) in a retrocecal position.

BIBLIOGRAPHY

Brown CM: Surgical issues of the gastrointestinal tract. In *Family Medicine* (House Officer Series). Edited by Rudy DR, Kurowski K. Baltimore, Williams & Wilkins, 1997, pp 235–254.

Test 15

Diseases of the Liver

DIRECTIONS (Items 1–12): Each of the numbered items or incomplete statements in this section is followed by answers or by completions of the statement. Select the ONE lettered answer or completion that is BEST in each case.

1. Diagnosis of acute hepatitis B is confirmed most characteristically by the presence of which of the following?

(A) HBsIGG antibodies
(B) HBsIGM and HbcAg antibodies
(C) HBsAg and HBcIGG antibodies
(D) HBsAg and HBcIGM antibodies
(E) HBcAg and HbcIGM antibodies

2. Which of the following indicates immunity to hepatitis B by normal response to earlier exposure?

(A) Absence of HBsIGG antibodies
(B) Presence of HBcIGM and HbsAg antibodies
(C) Absence of HBsAg and presence of HBcIGG and HBs antibodies
(D) Absence of HBsAg and presence of HBcIGM antibodies
(E) Presence of HbcAg and anti-HBcIGM antibodies

3. Which of the following is most characteristic of chronic active hepatitis B?

(A) HBsAG
(B) Anti-HBcIGM
(C) Anti-HBsIGG
(D) Persistence of HBsAg and HBeAg beyond 6 months
(E) Anti-HBcIGG

4. The second-ranking cause of transfusion-related hepatitis (after hepatitis B) is which of the following organisms?

(A) Hepatitis A
(B) *Entamoeba histolytica*
(C) Hepatitis C
(D) Hepatitis D
(E) Hepatitis E

5. Four months of alpha interferon therapy has been found to be effective in clearing hepatitic antigens in 65% of patients followed for 6 years after therapy. This statement applies to which of the following hepatitides?

(A) Hepatitis A
(B) Hepatitis B
(C) Hepatitis C
(D) Hepatitis D
(E) Hepatitis E

6. Your patient, a respected, 55-year-old, male college professor, has seemed stable in his professional life and marriage, and adequate in his role as a parent. A routine chemistry battery returns with surprise findings: gamma glutamyltransferase (GGT) = 255 U/L (normal = 5–40 U/L); serum aspartate aminotransferase = 199 U/L (AST, formerly SGOT, 1–36); and alanine aminotransferase 101 (ALT, formerly SGPT, 1–45). Alkaline phosphatase is normal at 75 U/L. Which of the following is a logical next step in this patient's diagnosis and management?

(A) Check for scleral icterus and order a hepatitis screen.
(B) Repeat the laboratory battery.
(C) Check for Murphy's sign and order a gallbladder ultrasound study.
(D) Order a consultation to obtain a liver biopsy.
(E) Recheck social history and check for spider angiomata.

7. Primary biliary cirrhosis (PBC) is diagnosed most specifically by which of the following?

(A) Endoscopic retrograde cholangiopancreatography (ERCP)
(B) Antimitochondrial antibody, anti-M_2
(C) The presence of pruritus
(D) The presence of portal hypertension
(E) Malabsorption of fat and fat-soluble vitamins

8. An African-American man has a 10-day history of jaundice in his sclerae accompanied by fever. He notes dark urine. The patient drinks no alcohol, and denies homosexuality and intravenous drug use. Physical examination is otherwise noncontributory. The gallbladder ultrasound study and hepatitis screen are negative. Serum alkaline phosphatase is 250 U/L (55–150); gamma-glutamyl transferase is 150 U/L (5–40). Total bilirubin is 2.1 mg/dl (0.3–1.1), while the conjugated bilirubin component is 1.4 mg/dl (0.1–0.4). A test for antimitochondrial antibodies is negative. A course of cefadroxil 250 mg 4 times per day for 10 days results in resolution of the symptoms within 48 hours of the first dose. Which of the following statements is true with regard to the most probable disease suggested by this picture?

(A) The Kayser-Fleischer ring may be present.
(B) Antimitochondrial anti-M_2 antibody is positive.
(C) Inflammatory bowel disease is frequently associated.
(D) The majority of cases are in Caucasian women.
(E) A ratio of iron to total iron binding capacity (TIBC) $\geq 62\%$ can make the diagnosis.

9. Autoimmune hepatitis, as distinguished from primary biliary cirrhosis and primary sclerosing cholangitis, accounts for approximately what percentage of chronic liver disease?

(A) 10%
(B) 25%
(C) 40%
(D) 55%
(E) 75%

10. A 50-year-old male patient presents with peripheral edema and ascites. In this patient, which finding would be most indicative of cirrhosis as the basis for ascites?

(A) A blood urea nitrogen (BUN) of 9
(B) A serum albumin to peritoneal fluid albumin ratio of 1:1
(C) Angiectasis visible on the cheeks
(D) A clinical response to spironolactone
(E) A peritoneal fluid glucose to blood glucose ratio of < 1

11. An alcoholic, 50-year-old, male patient has had palmar erythema, numerous spider angiomata over the anterior chest, and ascites. Now he presents with fever of 101°F (38.3°C), leukocytosis, and abdominal pain and tenderness. Which is the most logical next step?

(A) Diagnostic peritoneal tap and complete blood cell count
(B) Three blood cultures from samples drawn 5 minutes apart
(C) Abdominal x-ray
(D) Test for occult blood in stool
(E) Ventilation-perfusion lung scan

12. The most dreaded complication of cirrhosis in terms of prognosis, rapidity of development, and frequency of occurrence is

(A) Liver failure
(B) Bleeding internal hemorrhoids
(C) Spontaneous bacterial peritonitis
(D) Refractory ascites
(E) Bleeding esophageal varices

DIRECTIONS (Item 13): The incomplete statement in this section is negatively phrased, as indicated by the capitalized word, EXCEPT. Select the one lettered completion that is best.

13. With regard to the effects of ethanol on the liver, all of the following statements are true EXCEPT

(A) Four to six drinks per day significantly increases the risk of liver damage.
(B) Ethanol can aggravate existing liver disease.
(C) Women are more susceptible to alcoholic liver disease than men.
(D) The majority of alcoholics develop chronic alcoholic liver disease.
(E) Spider angiomas result from failure of hepatic metabolism of circulating estrogens.

DIRECTIONS (Items 14–18): For each numbered hepatitis type in these matching questions, select the letter of the mode of transmission. (Knowledge of incubation periods and portals of entry of the five identified hepatitides is critical for prognosticating and preventing spread of cases.)

(A) Transmitted by body fluids other than gastrointestinal; carries high risk of chronic hepatitis and high risk of sexual transmission.

(B) Transmitted mainly by feco-oral contamination; carries little risk of complications except in the third trimester of pregnancy.

(C) May be transmitted by percutaneous or nonpercutaneous means; requires the presence of hepatitis B in order to reproduce.

(D) Transmitted by body fluids other than gastrointestinal; carries very high risk of chronic hepatitis; figures prominently in transfusion-induced hepatitis; carries relatively low risk of sexual transmission and transmission by accidental needle stick.

(E) Transmitted mainly by feco-oral contamination; generally carries little risk of complications.

14. Hepatitis A

15. Hepatitis B

16. Hepatitis C

17. Hepatitis D

18. Hepatitis E

ANSWERS AND EXPLANATIONS

1. The answer is D. The diagnosis of acute hepatitis B is confirmed most characteristically by the combination of HBsAg and HBcIGM antibodies. During the acute phase, the hepatitis B surface antigen (HBsAg) is present (and accessible for testing), as is the rapidly rising IGM antibody to the core antigen (HbcIGM). The combination of positive tests depends on an immunologically normal response to the infection.

2. The answer is C. Normal response to earlier exposure to hepatitis B virus and immunity to hepatitis B includes a negative finding for HBsAg and a positive finding for HBcIGG antibodies.

3. The answer is D. The presence of HBsAg and HBeAg is most characteristic of chronic hepatitis B (HB). While chronic persistent HB manifests HBsAg, chronic active HB, fraught with a high incidence of cirrhosis, is characterized by intermittent or persistent presence of HBeAg as well.

4. The answer is C. Hepatitis C is responsible for the majority of transfusion-related non-A/non-B hepatitis. However, the risk of infection from parenteral exposure (i.e., needlestick) to an HCV-infected patient is apparently less than 10% of the risk of infection with HBV after such exposure to an HBV-infected patient. Hepatitis D, while often involved, requires prior infection by HBV in order to exist. Hepatitides A and E are generally not passed parenterally. Entamoeba histolytica is a protozoan disease which attacks the liver after ingestion.

5. The answer is B. In 65% of hepatitis B cases, 4 months of alpha interferon therapy has been found to be effective in clearing HBeAg and HBsAg for 6 years following therapy.

6. The answer is E. Recheck the social history of this patient and check for spider angiomata. The elevation of GGT in the presence of a normal alkaline phosphatase indicates a significant amount of recent alcohol intake, until proven otherwise. The elevation of serum aspartate aminotransferase (AST) out of proportion to alanine aminotransferase (ALT) [e.g., 2:1] is strongly suggestive of alcoholic hepatitis as opposed to viral hepatitis. Examining for the stigmata of cirrhosis (i.e., spider angiomata, palmar erythema, testicular atrophy, distended flank veins) is appropriate.

7. The answer is B. The presence of antimitochondrial antibody anti-M_2 is the most specific diagnostic criterion for primary biliary cirrhosis (PBC), a rare disorder, predominantly of Caucasian women. Endoscopic retrograde cholangiopancreatography (ERCP) also yields characteristic findings but they are not as specific. Pruritus is likely to be present, but it is a nonspecific accompaniment of cholestatic jaundice. Portal hypertension may be present, but it denotes the onset of fibrotic change that can occur with cirrhosis of any cause. Malabsorption of fat and fat soluble vitamins may occur, but it, too, is not specific for this condition.

8. The answer is C. Inflammatory bowel disease is associated in 60% of patients who have primary sclerosing cholangitis (PSC), the disease affecting this patient. This patient has obstructive jaundice, as confirmed by elevated alkaline phosphatase, elevated gamma glutamyl transferase and elevated total bilirubin (due predominantly to the conjugated form and bilirubinuria). Bile that occurs in the urine is always of the conjugated type; that is, any time urine is dark because of bilirubin, the jaundice is extra-hepatic (i.e., obstructive). The diagnosis of PSC is supported by the condition's responsiveness to antibiotics in the presence of obstructive jaundice, with no evidence of cholelithiasis. Suspected PSC is confirmed by endoscopic retrograde cholangiopancreatography (ERCP) [unlike the situation in primary biliary cirrhosis (PBC) in which ERCP is helpful, but not diagnostic]. With PSC, a 10% risk of hepatic carcinoma exists; thus liver transplantation should be considered. Portal hypertension may be present, but is neither sensitive (unless late in course) nor specific. Kayser-Fleischer rings are ocular limbal rings in Wilson's disease (a dominantly inherited inability to excrete copper); Wilson's disease does cause jaundice and may present as liver failure, but it does not present as febrile disease responsive to antibiotics. A transferrin saturation of 62% is diagnostic of hemochromatosis, caused by a hereditary excessive absorption of iron in the gastrointestinal tract. Hemochromatosis, which causes hepatocellular jaundice, heart disease, non-insulin dependent diabetes, and arthritis, is not characterized by cholangitis nor responsiveness to antibiotics. Caucasian women are not the predominant victims of PSC, but rather of PBC. Patients with AIDS may develop, as a result of *Cryptosporidium* infection, a cholangitis that is similar clinically to primary sclerosing cholangitis, but this patient has no risk factors for AIDS. Antimitochondrial anti-M_2 antibody is positive in PBC, but not PSC. While both are autoimmune diseases, in contrast to PBC, PSC is characterized by both intrahepatic and extrahepatic involvement.

9. The answer is A. Autoimmune hepatitis accounts for 10% of chronic liver disease. Autoimmune hepatitis is distinguished from primary biliary cirrhosis (PBC) and primary sclerosing cholangitis (PSC), although all three are classified in the broad category of autoimmune liver disease: Autoimmune hepatitis involves the parenchyma as opposed to the collecting system, whereas PBC and PSC involve the collecting system. Autoimmune hepatitis is more common than PBC and PSC. Approximately 75% of cases of autoimmune hepatitis afflict women under the age of 30. Two types of autoimmune hepatitis are known: Type I is characterized by the presence of antinuclear antibody and anti-smooth-muscle antibodies; Type II is characterized by the presence of anti-liver-kidney microsomal antibodies. Treatment with glucocorticoids is very effective in both types, which makes early diagnosis important.

10. The answer is B. A serum albumin to peritoneal fluid albumin ratio of about 1:1 (or more) is indicative of cirrhosis as the cause for ascites. Although serum albumin falls as a result of cirrhosis toward the transudative level found in ascitic fluid, the transudate in ascites that results from cirrhosis has a still lower albumin content. The only other common causes of ascites are malignant exudates and exudates caused by spontaneous bacterial peritonitis. These states are likely to cause a ratio of less than 1:1 as a result of the increase in ascitic fluid protein. An unexpectedly low blood urea nitrogen (BUN) of 9 may be a result of chronic imbibing leading to dilution; however, alcoholism is not associated with cirrhosis in more than 15% of cases. Angiectasias on the cheeks are usually seen when spider angiomata are also present, but, in themselves, can be signs of actinic keratosis or of "aging" in especially fair-skinned people. A clinical response to spironolactone is a nonspecific response to ascites of any cause, although spironolactone is usually more effective than other diuretics in the management of cirrhosis. A peritoneal fluid glucose to blood glucose ratio of less than 1 is a sign of bacterial infection in fluid-filled spaces (e.g., pleural and cerebrospinal fluids). Although bacterial peritonitis is a known complication of cirrhosis, it occurs in only 5% of cases, and the peritoneal to serum albumin ratio rises above 1:1.

11. The answer is A. A diagnostic peritoneal tap and complete blood cell count (CBC) should be performed in this patient, to test for spontaneous bacterial peritoni-

tis. Blood cultures are indicated, mainly for routine investigation of the fever. Plain abdominal x-rays would be indicated only in the presence of colicky pain (to rule out bowel obstruction) or rebound tenderness (to rule out perforated viscus). A ventilation-perfusion lung scan would be indicated if a pulmonary embolus were suspected. Spontaneous bacterial peritonitis, which occurs in about 5% of all cases of cirrhosis, would show cloudy fluid, with >300 WBCs/ml, mostly neutrophils, and a pH of < 3.5. Physical signs are more subtle than in peritonitis caused by perforated viscus.

12. The answer is E. Bleeding esophageal varices, a consequence of portal hypertension, as a result of opening up of potential collateral veins which provide bypass of the scarred liver, is the most dreaded complication of cirrhosis. The mortality rate remains 30%. With bleeding esophageal varices, hemorrhage may be brisk in the face of coagulation abnormalities as a result of the effect of liver disease on production of prothrombin. Although the ultimate prognoses for spontaneous bacterial peritonitis, liver failure, and persistent ascites are also poor, the course of each of these is slower than that of bleeding esophageal varices, giving more time for consideration of all therapeutic options and for establishing a therapeutic plan. Internal hemorrhoids, as another set of collaterals bypassing the liver, is a common complication of portal hypertension, but is more accessible to local measures.

13. The answer is D. The false statement is that the majority of alcoholics develop alcoholic liver disease. In fact, only 15% of them contract chronic liver disease, despite the fact that up to one third of patients who drink excessively develop fatty liver. Ethanol can aggravate existing liver disease. Women are more susceptible than men to alcoholic liver disease. Spider angiomas and small-vessel ectasias, presumptive signs of cirrhosis, are thought to result from elevated levels of estrogenic substances, inadequately metabolized by a chronically diseased liver.

14. The answer is E. Hepatitis A is transmitted mainly by feco-oral contamination. Generally, it carries little risk of complications.

15. The answer is A. Hepatitis B is transmitted by body fluids other than gastrointestinal. It carries high risks of chronic hepatitis and sexual transmission.

16. The answer is D. Hepatitis C is transmitted by body fluids other than gastrointestinal. It carries a very high risk of chronic hepatitis; approximately 50% of cases progress to chronic hepatitis. It is prominent in transfusion-induced hepatitis, but carries less risk of sexual transmission and only a 4% chance of transmission by accidental needle stick.

17. The answer is C. Hepatitis D may be transmitted by percutaneous or nonpercutaneous means. It requires the presence of hepatitis B in order to reproduce.

18. The answer is B. Hepatitis E is transmitted mainly by feco-oral contamination. It carries little risk of complications, except in the third trimester of pregnancy.

BIBLIOGRAPHY

Nidiry JJ: Diseases of the Liver. In *Family Medicine* (House Officer Series). Edited by Rudy DR, Kurowski K. Baltimore, Williams & Wilkins, 1997, pp 255–268.

SECTION VI

Problems of the Urinary Tract

Test 16

Urinary Tract Infections

DIRECTIONS (Items 1–14): Each of the numbered items or incomplete statements in this section is followed by answers or by completions of the statement. Select the ONE lettered answer or completion that is BEST in each case.

1. A 32-year-old man with no previous history of similar problems complains of 4 days of dysuria and arthralgias. He notices lower back pain and some difficulty starting and stopping his flow of urine. His temperature is 103°F (39.4°C); pulse is 106; blood pressure is 120/62. He appears ill and in mild distress. He has no peripheral joint erythema or tenderness and no costovertebral angle or abdominal tenderness. His prostate is mildly enlarged and very tender, but has no nodules. Which of the following is the next, most appropriate step in his treatment?

  (A) A transrectal prostate biopsy
  (B) A quinolone antibiotic daily for ≥ 2 weeks
  (C) Cystoscopy with a transurethral resection of the enlarged prostate
  (D) Sitz baths 4 times daily
  (E) Prostatic massage daily

2. You are evaluating a 34-year-old woman who has experienced five episodes of cystitis within the last year. Otherwise, she has been in good health and has not been taking medication. Which of the following is most likely responsible for the recurrences?

  (A) A cystocele
  (B) Duplicated ureters
  (C) A bladder diverticulum
  (D) Hydronephrosis
  (E) Rectal coliform bacteria

3. Which of the following uropathogens is most commonly associated with struvite (magnesium ammonium phosphate hexahydrate) stones?

  (A) *Escherichia coli*
  (B) *Staphylococcus saprophyticus*
  (C) *Proteus mirabilis*
  (D) *Enterococcus* species
  (E) *Chlamydia trachomatis*

4. A 32-year-old man develops the signs and symptoms of urethritis after having unprotected intercourse with a prostitute during a trip to Thailand. He has no allergies and is on no medication. Gram stain of a urethral smear reveals gram negative diplococci and many white blood cells. Which of the following would be the most appropriate empiric treatment?

  (A) Ciprofloxin
  (B) Penicillin
  (C) Ceftriaxone
  (D) Metronidazole
  (E) Ampicillin

5. You are choosing empiric therapy for a hospitalized, 50-year-old woman who developed cystitis 1 day after a Foley catheter was inserted. Which organism is most likely the causative one?

  (A) *Pseudomonas aeruginosa*
  (B) *Staphylococcus saprophyticus*
  (C) *Escherichia coli*
  (D) *Enterococcus*
  (E) *Staphylococcus epidermidis*

6. On a random urine analysis of a patient with cystitis, what is the sensitivity of the urinary nitrite test?

  (A) 5%
  (B) 10%
  (C) 20%
  (D) 30%
  (E) 60%

7. Which of the following statements is most helpful in the attempt to differentiate a patient's hemorrhagic cystitis from other causes of hematuria?

  (A) The hematuria of hemorrhagic cystitis is always minimal and microscopic.
  (B) Patients with hemorrhagic cystitis almost always have suprapubic pain.
  (C) More white blood cells than red blood cells are seen per high-powered microscopic field in hemorrhagic cystitis.
  (D) The patient experiences dysuria and/or frequency and urgency prior to, or concurrent with, the hematuria.
  (E) Hemorrhagic cystitis is seen in patients wiping back to front after defecation.

8. With respect to men who have urinary tract infections, which statement is correct?

(A) Most urinary tract infections in young adult men result from anatomic abnormalities in their urinary tract.

(B) Urinary tract infections in young adult men are seldom sexually acquired.

(C) Uncomplicated cystitis in young adult men is treated with a 3-day course of antibiotics.

(D) Urinary tract infections among infants are more likely to occur in uncircumcised males than in females or in circumcised males.

(E) Multiple urinary tract infections are usually experienced by men who are HIV positive with HIV helper cell count (CD 4 count) > 500/cm.

9. You are re-evaluating a 3-year-old girl with cystitis who has been on amoxicillin for 7 days with complete resolution of her symptoms. Which of the studies listed below would be most likely to demonstrate the most common urinary tract abnormality associated with a urinary tract infection in this age group?

(A) Radionuclide cystogram

(B) Renal ultrasound

(C) Cystoscopy

(D) Intravenous pyelogram

(E) Urodynamic study

10. With respect to acute bacterial cystitis, in patients in whom no family history of vesicoureteral reflux is known (and in whom a first urinary tract infection was not acute pyelonephritis), the physician should withhold evaluation for reflux and other anatomic abnormalities until at least two episodes of cystitis are documented in which of the following children?

(A) An infant girl

(B) A 2-year-old boy

(C) A 4-year-old girl

(D) A 6-year-old girl

(E) A 7-year-old boy

11. You have identified vesicoureteral reflux on the right during a radionuclide study of a 3-year-old boy who had cystitis 4 weeks earlier (E. coli culture was $> 10^5$ sensitive to all tested antibiotics). An intravenous pyelogram shows kidneys of normal size, with no scarring, and minimal hydroureter on the right. The most appropriate management option for the child is which of the following?

(A) Small, long-term, daily dosages of amoxicillin or trimethoprim plus sulfamethoxazole

(B) Urologic intervention to re-implant the right ureter

(C) Cystoscopy evaluation

(D) Urodynamic studies

(E) No therapy; close monitoring of the child for recurrent infections

12. In a patient presenting with a urinary tract infection, which of the following is a risk factor for subclinical pyelonephritis?

(A) Dysuria for 3 days before treatment is sought

(B) Gross hematuria that developed after 3 days of dysuria, frequency, and urgency

(C) Four episodes of cystitis in the last year, the last episode 1 month ago

(D) Development of dysuria and urgency 1 day after use of spermicidal jelly during intercourse

(E) Recurrence of symptoms 1 day after completion of a 3-day course of antibiotics for cystitis

13. In a patient with acute pyelonephritis, which is the MOST LIKELY presenting sign?

(A) Flank pain

(B) Nausea

(C) Fever

(D) Upper abdominal pain

(E) Hypotension

14. A 22-year-old man has had an inflammatory arthritis in his right ankle for 2 weeks. He denies any history of trauma or previous joint pain or swelling, and any family history of connective tissue disease. Which of the following is the most likely etiology?

(A) Rheumatoid arthritis

(B) Osteoarthritis

(C) Reflex sympathetic dystrophy

(D) Reiter's syndrome

(E) Systemic lupus erythematosus

DIRECTIONS (Item 15): The numbered item in this section is negatively phrased, as indicated by the capitalized word, NOT. Select the ONE lettered answer that is BEST.

15. Recurrent cystitis is common and has numerous predisposing factors. Which of the following is NOT associated with recurrent cystitis ($\geq$ 3 episodes per year)?

    (A) Urination after intercourse

    (B) Diabetes mellitus

    (C) Presence of postmenopausal atrophic vaginitis

    (D) Use of spermicidal jellies

    (E) Replacement of normal vaginal lactobacillus by coliform bacteria from the rectum

ANSWERS AND EXPLANATIONS

1. The answer is B. A quinolone antibiotic daily for ≥ 2 weeks is the next most appropriate step in this man's treatment, because the presentation is most consistent with acute bacterial prostatitis. The temporary enlargement caused by the infection will resolve with antibiotic therapy and does not require prostatic resection. Sitz baths, a mainstay of therapy for nonbacterial prostatitis, may afford transient symptom relief but are not a mainstay of therapy for bacterial prostatitis. Prostatic massage is contraindicated in the acute bacterial condition for fear it may cause bacteremia (although massage is sometimes useful in chronic prostatitis). Cystoscopy with transurethral resection of the prostate is sometimes necessary in cases of benign prostatic hypertrophy or localized prostatic carcinoma that cause significant prostatic urethral obstruction despite more conservative measures.

2. The answer is E. Rectal coliform bacteria that has replaced vaginal lactobacillus is responsible for the recurrences of this woman's cystitis. The absence of lactobacillus raises the vaginal pH and creates a more favorable vaginal and periurethral environment for the rectal coliform bacteria; the coliform bacteria now in the vagina easily ascends into the urethra. Cystoceles, bladder diverticula, and distended or duplicated ureters can all be associated with recurrent urinary tract infections, and the latter two with increased risk for pyelonephritis, but only about 1% of nongeriatric adult women with recurrent cystitis have an identifiable anatomic abnormality.

3. The answer is C. *Proteus mirabilis* is the uropathogen most commonly associated with struvite stones. These stones (magnesium ammonium phosphate hexahydrate with variable amounts of calcium phosphate) are seen only in the presence of infection in the urinary tract with organisms that commonly produce urease (*Proteus mirabilis,* as well as *Ureaplasma urealyticum* and some *Klebsiella* and *Pseudomonas* species). The urease hydrolyzes urea into ammonia and carbon dioxide, producing a very alkaline urine. On plain x-ray, the stones have a laminated pattern, and they often take on the form of the renal pelvis, producing the staghorn calculus. In addition to infection in the tract, the stones usually indicate at least partial obstruction. Treatment consists of antibiotics active against the associated organism, complete removal of the stone, and relief of any obstruction. *Escherichia coli, Staphylococcus saprophyticus, Enterococcus* species, and *Chlamydia trachomatis* usually produce no urease, and thus are not seen in association with struvite stones.

4. The answer is C. Ceftriaxone would be the most appropriate empiric treatment for this patient. His urethral smear shows many white blood cells, consistent with his presumptive diagnosis of urethritis and gram negative diplococci, which in men has an approximately 95% sensitivity for detecting gonorrhea. Gonorrhea originating in Southeast Asia (as well as many strains in most areas of the US) would have to be assumed to be resistant to penicillin and ampicillin. Ciprofloxin treatment is not appropriate because of the additional presence of quinolone-resistant gonorrhea in Southeast Asia. Metronidazole is not active against gonorrhea, but it is sometimes used in the treatment of pelvic inflammatory disease caused by anaerobes.

5. The answer is C. *Escherichia coli* is the organism most likely to cause cystitis in a female patient 1 day after insertion of a Foley catheter. Patients who have acquired their urinary tract infections (UTIs) iatrogenically in a hospital or nursing home environment or through instrumentation of the urinary tract are more likely to have resistant organisms, and these infections are therefore complicated. In complicated UTIs (which are also seen in patients with anatomically or functionally abnormal urinary tracts), the percentage of cases of cystitis caused by *E. coli* drops to about 35%, but it remains the most prevalent causative organism. *Staphylococcus saprophyticus* is a fairly common cause of uncomplicated cystitis, especially in young adult women, but it is not seen in complicated infections. The percentage of infections caused by *Proteus mirabilis, Enterococcus* species, and *Staphylococcus epidermidis* does increase in complicated UTIs, but *E. Coli* is still the most likely organism.

6. The answer is D. The sensitivity of the urinary nitrite test on a random urine analysis is 30%. This poor sensitivity is related to the incubation time needed to convert urinary nitrate to nitrite. Approximately 6 hours of incubation in the bladder with the bacteria enables urinary nitrate to be converted to nitrite, and improves the sensitivity to 60%.

7. The answer is D. The patient who has hemorrhagic cystitis experiences dysuria and/or frequency and urgency prior to, or concurrently with, the hematuria. Hemorrhagic cystitis may be gross or microscopic; and red blood cells can greatly outnumber white blood cells. Patients with hemorrhagic cystitis are not known to be any more likely than other cystitis patients to have suprapubic tenderness or a history of wiping back to front.

8. The answer is D. The incidence of UTIs in uncircumcised male infants exceeds that in female infants and in circumcised male infants in the first year of life. (Infancy is the only point in life in which the incidence of UTIs is greater in males than in females.) In adult men, uncomplicated cystitis is always treated with a 7-day antibiotic course, because 3-day antibiotic courses have not been tested in men. Anatomic abnormalities, although more frequent in males than in females with UTIs, are still quite unusual. A significant number of UTIs in young adult men are believed to be acquired through exposure to vaginal coliform colonization's during intercourse. HIV-positive men with adequate (> 500/cm) CD4 counts do not appear to be any more prone to urinary tract infection than men who do not have HIV.

9. The answer is A. A radionuclide cystogram would be most likely to demonstrate vesicoureteral reflux, the most likely urinary tract abnormality in the 3-year-old age group. A voiding cystourethrogram could be used, but a radionuclide study for reflux involves less radiation exposure and may be more sensitive. Renal ultrasound can be used in children to assess for congenital renal abnormalities and hydronephrosis. Cystoscopy is principally used to visualize the bladder mucosa directly for tumors and inflammation. The intravenous pyelogram allows visualization of the kidneys and ureter, and gives clues with respect to renal function, but has poor sensitivity in detecting bladder lesions. Urodynamic studies are typically used to assess bladder muscle tone, as well as bladder capacity and the response of bladder tonicity to increases in retained urine.

10. The answer is D. A 6-year-old girl with acute bacterial cystitis need not be evaluated for reflux and anatomic abnormalities unless at least two episodes of cystitis have been documented, the child's first urinary tract infection (UTI) was acute pyelonephritis, or a family history of vesicoureteral reflux is known. UTIs are less likely to be associated with reflux in female children older than age 5 than in younger girls. Multiple UTIs or acute pyelonephritis still warrant an anatomic work-up, even in girls older than age 5. The combination of vesicoureteral reflux and bacteriuria is associated with greater risk of renal damage in children of preschool age, of either sex.

11. The answer is A. A small, long-term, daily dosage of amoxicillin or trimethoprim plus sulfamethoxazole, follow-up urine cultures to verify that urine is sterile, and a repeat radionuclide study in 1 year constitute the most appropriate management option for this child. Most children with vesicoureteral reflux can be managed with small, daily, prophylactic antibiotics and monitored for breakthrough infections. Most children of preschool age who have reflux will naturally stop refluxing within a year. Surgical ureteral re-implantation is reserved for children who continue to experience urinary tract infections despite prophylaxis and for children with renal scarring or megahydronephrosis. "No therapy" is not an option, because recurrent infections in the face of reflux in children of preschool age can be associated with renal scarring. Cystoscopy, which permits direct visualization of the urethra and bladder, is invasive and is not effective in identifying reflux. Urodynamic studies, used to determine bladder tone and responses to urine volume, are not useful with respect to vesicoureteral reflux.

12. The answer is E. Relapse after recent antibiotic treatment for cystitis is a risk factor for subclinical pyelonephritis in a patient presenting with a urinary tract infection. Failure to seek treatment after 1 week of cystitis symptoms is also a risk factor. Hemorrhagic cystitis and recurrent cystitis are not risk factors. Spermicidal jellies can destroy protective vaginal lactobacillus and thus increase the risk for cystitis, but they do not make the patient any more specifically prone to upper tract infections.

13. The answer is C. Fever is the sign MOST LIKELY to be present in a patient with acute pyelonephritis; however, the signs listed in the other answer choices (flank pain, nausea, upper abdominal pain, and hypotension) can also be seen.

14. The answer is D. Reiter's syndrome is the most common etiology for an acute inflammatory arthritis in a young adult. Arthritis is one of a classic tetralogy of signs of Reiter's syndrome. The other three signs, which are urethritis, conjunctivitis, and dermatitis, may be absent. Approximately 1%–2% of all chlamydia urethritis infections (which are fairly common) results in Reiter's syndrome.

15. The answer is A. Urinating after intercourse is NOT associated with recurrent cystitis. Voiding after intercourse may actually diminish the risk of recurrent urinary tract infection (UTI), especially in women whose episodes tend to be associated with intercourse. An alteration in the normal lactobacillus of the vagina, such as occurs with spermicide use, atrophic vaginitis, or antibiotic use, predisposes the woman to UTIs. Diabetes mellitus is also a predisposing factor.

BIBLIOGRAPHY

Kurowski K: Urinary tract infections. In *Family Medicine* (House Officer Series). Edited by Rudy DR, Kurowski K. Baltimore, Williams & Wilkins, 1997, pp 269–284.

Test 17

Noninfectious Diseases of the Urinary Tract

DIRECTIONS (Items 1–13): Each of the numbered items or incomplete statements in this section is followed by answers or by completions of the statement. Select the ONE lettered answer or completion that is BEST in each case.

1. In the chemical test for hematuria, which of the following produces a false-positive result?

(A) Microscopic hematuria
(B) Gross hematuria
(C) Highly concentrated urine
(D) Dilute urine
(E) Myoglobinuria

2. On a company physical examination, a 30-year-old woman had positive chemical and microscopic test results for hematuria. She has been feeling well and has no urinary complaints nor weight loss. Which of the following personal exposures in her history would prompt you to recommend cystoscopic examination early in her evaluation?

(A) Radiographic contrast dye
(B) Indomethacin
(C) Warfarin
(D) Inhaled cigarette smoke
(E) Danazol

3. You palpate a smooth, nontender mass, deep in the right upper quadrant of a male newborn, whose birth was by normal, spontaneous vaginal delivery and who required no resuscitation. The most likely diagnosis is which of the following?

(A) Lymphoma
(B) Wilm's tumor
(C) Rhabdomyosarcoma
(D) Hepatocellular carcinoma
(E) Polycystic kidney disease

4. Which best describes the mechanism of exercise-induced proteinuria?

(A) High urine concentration secondary to dehydration
(B) Defective protein retention
(C) Defective protein reabsorption
(D) Increased protein filtration
(E) Increased protein production

5. The presence of hyaline casts in the urine analysis suggests

(A) Glomerulonephritis
(B) Dehydration
(C) Acute pyelonephritis
(D) Acute cystitis
(E) Interstitial nephritis

6. The nephrotic syndrome (nephrosis) is defined as at least how many grams of protein in the urine in a 24-hour period?

(A) 1 g/24 hr
(B) 2 g/24 hr
(C) 3.5 g/24 hr
(D) 5 g/24 hr
(E) 7.5 g/24 hr

7. You have just diagnosed renal cell carcinoma in a 60-year-old woman. With respect to her diagnosis, which of the following statements is correct?

(A) It is more common in women than in men.
(B) It is more common in patients with a history of alcohol abuse than those without this history.
(C) Hematuria is associated and usually intermittent.
(D) Most patients live more than 5 years after diagnosis.
(E) Most patients have distant metastases at the time of diagnosis.

8. While examining a 4-year-old boy, you notice a large mass (approximately 20 cm) in the left abdomen. The mass is smooth and nontender. No cervical nor supraclavicular adenopathy is present. Which is the most likely cause of this mass?

(A) Renal cell carcinoma
(B) Urothelial cell carcinoma of the renal pelvis
(C) Lymphoma
(D) Polycystic kidney disease
(E) Wilm's tumor

9. You are evaluating a 30-year-old man who complains of severe right flank pain and hematuria which started 6 hours ago. Otherwise, he has been in good health and is taking no medications. He is afebrile; his blood pressure is 150/90, and his pulse is 90. An intravenous pyelogram shows a radiopaque stone approximately 3 mm in size in the distal right ureter. Only minimal hydronephrosis of the right ureter is present. BUN and creatinine levels are normal. Which of the following should you recommend?

(A) Urgent extracorporeal shock wave lithotripsy (ESWL)
(B) Urgent endourological stone extraction
(C) Urgent stent placement
(D) Narcotic analgesics and intravenous fluids
(E) Open surgical stone extraction

10. What percentage of urinary calculi consist of uric acid stones?

    (A) 1%
    (B) 2%
    (C) 6%
    (D) 15%
    (E) 30%

11. A 30-year-old man complains that his face, feet, and hands have been "puffy" for the last 2 weeks. His BUN is only 15 mg/dl (normal = 10–20 mg/dl); creatinine is 1.0 mg/dl (normal = 0.5–1.3 mg/dl); serum protein is low at 5.2 g/dl (normal = 6–8 g/dl); serum albumin is low at 2.4 grams/dl; and he is excreting 5 g/day of protein in his urine. His urine is 3+ for protein, but glucose, leukocyte esterase, and blood checks are all negative on urine analysis. Which of the following is a potential cause for his condition?

    (A) Dehydration
    (B) Focal segmental glomerulonephritis
    (C) Hyperglobulinemia secondary to multiple myeloma
    (D) Osteoarthritis
    (E) Exercise proteinuria

12. A 40-year-old man has membranoproliferative glomerulonephritis and you want to calculate his creatinine clearance. He weighs 72 kg and his plasma creatinine is 2.0 mg/dl. What is his clearance?

    (A) 50 ml/min
    (B) 75 ml/min
    (C) 100 ml/min
    (D) 125 ml/min
    (E) 150 ml/min

13. What is the significance of microalbuminuria (100–300 mg/24 hr)?

    (A) It is usually an early marker for primary glomerular disease.
    (B) It is an early feature of nephrosis.
    (C) Along with hematuria and renal failure, it defines nephritis.
    (D) It is produced by postural changes.
    (E) It may be early evidence of diabetic nephropathy in diabetes mellitus.

DIRECTIONS (Items 14–15): Each of the numbered items or incomplete statements in this section is negatively phrased, as indicated by a capitalized word such as NOT, LEAST, or EXCEPT. Select the ONE lettered answer or completion that is BEST in each case.

---

14. Which of the following is NOT commonly associated with hematuria?

    (A) Uncontrolled malignant hypertension
    (B) Transitional cell carcinoma of the bladder
    (C) Sickle cell anemia
    (D) Glomerulonephritis
    (E) Alport's syndrome

15. All of the following are part of the nephrotic syndrome (nephrosis) EXCEPT

    (A) Edema
    (B) Hematuria
    (C) Proteinuria greater than 3.5 g/day
    (D) Hypoalbuminemia
    (E) Hyperlipidemia

ANSWERS AND EXPLANATIONS

1. The answer is E. Myoglobinuria produces a false-positive result in a chemical test for hematuria. Myoglobin reacts positively with the chemical test for urine hemoglobin. Gross and microscopic hematuria represent true positives not false positives. High urine concentration effects specific gravity, but does not produce a false positive dipstick for hematuria.

2. The answer is D. If this woman has a history of inhaled cigarette smoke, which significantly increases the risk of transitional cell carcinoma of the bladder, you would recommend cystoscopic examination early in her evaluation. Cystoscopic evaluation is the most appropriate study to assess for bladder carcinoma. Cystograms and intravenous pyelograms have poor sensitivity in detecting bladder neoplasms (even the larger ones). Aniline dye exposure also increases the risk, but contrast dye does not. NSAIDs (e.g., indomethacin), anticoagulants (e.g., warfarin), danazol, and rifampin are sometimes associated with hematuria, but are not known to cause bladder carcinoma. Textile, rubber, and printing workers exposed to aromatic amine are at increased risk for bladder carcinoma.

3. The answer is E. Polycystic kidney disease, along with congenital hydronephrosis, accounts for most abdominal masses in newborns. Wilm's tumor and rhabdomyosarcoma (the most common soft tissue sarcoma in children) are common causes of abdominal masses in small children, but not in newborns. Pyloric stenosis, the most common cause of abdominal masses in infants, is not seen before an infant's third day of life, nor does it typically become symptomatic until an infant is 2–8 weeks of age. The mass seen with pyloric stenosis is olive-shaped, muscular, and palpable in the right upper quadrant, especially after the child has been vomiting. Non-Hodgkin's lymphoma is also a common cause of abdominal masses in children, but its peak incidences are at 5–7 years of age and during the teen years; it is almost never seen in children younger than 5 years. Hepatocellular carcinoma typically presents with an abdominal mass, but it is strongly linked with hepatitis B infection and is not seen in children younger than 4 years.

4. The answer is D. Increased protein filtration best describes the mechanism of exercise-induced proteinuria. Smaller proteins are freely filtered by the glomerulus and then mostly reabsorbed by the tubules, normally resulting in < 150 mg per day excreted in the urine. Exercise, orthostatic changes, and fever increase glomerular filtration, which overwhelms tubular resorption and leads to transient proteinuria. (Although dehydration produces a more concentrated urine in a normal individual, the *net* excretion of protein does not increase.) Increased protein production is seen in multiple myeloma (immunoglobulin) and in leukemia. Proteins as large as, or larger than, albumin are not normally filterable through the glomerular capillary. This protein retention is disrupted by inflammatory disorders of the glomerulus (e.g., glomerulonephritis). Tubular resorption can also be affected by toxic nephropathies, renal failure, and other conditions.

5. The answer is B. Dehydration or diuretic therapy, or both, are suggested by the presence of hyaline casts in the urine. Hyaline casts are not associated with renal parenchymal disease. Casts are small masses of agglutinated material formed in the renal tubules. Hyaline casts are formed from a low-molecular-weight mucoprotein from the kidney. In response to dehydration or diuretics, urinary sodium excretion is decreased, and the lower urinary sodium concentration promotes precipitation of protein and the formation of hyaline casts. Glomerulonephritis is associated with red blood cell casts and, occasionally, white blood cell casts. Red blood cell casts can be seen with acute tubular necrosis. Casts are not seen in cystitis. Pyuria is seen in cystitis, but the absence of renal involvement precludes agglutination within the tubules. Pyelonephritis and interstitial nephritis are associated with the presence of white blood cell casts.

6. The answer is C. At least 3.5 g of protein must be present in the urine in a 24-hour period to meet the definition of nephrotic syndrome (nephrosis). This degree of proteinuria is usually seen with significant glomerular disease. Urine protein of 150 mg/24 hr to 1 g/24 hr is called "low-grade" proteinuria. (Less than 150 mg/24 hr is normal.) Prognosis in the face of nephrotic syndrome and persistence of this syndrome depends upon the cause. Patients with nephrotic syndrome are at increased risk for edema secondary to the hypoalbuminemia; malnutrition; sepsis (including peritonitis); and thromboembolism secondary to increased coagulation.

7. The answer is C. Hematuria is associated with renal cell carcinoma, and is usually intermittent. Renal cell carcinoma is more common in men than in women by a 3:1 ratio. The incidence of this carcinoma is increased in patients who smoke, but not in those who abuse alcohol. Only 45% of patients are alive 5 years after diagnosis. Only 25% of patients have distant metastases at the time of diagnosis.

8. The answer is E. Wilm's tumor is the most likely cause of the mass in this boy's left abdomen. Although the diseases listed in all of the answer choices (renal cell carcinoma, urothelial cell carcinoma of the renal pelvis, lymphoma, and polycystic kidney disease) could present with an abdominal mass, the patient's age of 4 years makes Wilm's tumor (which has a peak incidence of approximately 3 years of age) the most likely etiology. (Neuroblastoma is another possibility, although it more typically affects children within the first 2 years of life.) Wilm's tumor, the most common renal neoplasm of childhood, and bilateral in only a little more than 5% of cases, may present as an enlarging abdominal girth or as an asymptomatic mass which parents first notice when they are bathing the child. Gross hematuria is present in only approximately 20% of cases, and hypertension and polycythemia are rarely seen. Wilm's tumor is often associated with genitourinary syndromes (e.g., hypospadias, cryptorchidism) or with hemihypertrophy. More than 90% of cases can be cured by a combination of nephrectomy and chemotherapy.

9. The answer is D. For this man with renal colic, right flank pain, and gross hematuria, you should recommend narcotic analgesics and intravenous fluids. Approximately 85%–90% of stones smaller than 4 mm, as well as most stones up to 6 mm in diameter, pass spontaneously within 24–48 hours, especially if the patient is on IV fluids. A distal ureteral stone can usually be manipulated out, but only after more conservative measures have failed. Stent placement is usually performed prior to ESWL, but only after the stone fails to pass spontaneously. Open surgical stone extraction is now almost never performed: It carries a significant morbidity, and less invasive methods are usually successful.

10. The answer is C. Of urinary calculi, 6% are uric acid stones. Most urinary calculi (75%) are calcium-containing stones. Uric acid stones occur when the urine is particularly concentrated, or when the kidneys excrete increased levels of uric acid, or both. Acidic urine also promotes uric acid stone formation. Uric acid stones are commonly seen in patients with gout or with myeloproliferative or neoplastic disorders where increased cell turnover is present. Patients with neoplasms under treatment with cytolytic chemotherapy release even more uric acid and have an even greater risk for uric acid stones. In contrast to calcium-containing stones, uric acid stones are radiolucent. Although not directly visible, obstruction (if it is present) is evident on an intra-

venous pyelogram or a renal ultrasound. Uric acid stones (even large ones) are more likely than calcium-containing stones to respond to dissolution therapy. Large intake of oral fluids with alkali (e.g., sodium bicarbonate) may produce dissolution. Oral allopurinol is effective in patients who are producing too much acid.

11. The answer is B. Focal segmental glomerulonephritis is a possible cause of this man's condition. This case demonstrates a typical clinical presentation of acute glomerulonephritis but does not allow you to differentiate between the many potential causes, such as postinfectious, minimal-change disease, membranoproliferative, focal segmental, and mesangial proliferative. Dehydration first elevates (not lowers) the blood urea nitrogen (BUN) and induces a concentrated urine, but not one with excessive protein loss. Multiple myeloma is associated with elevated (not lowered) serum protein (globulin) levels, and produces no edema. Rheumatoid arthritis and lupus can produce nephrosis, but osteoarthritis does not. Exercise proteinuria is never associated with hypoalbuminemia, edema, or any other sign or symptom, and does not increase the daily urinary protein excretion.

12. The answer is A. The creatinine clearance is 50 ml per minute. Ccr = (140—age × wt in kg) ÷ (Serum creatinine × 72). This computes to (100 × 72) ÷ (2 × 72), which equals 50 ml/min. (To calculate clearance in women, use the same formula, but multiply the result by 0.85.)

13. The answer is E. Microalbuminuria may be early evidence of diabetic nephropathy in patients with diabetes mellitus, and it can also be an early marker of hypertension. Angiotensin-converting enzyme (ACE) inhibitors can ameliorate the proteinuria of diabetic nephropathy and can help to preserve renal function but are contraindicated if the serum creatinine is > 2.5 mg/dl. Isolated proteinuria < 2 g/24 hr does not usually predict primary glomerular disease such as nephrosis or nephritis. Postural change could increase urine protein on a random urine analysis, but no significant increase in proteinuria would occur on a 24-hour analysis. In testing for microalbuminemia, care must be taken not to confuse 24-hour urine protein with 24-hour albumin.

14. The answer is A. Uncontrolled malignant hypertension, even if severe, does NOT produce hematuria, although severe hypertension can lead to hypertensive neuropathy and even renal failure. The most common symptomatic presentation of transitional cell carcinoma of the bladder is episodic, painless hematuria. Sickle cell crises may result in renal infarctions and hematuria. Glomerulonephritis is characterized by proteinuria, hematuria (with red blood cell casts visible microscopically), and usually some reduction in renal function that leads to sodium and water retention and hypertension. Alport's syndrome is a hereditary disorder in which a defect exists in a structural protein common to the basement membrane of the kidneys, the anterior lens of the eye, and the organ of Corti. The syndrome causes neural hearing loss, ocular defects, the development of hematuria, and, later, renal failure.

15. The answer is B. Hematuria is NOT part of the nephrotic syndrome. The nephrotic syndrome is a grouping of signs and symptoms seen in patients with glomerular disease which involves increased renal capillary permeability to serum protein that results in severe proteinuria, hypoalbuminemia, and edema. Increased hepatic synthesis occurs, along with decreased catabolism of cholesterol, triglyceride, and lipoprotein. Inflammatory glomerular changes (and, thus, hematuria) are not characteristic of pure nephrotic syndrome, but are seen in the nephritic syndromes.

BIBLIOGRAPHY

Suchomski GD: Noninfectious diseases of the urinary tract. In *Family Medicine* (House Officer Series). Edited by Rudy DR, Kurowski K. Baltimore, Williams & Wilkins, 1997, pp 285–296.

SECTION VII

Problems Unique to Females

Test 18

Gynecology in Primary Care

DIRECTIONS (Items 1–15): Each of the numbered items or incomplete statements in this section is followed by answers or by completions of the statement. Select the ONE lettered answer or completion that is BEST in each case.

1. A 26-year-old woman complains of amenorrhea which began 3 months earlier when she stopped taking her birth control pills, which she had been taking for 18 months. In the past, she always had normal menses, with a 29-day interval and 5 days of mild-to-moderate flow. She denies feeling ill, and says she has not been sexually active since she stopped taking her birth control pills. Many causes are possible. Which of the following must be investigated and ruled out first?

(A) Hypothyroidism
(B) Prolactin-secreting pituitary adenoma
(C) Hypopituitarism
(D) Pregnancy
(E) Weight loss associated with competitive athletics

2. A woman with secondary amenorrhea is given medroxyprogesterone acetate 10 mg per day by mouth for 5 days, and she is monitored for the onset of bleeding after progesterone withdrawal. A positive (bleeding upon withdrawal) response to this challenge will be produced by which of the following causes of amenorrhea?

(A) Asherman's syndrome
(B) Anovulatory cycle
(C) Gonadal agenesis
(D) Ovarian failure
(E) Menopause

3. You are evaluating a 38-year-old woman who has been experiencing amenorrhea for the last 8 months. She has normal secondary sexual development and shows no evidence of virilization. Her pelvic exam shows a normal cervix and fundus, and no adnexal masses. Her urine beta HCG (human chorionic gonadotropin) is negative. Thyroid-stimulating hormone (TSH) and serum prolactin levels are normal. She does not have uterine bleeding during the withdrawal phase of a progestin challenge, but does bleed after being on conjugated estrogen (1.25 mg) for 21 days with a progestin agent added on the last 5 days. Follicle-stimulating hormone and luteinizing hormone are both elevated. Which of the following is the most likely diagnosis?

(A) Hypothalamic amenorrhea
(B) Asherman's syndrome
(C) Premature ovarian failure
(D) Anovulatory cycle
(E) Polycystic ovarian syndrome

4. Which of the following is associated with hypothalamic amenorrhea?

(A) Elevated serum estrogen level
(B) Osteoporosis
(C) Sedentary lifestyle
(D) Obesity
(E) Elevated follicle-stimulating hormone and luteinizing hormone levels

5. A 40-year-old woman whose menstrual periods previously lasted for 5 days and involved the passing of clots, complains that her menses are now heavy (soaking several pads each day), still involve the passage of clots, and last for 7 days. The 30-day interval between her menses has not changed. This development is best described by which of the following terms?

(A) Oligomenorrhea
(B) Menorrhagia
(C) Polymenorrhea
(D) Metrorrhagia
(E) Dysmenorrhea

6. Which of the following is associated with primary dysmenorrhea?

(A) Infertility
(B) A palpable, smooth, nontender, 3-centimeter uterine mass
(C) Symptoms that fail to improve during a 6-month trial of ibuprofen
(D) Onset of symptoms 6–12 months after menarche
(E) Pelvic pain unassociated with menstruation

7. Which of the following is associated with bacterial vaginosis?

(A) Macrosomia in newborns born to infected women
(B) A vaginal pH of 4.0
(C) Large numbers of leukocytes on saline vaginal smear
(D) An overgrowth of vaginal lactobacillus
(E) An increased risk of endometritis after abortions

8. Which of the following is associated with *Chlamydia trachomatis* infections of the genitourinary tract?

(A) Dysuria or pelvic pain experienced by most infected patients
(B) Spontaneous abortion during pregnancy
(C) Patient age of 30–50 years
(D) Macrosomia in newborns of infected mothers
(E) Incubation period of 48 hours

9. A 28-year-old woman, who was treated for bacterial vaginosis 6 years ago, was informed 2 years ago that her Pap test revealed changes typical of human papillomavirus (HPV) on her cervix. She was not compliant with follow-up recommendations. She denies any pelvic pain, dysuria, vaginal bleeding, or discharge. Her last menstrual period was 16 days ago. Pelvic examination reveals no pelvic mass nor uterine enlargement, and her cervix appears normal. A Pap smear reveals a high-grade squamous intraepithelial lesion. Which of the following is the most appropriate next step in her management?

(A) Obtain a repeat Pap smear in 6 months.
(B) Obtain a KOH (potassium hydroxide) vaginal smear.
(C) Order colposcopy with directed biopsies.
(D) Order a DNA hybridization probe for HPV.
(E) Order laser surgery or cryosurgery of the involved areas of the cervix.

10. With respect to primary symptomatic genital herpes, which statement is correct?

(A) The primary episode is shorter than recurrent outbreaks.
(B) Malaise and headache are commonly associated with it.
(C) Herpes simplex II virus causes approximately 60% of cases.
(D) A viral culture taken within the first 2 days of the outbreak is about 95% sensitive in detecting the responsible virus.
(E) About 50% of patients experience a recurrence within 1 year of follow-up.

11. Which of the following is most accountable for the acquisition of human immunodeficiency virus (HIV) by women in the United States?

(A) Heterosexual contact
(B) Homosexual contact
(C) Needle injury to skin during surgical procedures
(D) Receipt of contaminated blood
(E) Receipt of contaminated plasma

12. You notice a painless, indurated ulcer with a slight, clear, overlying exudate on the vulva of a 25-year-old woman who has nontender inguinal adenopathy. Which of the following tests is the most appropriate next step in her evaluation?

(A) Venereal Disease Research Laboratory (VDRL) test
(B) Rapid plasma reagin (RPR) test
(C) Dark-field microscopy examination of exudate
(D) Fluorescent treponemal antibody absorption (FTA-ABS) test
(E) Aerobic culture of cervix

13. A 30-year-old woman has a Pap smear that shows some mild inflammation. She has no complaints, and she specifically denies pelvic pain, bleeding, or dyspareunia. She has been in a monogamous relationship for 10 years, with no reported high-risk activity for HIV acquisition in herself or her partner. Her last Pap smear, 2 years ago, was normal. Findings in her pelvic exam are normal, including a normal-appearing cervix. No adnexal masses or uterine masses are found. Your recommendation should be

(A) A repeat Pap smear in 6–12 months
(B) A colposcopy
(C) A hysterectomy
(D) A DNA hybridization probe for human papilloma virus
(E) A 5% acetic acid application to the cervix

14. Which of the following is an indication that a patient with pelvic inflammatory disease (PID) needs to be hospitalized?

(A) The patient has multiple sex partners.
(B) The infection, on culture, is polymicrobial.
(C) The patient has an elevated sedimentation rate.
(D) Gram stains show intracellular gram-negative diplococci.
(E) The patient is pregnant.

15. With regard to infection with the human papilloma virus (HPV), which of the following statements is correct?

(A) It is considered the causative agent of cervical cancer.
(B) Patients with a clinical history of venereal warts (condylomata acuminata) are at greatest risk for cervical dysplasia.
(C) A woman with a sexual history of unprotected intercourse with only three different male partners is unlikely to be infected with HPV.
(D) Approximately 20% of sexual partners of an HPV-positive individual acquire the infection.
(E) Most mild, HPV-associated cervical dysplasia leads to invasive cervical carcinoma if not treated during the early stages.

DIRECTIONS (Item 16): The question in this section is negatively phrased, as indicated by the capitalized word NOT. Select the ONE lettered answer that is BEST.

16. A 37-year-old woman, who denies the use of contraceptives, is experiencing dysfunctional uterine bleeding secondary to anovulatory cycles for the last 18 months. She is a nonsmoker, is otherwise without health problems, and is taking no medications. Of the following tests and treatments, which is NOT initially indicated in her management?

    (A) Prolactin level
    (B) Pro-time and APTT
    (C) Endometrial biopsy
    (D) Iron supplementation in the presence of anemia
    (E) Oral contraceptive pills

ANSWERS AND EXPLANATIONS

1. The answer is D. Pregnancy, always the initial concern in any woman presenting with secondary amenorrhea, should be ruled out first. If she is not pregnant, she is probably experiencing post-pill amenorrhea (temporary cessation of menstruation experienced by some women after discontinuance of oral contraceptives), which may last up to 6 months. Hypothyroidism, prolactin-secreting pituitary adenoma, hypopituitarism, and weight loss associated with competitive athletics (the other answer choices) are all potential etiologies for secondary amenorrhea, although hypothalamic amenorrhea secondary to weight loss and prolactin-secreting adenomas are more common than amenorrhea secondary to hypothyroidism or hypopituitarism.

2. The answer is B. Anovulatory cycle will produce a positive response to this challenge. (Anovulatory cycle involves appropriate estrogen priming of the endometrium, but no egg release, and thus no progesterone phase and no menstruation.) If the patient has no obstruction to the outflow of menstrual blood, and if the endometrium has been sufficiently primed with estrogen, the exposure to and withdrawal of progesterone will induce uterine bleeding. This response will not occur in primary or secondary ovarian failure that results from lack of estrogen priming, nor in gonadal agenesis, which results in a barren, unprimed endometrium which cannot respond to progesterone withdrawal. In menopause, the estrogen and progesterone secretion is inadequate, and the unprimed endometrium cannot respond. Nor can a positive response occur in the presence of an obstruction to uterine outflow, such as Asherman's syndrome. The fibrous tissue in Asherman's syndrome develops in response to infection, endometrial instrumentation, or therapeutic abortion.

3. The answer is C. The most likely diagnosis of this woman's problem is premature ovarian failure. The failure to respond to the progestin challenge suggests a problem with estrogen stimulation of the endometrium, or an outflow obstruction in the uterus. Because the woman did bleed after reproduction of the estrogen/progestin cycle, outflow obstruction cannot be responsible. The cause must lie in the ovarian or pituitary axis regulating estrogen, causing inadequate serum estrogen level, but the increase in follicle-stimulating hormone and luteinizing hormone shows an appropriate pituitary response to these low estrogen levels; therefore, the difficulty must be ovarian failure. Patients who have polycystic ovary syndrome have amenorrhea secondary to anovulatory cycles

and will bleed upon progesterone withdrawal. These patients do not need exogenous estrogen, and the unopposed estrogen stimulation of their endometrium poses a risk for endometrial hyperplasia.

4. The answer is B. Osteoporosis is associated with hypothalamic amenorrhea, which is often a response to physical or psychological stress or to excessive exercise, weight loss, or both. The connection between osteoporosis and hypothalamic amenorrhea is partially explained by the lower serum estrogen levels present. Luteinizing hormone and follicle-stimulating hormone levels are also decreased or normal (rather than elevated) in hypothalamic amenorrhea.

5. The answer is B. Menorrhagia, an increase in the flow and duration of the menses, but not in the interval between the start of each cycle, best describes this patient's complaint. (Clots, mentioned in the vignette, form when increased amounts of blood are being lost from the endometrium.) Polymenorrhea and oligomenorrhea are a decrease and increase, respectively, in the interval between the start of each cycle. Metrorrhagia is the term used for irregular intervals between the start of each cycle. Dysmenorrhea is painful menstruation.

6. The answer is D. The symptoms of primary dysmenorrhea (painful or cramping menstruation without detectable pelvic pathology) usually develop 6–12 months after menarche, with the onset of ovulation. The condition is associated with increased prostaglandin synthesis, but the cause is unknown. Symptoms that develop more than 3 years after menarche suggest secondary dysmenorrhea, most commonly caused by endometriosis, but sometimes caused by intrauterine devices, adenomyosis, and uterine fibroids. Infertility, presence of a uterine mass, and failure of symptoms to improve during a 6-month trial of ibuprofen also suggest secondary, rather than primary, dysmenorrhea. (During the 6-month trial of ibuprofen, the woman experiences several menstrual cycles with the prostaglandin synthesis effected by the NSAID. If improvement occurs, more invasive procedures may not be necessary.) Long-standing pelvic pain, unassociated with menstruation, is defined as chronic pelvic pain, not dysmenorrhea.

7. The answer is E. Bacterial vaginosis, which is associated with a relative increase in *Gardnerella vaginalis, Mycoplasma hominis,* and anaerobes, as well as with a relative decrease in lactobacillus, carries an increased risk of endometritis after abortion. Infection in the mother is associated with preterm delivery and low birth weight, rather than with macrosomatia (abnormally large size), in newborns. A pH greater than the normal vaginal pH of 3.5–4.0 occurs, but little or no vaginal inflammation, and, thus, no dysuria and no increased white blood cells on vaginal smears. In addition, clue cells (vaginal epithelial cells stippled with bacteria), which are present normally on occasion, signify bacterial vaginosis if they are abundant. Bacterial vaginosis is treated with oral or intravaginal metronidazole, which does not appear to be teratogenic (i.e., does not tend to produce physical defects in embryos or fetuses).

8. The answer is B. Spontaneous abortion during pregnancy is associated with *Chlamydia trachomatis*. Fetuses of women who developed active chlamydial infections during pregnancy are at increased risk for premature rupture of membranes, premature birth, smaller-than-normal size at birth, spontaneous abortion, and intrauterine death. The greatest incidence of *Chlamydia trachomatis* is seen in young women of 15–20 (rather than 30–50 years of age. Most cases (70%) of chlamydial genitourinary infection are asymptomatic and have an incubation period of about 1 week (rather than 48 hours).

9. The answer is C. Colposcopy with directed biopsies is the most appropriate next step in the management of this woman's condition. Her Pap smear indicates moderate or severe dysplasia, and confirmation of this screening result requires deeper biopsy material. Repetition of the Pap smear in 6 months is inappropriate in cases of high-grade squamous epithelial lesion, although it is appropriate in cases of low-grade squamous epithelial lesion (especially those in which the changes are mild cellular atypia thought to be inflammatory). The patient's present status with respect to bacterial vaginosis or papillomavirus will not affect the immediate investigation or therapy. If the biopsies performed during the colposcopy examination reveal severe dysplasia, or even carcinoma in situ confined to the ectocervix, cryosurgery or laser therapy are alternatives.

10. The answer is B. Associated malaise and headache, along with fever and tender inguinal adenopathy, are common in primary symptomatic genital herpes. Primary symptomatic infections produce severer, longer lasting symptoms (not shorter episodes) than recurrences produce. Of primary symptomatic infections, 70%–90% (not 60%) are caused by herpes simplex virus II (HSV-II). HSV-1 is less likely to result in recurrence. Even with a freshly unroofed vesicle, viral culture is only about 80% (not 95%) sensitive. Almost 90% (rather than 50%) of patients experience a recurrence within a year.

11. The answer is A. Among the answer choices, heterosexual contact is the most likely mode of acquisition of the HIV virus by women in the US. In 1994, intravenous drug use was responsible for 41% of cases and heterosexual contact for 38% of cases among US women. Blood product exposure was responsible for only 2% and needle sticks for less than 1% of cases.

12. The answer is C. Dark-field microscopy examination of serous exudate from the lesion should be undertaken next to assess for syphilis. The lesions of syphilis usually team with spirochetes that can be detected via dark field microscopy or direct fluorescent antibody slides. Standard culture techniques will not grow *Treponema pallidum*. The Venereal Disease Research Laboratory (VDRL), rapid plasma reagin (RPR), and fluorescent treponemal antibody absorption (FTA-ABS) tests are not indicated in *primary* syphilis because the patient must be approximately 4 weeks past exposure for them to become positive.

13. The answer is A. A repeat Pap smear in 6–12 months is all that is indicated in this case. More intense inflammation would require evaluation and possible treatment for cervicitis. Mild dysplasia may also be followed with a Pap smear every 6 months, but colposcopy is indicated if it persists or develops into a high-grade squamous intraepithelial lesion. Colposcopy would also be indicated if the last Pap smear showed mild or greater dysplasia, or if the patient is HIV positive. Hysterectomy, which is frequently part of the treatment for invasive cervical carcinoma, is not appropriate for cervical dysplasia. Although the presence of human papillomavirus is strongly linked to cervical dysplasia and carcinoma, its identification here will not effect therapy or follow-up.

14. The answer is E. Pregnancy is one indication that a patient with pelvic inflammatory disease needs to be hospitalized. Other indications are the presence of an associated abscess or peritonitis, or a lack of response to outpatient treatment. Many pelvic inflammatory infections are polymicrobial and many are secondary to gonorrhea; however, the presence of these organisms does not indicate the need for hospitalization. Fevers and elevated sedimentation rates, seen in many patients with pelvic inflammatory disease, also do not indicate the need for hospitalization.

15. The answer is A. HPV is considered to be the causative agent of cervical cancer. Possibly, in the near future, women who have no evidence of HPV and no increased risk for HPV acquisition will not require Pap-smear screening. HPV virus subtypes that produce the visible condylomata acuminata are not the same subtypes as those associated with cervical dysplasia and cancer. HPV infection is extremely prevalent; the majority of college-age women who have unprotected intercourse with two different partners are estimated to acquire the infection. Once acquired, the infection is usually lifelong. Approximately 60%–90% of the sexual partners of an infected individual also become infected. Fortunately, most of the infected patients do not develop invasive cervical cancer, even if they have mild dysplasia. Some lesions regress spontaneously.

16. The answer is B. Pro-time and APTT are NOT initially indicated in this woman's management. Bleeding disorders are more commonly associated with ovulatory menorrhagia, and, in dysfunctional uterine bleeding secondary to anovulatory cycles, coagulation studies would not be indicated initially, unless the patient was not responding to therapy. Unopposed estrogen stimulation to the endometrium, such as occurs with anovulatory cycles, can lead to endometrial hyperplasia; therefore, endometrial biopsy is usually indicated if this situation has been present 1 year or more. Serum prolactin levels to exclude a prolactin-secreting pituitary adenoma are appropriate in a 37-year-old woman experiencing dysfunctional uterine bleeding with anovulatory cycles for as long as she has. (The likelihood of this type of adenoma producing her symptoms would be higher if she also had galactorrhea.) Iron supplementation is indicated for uterine bleeding of any cause if iron deficiency develops (evidence includes microcytic anemia, microcytosis, low serum ferritin level). Low-dose oral contraceptive pills are a mainstay of the treatment of dysfunctional uterine bleeding secondary to anovulatory cycles. This patient has no history of premature atherosclerosis; she does not smoke; and she has no identifiable contraindications to this therapy. If she wants no contraception, the therapy could be discontinued after 3–6 months.

BIBLIOGRAPHY

Bauman KA, Brown DR: Gynecology in primary care. In *Family Medicine* (House Officer Series). Edited by Rudy DR, Kurowski K. Baltimore, Williams & Wilkins, 1997, pp. 297–328.

Test 19

Problems of the Female Climacteric

DIRECTIONS (Items 1–10): Each of the numbered items or incomplete statements in this section is followed by answers or by completions of the statement. Select the ONE lettered answer or completion that is BEST in each case.

1. By liberally accepted standards, diagnoses of ovarian failure or menopause are secure when the level of follicle-stimulating hormone (FSH) is above

- (A) 20 IU
- (B) 30 IU
- (C) 40 IU
- (D) 50 IU
- (E) 60 IU

2. A 49-year-old Caucasian woman complains of several symptoms: 3 weeks of deep depressive bouts that begin rapidly and remit within 12–24 hours; drenching sweats without measurable fever; and intermittent muscular aches in the shoulders, hips, and low back. Her last menstrual period was 6 weeks ago. Her cycle has normally been 28–30 days until 6 months ago when it began varying between 3 and 8 weeks. She always slept well until 3 weeks ago, when she began awakening with depression or attacks of diaphoresis. Which of the following is your best next course of action?

- (A) Obtain the patient's follicle-stimulating hormone (FSH) level.
- (B) Schedule the patient for a dilatation and curettage (D&C) to rule out endometrial carcinoma.
- (C) Treat the patient for depression.
- (D) Prescribe for the patient's insomnia.
- (E) Order electrical studies of the patient's upper and lower extremities.

3. For a woman such as the one in the previous question, which is the medication that gives effective and rapid symptomatic relief?

- (A) Sertraline
- (B) Paroxetine
- (C) Conjugated equine estrogen
- (D) Diazepam
- (E) Ibuprofen

4. Which dosage of conjugated equine estrogen (CEE) is necessary to prevent osteoporosis?

- (A) 0.3 mg
- (B) 0.625 mg
- (C) 1.25 mg
- (D) 3 mg
- (E) 625 mg

5. Surgical menopause is most likely to differ from physiologic menopause in suddenness of onset. Which of the following is also true?

- (A) Depression is more of a problem after surgical than after physiologic menopause.
- (B) Atrophic vaginitis is more severe after surgical than after physiologic menopause.
- (C) Osteoporosis is a greater issue after physiologic than after surgical menopause.
- (D) Heart disease is a greater risk after surgical than after physiologic menopause.
- (E) Loss of libido is more likely after surgical than after physiologic menopause.

6. The ranking cause of death in postmenopausal women is

- (A) Coronary artery disease
- (B) Endometrial carcinoma
- (C) Carcinoma of the breast
- (D) Hip fracture
- (E) Stroke

7. Which of the following is the most significant predicted benefit of estrogen replacement therapy/hormone replacement therapy from the point of view of public health and longevity?

- (A) A 50% reduction in deaths from coronary artery disease
- (B) A 50% reduction in deaths from hip fracture
- (C) A reduction in the mortality caused by breast cancer
- (D) A reduction in the mortality caused by endometrial cancer
- (E) A reduction in the mortality caused by vulvar cancer

8. During a routine preventive examination, a 47-year-old Caucasian woman of English and Irish heritage and of slender build reported that her periods became irregular in the past 8 months. She noticed intermenstrual mid-cycle spotting, two completely missed periods, and prolonged bleeding (8 days of significant flow, compared to her normal 3 days). Her last menstrual period was 3 months ago. She also noted emotional lability and unpredictable bouts of sweating. She has no family history of breast cancer nor personal history of major surgery. After the results of routine pelvic examination, pap smear, and scheduled baseline mammogram are found to be normal, what is the best course you should take in her routine care?

(A) Make the presumptive diagnosis of normal menopause, and observe for permanent cessation of periods during the next 12 months.

(B) Prescribe estrogen replacement therapy (ERT) with 0.625 mg conjugated equine estrogens (CEE) daily for 25 days per month.

(C) Conduct a diagnostic/therapeutic trial with 0.3 mg CEE, and, if the patient's hot flashes respond to this regimen, diagnose estrogen deficiency.

(D) Obtain a follicle-stimulating hormone level, and, if it is ≥ 20, start the patient on hormone replacement therapy.

(E) Reassure the patient that her symptoms are based on stress, and prescribe a benzodiazepine agent.

9. Which statement is correct with respect to the detrimental effect of regular smoking on bone density?

(A) It is 10% as strong as the beneficial effect of estrogen.

(B) It is 25% as strong as the beneficial effect of estrogen.

(C) It is equally as strong as the beneficial effect of estrogen.

(D) It is twice as detrimental as estrogen is beneficial.

(E) Smoking is irrelevant if a postmenopausal patient is on a hormone replacement regimen.

10. A woman who began hormone replacement therapy 8 months ago reports that she still has mild uterine bleeding. After obtaining hemoglobin and hematocrit and/or measuring thyroid function, which further step should you take?

(A) Discontinue the patient's hormonal therapy.

(B) Double the patient's dosage of estrogen.

(C) Adjust the patient's dosage of progesterone.

(D) Refer the patient for dilatation and curettage (D&C).

(E) Refer the patient for endometrial biopsy.

DIRECTIONS (Items 11–15): For each numbered candidate for hormone therapy in these matching questions, select the letter of the correct regimen. Each lettered option may be selected once, more than once, or not at all.

(A) Conjugated equine estrogens (CEE) 0.625 mg and medroxyprogesterone acetate 2.5 mg daily

(B) Conjugated equine estrogens (CEE) 0.625 mg daily

(C) Transdermal estradiol 0.1 mg twice weekly

(D) Observation and periodic measurement of FSH levels

(E) Alendronate 10 mg daily

11. A 33-year-old Caucasian woman who underwent an ovary-sparing hysterectomy.

12. A slim, 40-year-old woman of northern European heritage who has early, physiologic menopause and who smokes a pack of cigarettes per day.

13. A 55-year-old Caucasian woman who underwent physiologic menopause at the normal age and whose mother and maternal aunt suffered hip fractures, one of which resulted in death within the first year.

14. A 40-year-old woman who underwent total hysterectomy and has no history of carcinoma of the breast, cervix, or ovary.

15. A 50-year-old woman who had a total hysterectomy, is free of evidence of breast cancer disease 10 years after mastectomy and radiation therapy, and recently suffered two fractures of distal radii and a wedge fracture of thoracic vertebra T10.

ANSWERS AND EXPLANATIONS

1. The answer is A. By liberal standards, a level of follicle-stimulating hormone greater than 20 IU confirms a diagnosis of ovarian failure, whether the failure is premature or associated with the female climacteric. (Although some authorities recognize a more conservative cutpoint of 40 IU, the level of 20 IU permits a lower threshold for commencement of hormone replacement therapy (HRT) after menopause.) The term "climacteric" is used broadly for physiological changes that occur with advancing age in both men and women. The most dramatic aspect of the climacteric is the menopause in women.

2. The answer is A. This woman's follicle-stimulating hormone (FSH) level should be determined to confirm acute menopause, the condition strongly suggested by her symptoms. An FSH level greater than 40 international units (IU), a conservative cutpoint, provides a secure diagnosis. Although the patient's recent history of irregular periods constitutes dysfunctional uterine bleeding, early diagnosis and treatment of acute menopause will probably resolve the irregular menses quickly. And, although sleep disturbance and subjective symptoms of depression may indicate depression, symptoms are likely to resolve with empiric treatment for acute menopause. With or without confirmation of acute menopause, treatment of insomnia with sedatives is seldom wise, except for very brief transitional periods. Muscular symptoms (such as this woman's) often occur as nonspecific manifestations of acute estrogen deficiency.

3. The answer is C. In a case of acute menopause, the conjugated equine estrogen (minimum, 0.3 mg) component in hormone replacement therapy (HRT) is required to prevent symptoms of acute estrogen insufficiency, including hot flashes, depression, muscular aches, and emotional lability. HRT includes both estrogen and a progestogen, but the estrogen content is solely responsible for relief of symptoms. Antidepressants (e.g., sertraline, paroxetine), bedtime sedatives (e.g., diazepam), muscle relaxants, and nonsteroidal anti-inflammatory drugs (e.g., ibuprofen) each treat only one aspect of the total syndrome.

4. The answer is B. A dosage of 0.625 mg of conjugated equine estrogen (CEE) is necessary to prevent osteoporosis. This dosage (or its equivalent in other types of estrogen preparations) is estimated to prevent up to 50% of hip fractures in postmenopausal women. (It may eventually prevent 50% of postmenopausal heart disease deaths as well because of its effects on serum lipids.)

5. The answer is E. Loss of libido is more likely after surgical than after physiologic menopause, even with hormone replacement therapy. "Total hysterectomy" (which includes oophorectomy) removes the source of secondary testosterone. Even ovary-sparing hysterectomy may cause loss of libido, possibly because of compromise of ovarian blood supply during surgery.

6. The answer is A. Coronary artery disease (CAD) is the first-ranking cause of death among postmenopausal women, whether the women are on hormone replacement therapy (HRT) or not.

7. The answer is A. A 50% reduction in deaths from coronary artery disease (CAD) is the most significant predicted benefit of hormone replacement therapy (HRT) and estrogen replacement therapy (ERT). In women on HRT, the prediction is that CAD deaths will be reduced from approximately 10,500 per 100,000 to 5250 per 100,000. First-year hip-fracture mortality will also be reduced about 50% (from about 938 per 100,000 to roughly 419 per 100,000). [See Table 19.1 in *Family Medicine* (House Officer Series)]. An increase in predicted breast cancer deaths from 1406 per 100,000 to 2250 per 100,000 will be more than offset by lives saved in the other two categories. Endometrial carcinoma, while more incident in women whose estrogen replacement therapy includes no opposing progestogen, is predicted to be reduced by more than 75% in women on HRT. ERT is contraindicated when the uterus is present. Carcinoma of the vulva, an unusual and seldom-fatal sequela of the postmenopausal (hormone-deprived) state, is presumably prevented by replacement therapy.

8. The answer is D. Obtain a follicle-stimulating hormone (FSH) level for this patient, whose symptoms and setting suggest natural menopause. If the diagnosis is confirmed by an FSH level of 20 IU or more, and if history and evidence of cervical or breast cancer are absent, start the patient on hormone replacement therapy (HRT). Her northern European (including Celtic) heritage confers a greater-than-average risk of osteoporosis. Do not wait for 1 year of amenorrhea before you start this patient on treatment: HRT would prevent probable, measurable bone loss that could occur during that time. Unopposed estrogen is contraindicated in the presence of the patient's intact uterus because of the attendant risk of endometrial carcinoma. Stress is not an appropriate diagnosis for the symptoms in this setting, so you would not prescribe a benzodiazepine agent.

9. The answer is C. The detrimental effect of regular smoking on bone density is equally as strong as the beneficial effect of estrogen. Thus, a woman on hormone replacement therapy (HRT) or estrogen replacement therapy (ERT) who continues to smoke sacrifices the benefit she should obtain from HRT. Of course, if she smokes and receives no HRT or ERT, she is much more at risk for osteoporosis.

10. The answer is E. Refer this patient for endometrial biopsy, the course generally recommended in cases where bleeding persists more than 6 months after the patient begins hormone replacement therapy (HRT, estrogen/progesterone). This situation is of low urgency because HRT confers a negative risk for endometrial carcinoma, and bleeding often persists for up to 9 months with no pathological basis. [The relative risk of endometrial carcinoma with HRT is 0.2. See Table 19.1 in *Family Medicine* (House Officer Series). ERT (estrogen without accompanying progesterone) increases the risk for endometrial carcinoma. For that reason, ERT is contraindicated in the presence of an intact endometrium.] Nevertheless, postmenopausal bleeding is the hallmark of endometrial carcinoma, the most common uterine cancer. Discontinuance of HRT is not recommended at this time because the findings of most biopsies are benign. Once endometrial carcinoma is ruled out, the dosage of either the estrogen or progesterone may be adjusted upward. Dilatation and curettage (D&C), a more aggressive procedure than endometrial biopsy for obtaining biopsy tissue, is not necessary.

11. The answer is D. Observation and periodic measurement of follicle-stimulating hormone (FSH) levels is appropriate for this patient. Until she undergoes physiologic ovarian involution, you may presume that a young Caucasian woman who has undergone ovary-sparing hysterectomy is producing sufficient estrogen. In the absence of menstrual periods and symptoms, only a rise in FSH will confirm humoral menopause.

12. The answer is A. Conjugated equine estrogens (CEE) 0.625 mg and medroxyprogesterone acetate 2.5 mg daily is an appropriate regimen for the 40-year-old woman with early, physiologic menopause. She should be informed that her pack-a-day smoking habit cancels out the benefit of HRT, and she should be encouraged to quit. In addition, supplementation with calcium and magnesium, along with vitamin C, which are now known to help protect bone density, should be part of her regimen.

13. The answer is A. Conjugated equine estrogens (CEE) 0.625 mg and medroxyprogesterone acetate 2.5 mg daily is appropriate for the 55-year-old menopausal Caucasian woman who is assumed to be at high risk for osteoporosis. In addition, supplementation with calcium, magnesium, and vitamin C should be part of her regimen.

14. The answer is B. Conjugated equine estrogens (CEE) 0.625 mg daily (estrogen replacement therapy "unopposed" by a progestogen) is appropriate for this woman, in the presence of a total hysterectomy (which precludes the danger of endometrial cancer) and in the absence of a history of carcinoma of the breast, cervix, or ovary.

15. The answer is E. Alendronate 10 mg daily, taken 30 minutes before breakfast, is a choice for the 50-year-old woman who underwent total hysterectomy, has a history of breast cancer, and recently suffered several fractures. The history of breast cancer is a contraindication for treatment with hormone replacement therapy. (Note: Alendronate is less irritating to the gastrointestinal tract than earlier diphosphonates but causes esophagogastritis in a significant number of cases.) Tamoxifen or raloxifene could also be considered as supplemental agents. Tamoxifen and, more so, raloxifene, effectively block estrogen receptors in the breast, thus suppressing estrogen receptor positive breast tumors, and retain enough estrogenic properties to retard the progress of osteoporosis. Raloxifene inhibits the progress of atherosclerosis as well. Supplementation with calcium, magnesium, and vitamin C should also be part of this woman's regimen.

BIBLIOGRAPHY

Rudy DR: Problems of the female climacteric. In *Family Medicine* (House Officer Series). Edited by Rudy DR, Kurowski K. Baltimore, Williams & Wilkins, 1997, pp 329–340.

Test 20

Diseases of the Breast

DIRECTIONS (Items 1–12): Each of the numbered items or incomplete statements in this section is followed by answers or by completions of the statement. Select the ONE lettered answer or completion that is BEST in each case.

1. Use of routine mammography has produced the most verifiable reduction in deaths from breast cancer in which age group?

(A) Menarche to menopause
(B) 20–40 years
(C) All ages beyond 40 years
(D) 50–65 years
(E) All ages beyond 60 years

2. A 25-year-old woman with a history of two pregnancies and deliveries complains of sore breasts during the 5–7 day interval that precedes her menstrual period. Which initial course should you follow?

(A) If you find no mass in the patient's breasts, reassure the patient and schedule a visit in 1 year.
(B) Prescribe an NSAID (e.g., ibuprofen); reassure the patient; and schedule a visit in 1 year.
(C) If you find no mass in the patient's breasts, ascertain that the patient's bra fits correctly; prescribe a trial diet of lower fat and caffeine content; and schedule a visit in 1 month.
(D) Prescribe natural progesterone during the period of symptoms.
(E) Prescribe chlorotrianisene (TACE) for 10 days.

3. Your examination of the patient in Question 2 revealed no mass in her breasts, but the initial measures resulted in no relief. Now, 3 months later, she complains of worsening pain. What is the best next step you should take?

(A) Prescribe birth control pills for 3 monthly cycles, and schedule a return visit for the end of that interval.
(B) Prescribe ice packs for pain, daily as needed.
(C) Prescribe danazol (a mild androgen) 100 mg twice daily.
(D) Order a CT scan of the sella turcica.
(E) Institute 10 days of medroxyprogesterone acetate, 100 mg daily, followed by abrupt withdrawal.

4. Of the following breast complaints, which warrants the closest and most persistent evaluation?

(A) Bilateral nipple discharge that has a milky appearance
(B) Cyclic occurrence of bilateral tenderness with irregular, palpable masses
(C) Unilateral, purulent, nipple discharge accompanied by tenderness
(D) Bilateral nipple irritation during nursing
(E) Unilateral, bloody, nipple discharge

5. A 26-year-old woman complains of a breast lump, which you find to be approximately 1 cm in diameter and tender. She reports that the lump is tenderer this week than last week; also, it has been tender several times in the past 3 months, each time for approximately 1 week. Which of the following is your best first step?

(A) Refer the patient for mammography.
(B) Refer the patient for biopsy.
(C) Examine the patient monthly during the next 3 months.
(D) Perform, or refer the patient for, needle aspiration.
(E) Assure the patient that breast cancer is unlikely in her age group.

6. A female patient in her mid-twenties complains of a breast lump of 2 weeks duration, which you find to be about 1 centimeter in diameter. The patient reports the incidence of some trauma to the area that occurred approximately 2 weeks ago. Which of the following is your best next step?

(A) Refer the patient for mammography this week.
(B) Refer the patient for breast biopsy.
(C) Examine the patient monthly during the next 3 months.
(D) Perform, or refer the patient for, needle aspiration.
(E) Assure the patient that breast cancer is unlikely in her age group.

7. In which of the following age groups in the US do the largest proportion of breast cancers occur?

(A) Menarche to 25 years
(B) 20–40 years
(C) Menarche to 50 years
(D) 50–65 years
(E) 65 years and older

8. For primary prevention of breast cancer in individuals with a strong genetic tendency for this disease, which of the following agents should be considered?

(A) Conjugated equine estrogens (CEE)
(B) CEE combined with a progesterone (e.g., medroxyprogesterone acetate) overlapping monthly
(C) Cisplatin
(D) Tamoxifen
(E) Ethinyl estradiol

9. The most common cause of complaint of breast pain is

(A) Fibrocystic breast disease
(B) Costochondritis
(C) Trauma
(D) Breast abscess
(E) Intraductal carcinoma

10. Mammography shows a lesion 7 centimeters in diameter, which proves to be cancer, in a 55-year-old Caucasian woman. Examination reveals no palpable lymph nodes. Liver battery and chest x-ray are negative for metastases. The woman expresses a preference for lumpectomy and radiation of regional lymph nodes rather than a radical mastectomy. Your appropriate response is which of the following?

(A) You concur because lumpectomy and irradiation give overall cure rates that are comparable to radical mastectomy.
(B) You concur because of the size of the primary lesion.
(C) You disagree and counsel against lumpectomy because radical mastectomy offers a better overall cure rate.
(D) You disagree because irradiation interferes with the wound-healing process.
(E) You disagree and counsel against lumpectomy because of the size of the primary lesion.

11. A 46-year-old Caucasian woman complained of a breast lump that she first noticed 1 week earlier, 2 days before the onset of her menstrual period (which occurred at the expected time). You palpated a 2-centimeter mass in the superolateral quadrant of the left breast. A mammogram, obtained within 5 days and reported 1 week after the examination, failed to show an abnormality. An attempt at aspiration yielded no fluid. Which is the most appropriate next course of action?

(A) Reassure the patient that the lump is a cyst, exacerbated by the menstrual period.
(B) Instruct the patient to perform self-examination and to compare the size of the lump two weeks before, as well as during, the next three periods.
(C) Perform, or refer the patient for, a thin-needle biopsy.
(D) Request a repeat mammography for the patient for 1 month from now.
(E) Prescribe a low-fat, no-caffeine diet, and re-examine the patient in 1 month.

12. After a routine annual Pap smear (negative) and normal breast examination of a 55-year-old African-American woman who has no family history of breast cancer, you learn that the routine mammogram you ordered shows she has a lesion 1.5 centimeters in diameter with calcifications of vague description. The radiologist describes a few radiation spicules in a pattern otherwise consistent with chronic inflammation. You re-examine the patient and are still unable to palpate a nodule. Which of the following options is most appropriate at this time?

(A) Attempt fluid aspiration by stereotactic approach.
(B) Instruct the patient to perform self-examination before and during the next three menstrual periods and note the relative size of the nodule.
(C) Perform, or refer the patient for, thin needle biopsy.
(D) Order repeat mammography for 1 month from now.
(E) Prescribe a low-fat, no-caffeine diet, and re-examine the patient in 1 month.

DIRECTIONS (Items 13–17): For each numbered condition in these matching questions, select the letter of the most appropriate finding. Each lettered option may be used once, more than once, or not at all.

(A) Conveys a worse prognosis
(B) Known to be associated with autoimmune disease
(C) Interferes with adequate examination
(D) Present in 15% of breast cancer cases
(E) Most likely cause of a solid mass in a 25-year-old woman

13. Primary breast lesion larger than 2 centimeters, compared with smaller lesion

14. Silicone breast implants

15. Bloody nipple discharge, compared with clear or milky discharge

16. Family history of breast cancer

17. Fibroadenoma

ANSWERS AND EXPLANATIONS

1. The answer is D. In the age group of 50–65 years, a reduction in mortality from breast cancer as a result of routine mammogram has been found in several prospective studies of screened versus unscreened women. Women younger than 50, who have more fibrous, and less fatty, tissue in their breasts have not benefitted as much because mammograms of such tissue are less accurate. Women younger than forty tend to contract more aggressive cancers than do older women, so biannual screening may not be frequent enough to improve the survival rate. A study in 1996 by Kerlikowske, et al (see Bibliography), found that more frequent screening also improves mortality in women 40–50, a group in whom the benefits have been less clear. [This finding was not reflected in the discussion in *Family Medicine* (House Officer Series)].

2. The answer is C. For the 25-year-old woman with cyclic, premenstrual mastalgia, you should first ascertain that the patient's bra fits correctly; prescribe a trial diet that is lower than usual in caffeine, other xanthine derivatives (e.g., theobromine found in chocolate), and fat; and, if no mass is found during your examination of the breasts, reassure the patient about the nature of the breast lump, and schedule a visit in 1 month. (The relationship between xanthines and fibrocystic disease of the breast is known statistically and empirically.) If these measures do not suffice, a trial course of low-dose birth-control pills can be prescribed during the period of symptoms. Natural progesterone is being prescribed for premenstrual tension, which sometimes underlies premenstrual mastalgia, but does not necessarily do so. Waiting a year for the next appointment is inappropriate; the success or failure of the measures taken should be ascertained much sooner. A 10-day prescription of chlorotrianisene, an old remedy for suppressing lactation after childbirth in painful breasts of nonbreastfeeding mothers, is not used in premenstrual mastalgia.

3. The answer is A. Prescribing birth control pills for three monthly cycles and following up with a re-examination is the best next step in the treatment of this patient. Danazol, bromocriptine, tamoxifen, or a GnRH agonist, capable (in varied ways) of inhibiting the pituitary or otherwise blunting the affects of estrogen to reduce stimulation of the breast tissue, would be prescribed only in an extreme case. Conducting a "medical D&C" by medroxyprogesterone acetate withdrawal is inappropriate for this patient: It is used in the diagnosis and management of dysfunctional uterine bleeding (abrupt withdrawal of the progestogen results in shedding of proliferative or secretory endometrium).

4. The answer is E. Unilateral bloody discharge, the most likely of the breast complaints to be a sign of cancer (most breast cancers begin as intraductal carcinomas), is caused by cancer in one out of three cases and warrants the closest and most persistent evaluation. A bilateral, milky-looking nipple discharge is galactorrhea, which has a variety of causes, including pregnancy, mechanical stimulation, pituitary adenoma (prolactinoma), hypothyroidism, Cushing's disease, and chronic renal failure. The cyclic occurrence of bilateral tenderness with irregular palpable masses is caused by fibrocystic disease; it is seen commonly in primary care practice. Tenderness accompanying purulent discharge represents an infection, often in a lactating woman.

5. The answer is D. Your next step should be to perform, or refer this patient for, needle aspiration, to determine whether the condition suggested by the cyclically tender breast lump is fibrocystic disease. If the nodule disappears as fluid is aspirated, cancer is extremely unlikely. Cytological examination of the fluid should be performed to eliminate any further doubt, and a mammogram may be obtained for baseline data. A mammogram as a first step is inappropriate in a 26-year-old woman: Cancer in this age group is unlikely; mammograms are less sensitive for cancer in women in their twenties and thirties because of the density of their breast tissue; and cancers are rarely painful or tender. A breast lump that fails to disappear with aspiration indicates the need for biopsy. Other breast lump symptoms and other settings require other first steps, including mammography, breast biopsy, or continued observation.

6. The answer is C. Examination of this patient monthly for the next 3 months is appropriate. The history of trauma to the area suggests a hematoma, which can persist for 6 weeks or longer before resolving. If the lump fails to resolve in 3 months, the patient can be referred for needle aspiration, ultrasound, breast biopsy, or more than one of these procedures. (An ultrasound is preferable to a mammogram for this patient because mammograms can be inaccurate in her age group.)

7. The answer is E. In the US, the largest percentage of breast cancer (almost 50%) occurs in women older than 65 years. Approximately 25% occurs in women of 50–65 years, and approximately 25% in women younger than 50 years. [Note: Because of mounting evidence that women younger than 50 tend to contract more aggressive cancers than do older women, yearly routine mammography is considered advisable for women of 40–49 years as well as for the older group. The conclusive report was not available in time for inclusion in *Family Medicine* (House Officer Series).]

8. The answer is D. Tamoxifen, a competitive inhibitor of estrogen, is the agent considered for use in primary prevention of breast cancer in individuals who have a strong genetic tendency for breast cancer. (However, tamoxifen shares many of the affects of estrogens, including the slightly increased risk of endometrial carcinoma.) The incidence of estrogen-receptor-positive breast cancer has increased in the past 15 years, but mortality from this disease has not accompanied the increase, possibly because of the better differentiated cell type of this cancer as well as earlier diagnosis (the result of increased screening). Conjugated equine estrogens (CEE) combined with a progesterone (e.g., medroxyprogesterone acetate) is a standard hormone replacement protocol, which is not protective against breast cancer, and is still being investigated as a possible risk for it. CEE and ethinyl estradiol are estrogenic substances, contraindicated in the presence of a history of breast cancer; they may be risk factors, especially in women with strong family histories of breast cancer. Cisplatin, a chemotherapeutic agent used in breast cancer (among other cancers) is not used as a preventive agent.

9. The answer is B. Costochondritis is the most common cause of "breast pain" complaints, despite the non-mammary origin. Fibrocystic disease, abscesses, and trauma are other, less common causes of breast pain. Intraductal carcinoma is unlikely to be painful or tender in the early stages.

10. The answer is E. This patient should be counseled against lumpectomy and radiation, which are contraindicated for a primary breast cancer lesion ≥ 5 centimeters in diameter. Radical mastectomy is appropriate for her 7-centimeter lesion. Other contraindications for breast-conserving therapy are multifocal cancerous lesions and lesions with an extensive intraductal component. Intraductal carcinomas are the most common of the aggressive breast tumors. Lumpectomy and node dissection, followed by irradiation, give results comparable to radical mastectomy in breast cancers that are smaller than 5 centimeters, not multifocal, and without an extensive intraductal component. Wound healing is not impeded by irradiation if it is delayed for 10–14 days after surgery.

11. The answer is C. A needle biopsy of this patient's palpable nodule is required within 3 months, despite the negative results of mammography. Failure of aspiration to produce fluid indicates that you cannot assume the nodule is a benign cystic lesion, despite the seeming association of the lump with the time of the month. If aspiration had produced fluid, or, perhaps, if the patient were younger than 40 years, 3 months of cyclic follow-up and self-examination would be appropriate to confirm the presence of cystic changes. If the evidence pointed more strongly to fibrocystic disease, prescription of a low-fat, no-caffeine diet would be appropriate. Repeat mammography would not be appropriate, because it would probably produce findings similar to those of the original mammography. This patient's Caucasian race is mentioned because Caucasian-Americans have a higher rate of breast cancer than do Americans of other races.

12. The answer is C. Perform, or refer this patient for, a thin-needle biopsy. An impalpable lesion seen on a mammogram requires a biopsy. Fluid aspiration (to rule out a cystic lesion) is impractical because the lesion is impalpable, and because a cystic lesion would have been identified as such on the mammogram. Self-examination of an impalpable lump is impossible. Repeat mammography is inappropriate, because it will contribute nothing more than before and will use time that may be crucial to treatment.

13. The answer is A. With respect to primary breast cancer, the prognosis of a lesion larger than 2 centimeters is considered measurably worse than that of a smaller one.

14. The answer is C. Silicone breast implants interfere with adequate breast examination. Despite class-action lawsuits that claim these implants cause autoimmune diseases (e.g., scleroderma, periarteritis), studies have found no evidence of such causation.

15. The answer is A. A bloody discharge from the nipple conveys a worse prognosis than a clear or milky one. A bloody discharge requires an evaluation for ductal carcinoma. A clear discharge is unlikely to be cancer; however, it is suspect, especially if it is unilateral, and must be examined microscopically to rule out the presence of red blood cells. A milky discharge is the least likely of the three types to signal cancer; its cause is most likely hormonal. It is most often bilateral, which almost always indicates benign lumps. Bilateral discharges are likely to be based on physiological dysfunction rather than on simultaneous development of cancers in both breasts.

16. The answer is D. Only 15% of all women with breast cancer have a first-degree family history of breast cancer. However, such a family history doubles a woman's lifetime risk for this disease.

17. The answer is E. Solid tumors in very young women (women in their twenties) are most likely to be fibroadenomas. Still, each of these tumors requires individual evaluation.

BIBLIOGRAPHY

Bowman MA, Szewczyk MB: Diseases of the breast. In *Family Medicine* (House Officer Series). Edited by Rudy DR and Kurowski K. Baltimore, Williams & Wilkins, 1997, pp 341–350.

Kerlikowske K, Grady D, Barclay MS, et al: Effect of age, breast density, and family history on the sensitivity of first screening mammography. *JAMA* 276(1):33–38,1996.

Angell M: Evaluating the health risks of breast implants: the interplay of medical science, the law, and public opinion (The Shattuck lecture). *N Engl J Med* 334(23):1513–1518, 1996.

SECTION VIII

Problems Unique to Males

Test 21

Genitourinary Problems of the Male

DIRECTIONS (Items 1–15): Each of the numbered items or incomplete statements in this section is followed by answers or by completions of the statement. Select the ONE lettered answer or completion that is BEST in each case.

1. By which of the following routes do viral infections (e.g., mumps) involve the testicle to produce orchitis?

(A) By contiguous spread
(B) By lymphatic spread
(C) From an infected epididymis
(D) Through the vas deferens
(E) By hematogenous spread

2. A 70-year-old, nursing-home resident, who developed a painful swelling of the right testicle 3 days ago, has a temperature of 102°F (38.8°C) and complains of dysuria. Examination reveals no tenderness at the costovertebral angle and no masses or tenderness in the abdomen. The patient's prostate is diffusely, mildly enlarged, without tenderness or palpable masses. The scrotum shows a firm, tender mass posteriorly on the right. The organism most likely responsible for this patient's symptoms is which of the following?

(A) *Escherichia coli*
(B) *Staphylococcus saprophyticus*
(C) *Enterococcus* species
(D) *Neisseria gonorrhoeae*
(E) *Chlamydia trachomatis*

3. A 19-year-old male patient says he has noted a mass in his right scrotum for the last 6 months. He has noted no dysuria, frequency, nor urethral discharge. On examination, you find an elongated, worm-like mass of approximately 2 centimeters in diameter in his right upper scrotum. The testicle, approximately 3.5 cm in size, is smooth and distinct from the mass. With respect to this type of scrotal mass, which of the following statements is correct?

(A) It is more common on the right side.
(B) It is sometimes associated with infertility.
(C) It produces a dull, scrotal pain.
(D) It diminishes in size during a Valsalva maneuver.
(E) Surgical repair in adolescence is recommended only when the involved testicle is smaller than the uninvolved testicle by 1 centimeter or more.

4. The use of a vacuum constriction device to improve potency is contraindicated in a patient who has which of the following?

(A) Sickle cell disease
(B) Peripheral arterial occlusive disease
(C) Moderate emphysema
(D) Age greater than 65 years
(E) A history of stage B carcinoma treated by open prostatectomy

5. Patient-initiated penile self-injection with papaverine (for impotence) produces which of the following as a relatively common complication?

(A) Exacerbation of prostatic urethral obstruction from benign prostatic hypertrophy
(B) Systemic hypertensive response
(C) Central nervous system excitation
(D) Priapism
(E) Exacerbation of chronic, obstructive pulmonary disease

6. With respect to cancer death rates among American men, where does prostate cancer rank?

(A) First
(B) Second
(C) Third
(D) Fourth
(E) Fifth

7. The American Cancer Society recommends routine, annual, digital rectal examination and annual prostate-specific antigen (PSA) measurement in asymptomatic African-American men, starting at which age?

(A) Age 30
(B) Age 35
(C) Age 40
(D) Age 45
(E) Age 50

8. A 70-year-old man has nocturia, along with hesitancy and frequency of urination. His digital rectal examination reveals diffuse enlargement of the gland, but no nodules and no adjacent palpable masses. His prostate-specific antigen (PSA) level is 6.2. A biopsy and laboratory findings reveal some areas of well-differentiated adenocarcinoma of the prostate. A bone scan shows no abnormalities. With respect to this patient's prostate cancer, which of the following statements is true?

(A) The prostate-specific antigen (PSA) level determines the stage.
(B) A Gleason score would be at the high end of the scale.
(C) The cancer is in stage A.
(D) The cancer is in stage B.
(E) The cancer is in stage C.

9. Which age group would comprise the most realistic target for screening for testicular cancer?

(A) 10–15 years of age
(B) 15–35 years of age
(C) 35–55 years of age
(D) 55–75 years of age
(E) > 75 years of age

10. You cannot palpate a testis in the right scrotum of an 8-year-old boy, but you can palpate a 1-centimeter, slightly firm testis in the left scrotum. With respect to this patient's risk for development of testicular carcinoma, which of the following statements is correct?

(A) An increased risk is limited to the right (undescended) testicle.
(B) The malignancy that most commonly develops in a patient such as this one is a seminoma.
(C) Placement of the right testis into the scrotal sac by surgical correction greatly reduces the patient's risk.
(D) The majority of testicular carcinomas occur in patients with undescended testicles.
(E) The risk is higher if the missing testicle is in the inguinal canal than if it is in the intra-abdominal area.

11. In patients with testicular tumors, the most common presentation is

(A) A dull ache in the scrotum and lower abdomen
(B) Gynecomastia
(C) Symptoms of epididymitis
(D) Cough and shortness of breath from metastatic pulmonary involvement
(E) Absence of symptoms

12. In the afternoon, a 13-year-old boy complains that he developed right testicular pain and some nausea that morning. He denies any trauma or sexual activity, and he has no dysuria nor hematuria. On examination, his temperature is 99.0°F (37.2°C); his blood pressure is 118/80; his abdomen is soft, without tenderness or masses; and his right testicle is mildly tender and retracted upward. On this testicle, the epididymis is palpable anteriorly. The left testicle is normal in size, and nontender, but lies in the horizontal position within the scrotum. Which of the following tests would be most definitive in confirming the most likely diagnosis?

(A) Surgical aspiration and drainage
(B) Ultrasound imaging of the testes
(C) A voiding cystourethrogram
(D) Transillumination of the scrotum
(E) Testicular scintillation scan

13. A 53-year-old man complains of a 2-year history of gradually worsening nocturia (at present he needs to urinate four times per night), increasing hesitancy in initiating his urinary stream, and decreasing stream size. Your best first evaluative step is which of the following?

(A) Order an alkaline phosphatase test
(B) Order a bone scan
(C) Take a more careful history
(D) Perform a digital rectal examination
(E) Order a PSA test

14. Let us assume that, in your digital rectal examination of the patient in the preceding question, you find an enlarged, smooth prostate and an obliterated median depression where the raphe is located. The results of a prostate-specific antigen (PSA) test are 2.5 ng/ml. A medication (applicable to this case) that prevents conversion of testosterone to dihydrotestosterone is which of the following?

- (A) Finasteride
- (B) Terazosin
- (C) Prazosin
- (D) Doxazosin
- (E) Bethanechol

15. A 55-year-old man, who has smoked 45 pack years, complains of gross hematuria of several weeks duration, urinary frequency and urgency, and a week of incontinence involving loss of up to 0.5 ounce of urine on his way to the toilet. No fever nor flank pain are present, and no pain accompanies voiding. Examination is negative for costovertebral angle (CVA) tenderness, but mild to moderate suprapubic palpation produces a sense of urinary urgency in the patient. He denies hesitancy and a decrease in the size of his urinary stream. Routine and acid-fast cultures are negative. An intravenous pyelogram (IVP) is negative. The most logical next step or steps are which of the following?

- (A) Repeat the acid-fast smear and culture, and prescribe isoniazid, 300 mg daily, for 3 months.
- (B) Prescribe trimethoprim plus sulfamethoxazole, 160 mg/800 mg twice daily, for 2 weeks; repeat the urinalysis, culture, and sensitivity when this course of medication is finished.
- (C) Instruct the patient to strain his urine for 2 weeks while you treat him symptomatically.
- (D) Refer the patient for cystoscopy to examine the bladder mucosa.
- (E) Prescribe finasteride, 5 mg daily.

DIRECTIONS (Items 16–18): Each of the numbered items or incomplete statements in this section is negatively phrased, as indicated by a capitalized word such as NOT, LEAST, or EXCEPT. Select the ONE lettered answer or completion that is BEST in each case.

16. Which of the following is LEAST likely to be associated with erectile dysfunction?

- (A) Alcohol
- (B) Cimetidine
- (C) Theophylline
- (D) Propranolol
- (E) Antihistamine

17. A 74-year-old man complains of altered sexual function. You want to reassure him that many of the changes he has noted are normal for his age. All of the following are normally anticipated changes EXCEPT

- (A) Increase in time and stimulation needed to achieve an erection
- (B) Development of bilateral testicular atrophy
- (C) Increase in the refractory period needed to attain a second erection

- (D) Increase in the ability of fatigue to limit sexual arousal
- (E) Earlier loss of erection after stimulation stops

18. A routine prostate-specific antigen (PSA) test shows that a 52-year-old, African-American male patient has a mildly elevated PSA level at 7.0 ng/ml (normal, 0–4.0). In addition to cancer, all of the following may be associated with his elevated prostate specific antigen (PSA) level EXCEPT

- (A) Benign prostatic hypertrophy
- (B) Prostatic massage
- (C) Routine digital prostate examination
- (D) Transrectal prostate biopsy
- (E) Acute prostatitis

ANSWERS AND EXPLANATIONS

1. The answer is E. Hematogenous spread is the usual route by which viruses involve the testicle to produce orchitis. Bacterial orchitis can originate contiguously from epididymitis or hematogenously into testes damaged by trauma.

2. The answer is A. *Escherichia coli* is most likely the cause of this patient's symptoms; this is a typical clinical presentation of acute epididymitis. In patients younger than 35 years, *Chlamydia trachomatis* and *Neisseria gonorrhoeae* are the most likely organisms; but in the geriatric male, a coliform bacterium (e.g., *E. coli)* is more likely. *Enterococcus* species (a subset of Group D Streptococci that inhabit the large bowel and are contained in feces) and *Staphylococcus* species are not common causes of epididymitis.

3. The answer is B. A varicocele, the type of scrotal mass typified by the presentation in this case, is sometimes associated with infertility. A varicocele is a varicosity in the veins of the pampiniform plexus that forms a swelling that feels like "a bag of worms." It is present in up to one third of men evaluated for infertility. Varicoceles are more common on the left side than the right; they are usually asymptomatic; and they enlarge with a Valsalva maneuver. Adolescent surgical repair is recommended if the affected testicle is smaller than the other by 0.5 cm or more.

4. The answer is A. The use of a vacuum constriction device to improve potency is contraindicated in patients with sickle cell disease. Vacuum constriction devices draw blood into the penis, and the blood is held there with a type of tourniquet. The relatively hypoxic blood drawn into and held in the penis could sickle in a patient with sickle cell disease and cause ischemic injury to the penis. In moderate emphysema and in peripheral arterial disease, some relative hypoxia may already exist in the corpus cavernosum, but usually not enough to produce ischemia during the brief increase in hypoxia that results from use of the constriction device. Age greater than 65 years is not a contraindication to vacuum constriction. (Elderly patients are the most likely to need treatment for impotence.) Prostatectomy, which often produces impotence (even in "nerve-sparing" procedures), is not a contraindication for use of the device: Neurologic impotence is not adversely affected by the hypoxia produced by vacuum constriction.

5. The answer is D. Priapism (persistent penile erection that is not dependent on sexual desire) is a common complication of self-injection with papaverine. This therapy for impotence can induce local penile ischemia in men who have sickle cell disease (or trait), poor penile venous drainage, or hypotension. Even without the use of papaverine, priapism is a common complication of sickle-cell disease. Pooled, engorged penile blood becomes hypoxic and a sickling crisis may develop. Papaverine exacerbates the problem by relaxing vascular smooth-muscle tissue, resulting in increased local pooling and stagnation of penile blood, which can easily elicit a sickling crisis. This vaso-occlusive response prevents penile drainage and produces priapism. Treatments for priapism include: repeated ice-water enemas (sometimes helps); use of a sterile needle to drain the hypoxic blood trapped in the corpus cavernosa; intracavernous injection of alpha-adrenergic agents (usually effective); construction of a vascular shunt (in the case of prolonged priapism). Self-injection with papaverine is not contraindicated in men who have partial prostatic obstruction or chronic, obstructive pulmonary disease. Central nervous system (CNS) stimulation, the principal side effect of yohimbine, is not a side effect of papaverine.

6. The answer is B. The second highest death rate from cancer in American men is associated with prostate cancer, the most common cancer in American men. Lung carcinoma is associated with the highest cancer death rate.

7. The answer is C. Age 40 is recommended by the American Cancer Society for the start of routine, annual digital rectal examination and prostate-specific antigen (PSA) testing in asymptomatic African-American men. This population has a higher incidence of prostate cancer, and is more likely to have aggressive tumors, than do men of other races. In asymptomatic Caucasian men, age 40 is recommended for the start of digital rectal examinations, and age 50 for the start of PSA testing.

8. The answer is C. This patient's prostate cancer is in stage A, the stage in which the cancer is impalpable during a digital rectal examination and not seen on ultrasound, but is discovered microscopically (biopsy). Chances of survival are excellent if the malignancy is well differentiated, as in this case. The prostate-specific antigen (PSA) level does not determine stage, although a rough correlation exists between higher PSA levels and more advanced cancers. The PSA is most important for its ability to alert the physician to the need for biopsy, even when cancer is impalpable. It is also useful as a baseline to monitor treatment responses. Staging is accomplished through a combination of: digital rectal examination (DRE), including examination for palpable extension of cancer outside of the prostate; transrectal ultrasound (more sensitive examination than DRE); bone scan to assess for bony metastases; and CT or MRI to detect regional adenopathy. Stage B carcinomas have palpable nodules or diffuse induration within the prostate, but no extension outside of the prostate. Stage C carcinomas have local extension outside of the prostate (e.g., into the seminal vesicles, the surrounding fat, the bladder neck, the urethra). Stage D represents metastatic disease. A newer staging system is the TNM system, in which the tumor (T) is staged 0–4, representing size and extent of the tumor (T1-T4 are roughly equivalent to A-D, above); the grade is modified further by a lower case letter (a, b, or c) that represents the histologic grade; N indicates the level of lymph node involvement; and M indicates the level of metastasis. In addition to these grading systems, a Gleason score (ranging from 2–10) is assigned, based on histopathological examination of the biopsy samples: the higher the score, the less well differentiated (and the more aggressive) the tumor cell type. (A Gleason score for the well-differentiated cancer in this vignette would be low.)

9. The answer is B. The age group of 15–35 years is the one in which testicular cancer is most prevalent. Because of the relatively common occurrence of this tumor in young men, the instruction in testicular self-examination should ideally begin in high school, or even in junior high school. Approximately 35% of testicular tumors are seminomas, which are malignant neoplasms so radiosensitive that, if the tumor stage is low, radiation alone is used after transinguinal radical orchiectomy. Approximately 40% of testicular tumors are mixed-cell carcinomas, often containing components of seminoma or teratocarcinoma; 20% are embryonal cell carcinomas, including yolk-sac tumors that produce a great deal of alpha-fetoprotein (AFP); and 5% are teratomas that contain ectoderm-, mesoderm-, and endoderm-derived tissues. Less than 1% are choriocarcinomas that produce a great deal of human chorionic gonadotropin (hCG).

10. The answer is B. The testicular malignancy that develops most commonly in a patient with an undescended testicle (cryptorchidism) is a seminoma. Cryptorchidism is a little more common on the right side than the left. Approximately 10% of all testicular carcinomas (not the majority) develop in patients with a history of cryptorchidism, and 5%–10% of these develop in the contralateral (normally descended) testicle. The risk of a malignancy is greater if the undescended testicle is in the intra-abdominal area (approximately 1 in 20) than if it is in the inguinal canal (1 in 80). Surgical placement

of the undescended testicle into the scrotal sac offers no decrease in the risk, but it does permit earlier detection of malignancy.

11. The answer is E. Testicular tumors most commonly present with no symptoms. In most cases, by incidental palpation or self-examination, the patient finds a painless mass in the testicle. In 15%–20% (a minority) of cases, symptoms of epididymitis are present. Gynecomastia occurs with many endocrinologically active tumors, often with ectopic hormone production; however, the literature does not mention it as accompanying testicular tumor. Occasionally, testicular cancers may present with pulmonary metastases.

12. The answer is E. The testicular scintillation scan is the most definitive test to confirm the likely diagnosis of testicular torsion (to which the presentation points). Testicular torsion, which quickly leads to ischemic death of the testis, is a surgical emergency. The testicular scintillation scan with technetium is more than 90% specific in detecting torsion. The twisted testis is avascular and shows no uptake. The condition could appear to be epididymitis, but the latter usually occurs in a slightly older population (16–30 years), and produces no rotational changes in the testicle. An ultrasound test would show a swollen, solid, testicle but would probably fail to provide a clear differentiation from epididymitis. Color flow Doppler imaging would be superior to ordinary ultrasound imaging because, usually, it could demonstrate the absence of arterial flow to the twisted testis; however, it is less definitive than the testicular scan. Aspiration would be useless because torsion produces ischemia, with nothing to aspirate. Transillumination, which is useful in distinguishing a hydrocele within the scrotum, would not be helpful here. A voiding cystourethrogram, useful in diagnosing urinary retention or ureterovesical reflux, would not be useful here.

13. The answer is D. The digital rectal examination is the first evaluative step you should with regard to this patient, who has symptoms of prostatism (i.e., symptoms brought about by an enlarged prostate). The three main causes of prostatism include: (1) benign prostatic hypertrophy (most common cause), more accurately called benign prostatic hyperplasia, because the individual prostatic cells multiply rather than enlarging; (2) prostatitis, during which edema enlarges the gland (enlargement is reversed upon treatment or subsidence of the infection); (3) prostatic carcinoma (which may present as prostatism). Sometimes a combination of more than one of the three conditions is involved. Alkaline phosphatase, which is elevated in osteoblastic bone activity (as well as in hepatic obstruction), is elevated in prostatic cancer that has metastasized in an adult (also elevated in normally growing children), but testing for it would be premature in a patient who must first be examined. A bone scan, too, is useful in detecting bone metastases, but would be premature in this patient. The prostate-specific antigen (PSA) test follows the digital rectal test; The PSA test is sensitive but not perfectly specific for prostate cancer. Additional history is unnecessary; the information is sufficient to diagnose prostatism.

14. The answer is A. The applicable medication is finasteride. A diagnosis of benign prostatic hypertrophy (BPH) in this patient is based on symptoms of prostatism, symmetrical enlargement of the prostate (found by digital rectal examination), and a PSA level that is normal for the patient's age (see values below). Finasteride acts to prevent conversion of testosterone to dihydrotestosterone, the more potent form of the androgenic hormone. Prostatic hyperplasia is responsive to testosterone and subsides upon relative withdrawal of the hormone. Terazosin, prazosin, and doxazosin are examples of antihypertensive medications that have additional effects that reduce the smooth-muscle tone of the prostate and, in turn, the size of the gland. Bethanechol is a parasympathomimetic medication that assists a patient in bladder contraction when BPH is causing urinary retention. With respect to normal PSA numbers (ng/ml), the following are normal ranges and medians for men of 40–79 years:

40–49 years: 0.0–2.5 (median 0.7)

50–59 years: 0.0–3.5 (median 1.0)

60–69 years: 0.0–4.5 (median 1.4)

70–79 years: 0.0–6.5 (median 2.0)

15. The answer is D. Refer this patient for cystoscopy to examine the bladder mucosa. The presence of painless hematuria should trigger the differential diagnosis of tuberculosis, bladder cancer, hypercalciuria, and less common conditions (e.g., staghorn calculus, polycystic kidney disease). Cystoscopy to rule out transitional cell carcinoma of the bladder is the first priority. Isoniazid antituberculous therapy is not needed as indicated by the negative acid-fast culture (although repeat cultures would not be inappropriate). Empiric antituberculous therapy is inappropriate while the evaluation is underway. (Note that, if tuberculosis were a realistic possibility, a symptomatic patient would receive triple-drug therapy (e.g., isoniazid, ethambutol, and rifampin). Em-

piric medical therapy (finasteride) for benign prostatic hyperplasia is not indicated in the absence of hesitancy and decreased stream size. Treatment with trimethoprim with sulfamethoxazole for urinary infection (cystitis or pyelonephritis) is not indicated because clinical evidence (dysuria, fever, costovertebral-angle tenderness, positive routine urine culture) is lacking. Straining the urine is appropriate for confirming a diagnosis of ureterolithiasis, indicated by a positive intravenous pyelogram (IVP); however, this patient's IVP was negative. (In addition, in almost all cases, a ureteral stone causes a very severe colicky pain, not present in this patient.) Ordering the IVP before ordering cystoscopy is appropriate because the IVP is less invasive.

16. The answer is C. Of the five substances, theophylline is the LEAST likely to be associated with erectile dysfunction. Theophylline, a methylxanthine found in tea, is used for its bronchodilatory activity and is a central nervous system psychomotor stimulant. Alcohol is commonly implicated in erectile dysfunction. Many antihypertensives (especially beta-blockers, such as propranolol) and H2 antagonists (especially cimetidine), as well as antipsychotics, sedatives, and anticholinergics, have also been implicated in erectile dysfunction.

17. The answer is B. Bilateral testicular atrophy is NOT a normally anticipated change in geriatric men. Nor is decreased libido. Either occurrence warrants endocrine testing. Expected changes with respect to sexual function in geriatric men include the need for more time and stimulation in achieving an erection, the need for a longer refractory period until achievement of a second erection, the dampening effect of fatigue on sexual arousal, and the readier loss of erection after stimulation stops.

18. The answer is C. A routine digital prostate examination does NOT affect the prostate-specific antigen (PSA) level, although a more traumatic prostate massage does affect it. Increased PSA is seen for 6 weeks after a urinary tract infection or a prostate biopsy. Benign prostatic hypertrophy and acute prostatitis also elevate PSA levels.

BIBLIOGRAPHY

Strode SW: Genitourinary problems of the male. In *Family Medicine* (House Officer Series). Edited by Rudy DR, Kurowski K. Baltimore, Williams & Wilkins, 1997, pp 351–369.

SECTION IX

Musculoskeletal and Connective Tissue Problems

Test 22

Musculoskeletal Problems of the Neck and Back

DIRECTIONS (Items 1–13): Each of the numbered items or incomplete statements in this section is followed by answers or by completions of the statement. Select the ONE lettered answer or completion that is BEST in each case.

1. The single most common cause of neck pain is which of the following?

   (A) Playing football
   (B) Dancing
   (C) Practicing martial arts
   (D) Swimming
   (E) Motor vehicle accidents

2. Which of the following is most commonly associated with a whiplash injury to the neck?

   (A) Hyperextension of the neck
   (B) Hyperflexion of the neck
   (C) Contusion to the neck
   (D) Extreme rotation of the cervical spine
   (E) Strangulation

3. You are assessing a 40-year-old man with suspected cervical radiculopathy. Examination reveals diminished sensation over his middle finger, but normal sensation over the other fingers and hand; diminished triceps reflex, but normal biceps reflex; and some weakness of elbow extension, as well as wrist and finger extension. Which of the following cervical roots is most affected in this patient's radiculopathy?

   (A) C4
   (B) C5
   (C) C6
   (D) C7
   (E) C8

4. A 54-year-old man complains of neck, shoulder, and left arm pain, aggravated by certain neck movements. Which of the following would lead the most strongly to a diagnosis of cervical radiculopathy?

   (A) Atrophy of hand and arm muscle, which is present in chronic cases.
   (B) An electromyogram (EMG), which shows immediate signs of denervation in acute cases.
   (C) A history of recent, blunt neck trauma, which is usually associated.
   (D) An MRI of the neck, rather than cervical spine x-rays, which should begin the work-up.
   (E) Spurling's neck compression test, which is highly sensitive in confirming the diagnosis.

5. In patients younger than 50 years, the leading cause of disability is which of the following?

   (A) Upper respiratory tract infections
   (B) Depression
   (C) HIV infection
   (D) Heart disease
   (E) Lower back pain

6. A 38-year-old, afebrile woman complains of 2 days of lower back pain (with no radiation) that began after she did some heavy lifting. Some limitation to full flexion and rotation is present, but no spinal nor paravertebral tenderness. Findings in motor and sensory examinations of her legs are normal. In the straight-leg-raising test, you can raise each of her legs (with the knee in extension) 80° off the table without causing any radicular pain. Which of the following should you recommend?

   (A) An MRI of the lumbar spine
   (B) Strict bed rest for 1 week
   (C) Daily muscle relaxant for 1 week
   (D) Physical therapy (traction, massage, diathermy), 3 times per week for 2 weeks
   (E) Nonsteroidal anti-inflammatory drugs for 5–7 days

7. Most lumbar/sacral disc herniations occur at which two levels?

   (A) L_1–L_2 and L_2–L_3
   (B) L_2–L_3 and L_3–L_4
   (C) L_3–L_4 and L_4–L_5
   (D) L_4–L_5 and L_5–S_1
   (E) L_5–S_1 and S_1–S_2

8. You are evaluating a patient with right-leg sciatica, secondary to a posterolateral disc herniation. He has decreased sensation over his lateral heel, weak plantar flexion, and inability to toe-walk on his right foot. At what level is his disc herniation?

   (A) L_5–S_1
   (B) L_4–L_5
   (C) L_3–L_4
   (D) L_2–L_3
   (E) L_1–L_2

9. Which of the following is typical in a patient with cauda equina syndrome secondary to a centrally herniated lumbar disc?

(A) Sciatica involving only one leg
(B) Normal dorsiflexion and ventriflexion
(C) Fever
(D) Bladder dysfunction
(E) Weight loss

10. You are examining a 50-year-old man who has been experiencing lower back pain and RIGHT leg sciatica for 2 weeks. With his left knee in extension, you raise his LEFT leg to 40°. This causes the patient to complain of pain in his lower back that radiates into his RIGHT calf. With respect to this finding, which of the following statements is true?

(A) The result shows that the patient is not malingering.
(B) A positive straight-leg-raising test is more specific for nerve-root compression on the contralateral side than on the ipsilateral side.
(C) The result is pathognomonic for sacroiliac (SI) sprain syndrome.
(D) It indicates the presence of the cauda equina syndrome.
(E) It indicates the need for surgical intervention to correct radiculopathy.

11. What percentage of patients with herniated discs experience spontaneous resorption of the nucleus pulposus material and resolution of their radicular pain?

(A) 10%
(B) 30%
(C) 50%
(D) 75%
(E) 95%

12. A 28-year-old woman who is pregnant (30 weeks gestation) complains of a 2-week history of right lower back pain that sometimes radiates to her right groin. She experienced no falls nor trauma and has no previous history of back pain. Her pain increases with spine rotation. She is afebrile. Physical examination reveals tenderness of her right sacroiliac joint; also pain in the joint with flexion, abduction, and external rotation of the right hip. Which of the following statements is correct with respect to this condition?

(A) Approximately 90% of afflicted patients are positive for HLA B-27.
(B) Approximately 5% of afflicted patients require surgery.
(C) Most afflicted patients experience resolution of pain within 4–6 weeks.
(D) The afflicted patient can lean forward more easily in the standing position than in other positions.
(E) The pain intensifies when the patient reclines on the unaffected side.

13. An indication for surgical intervention exists in which of the following cases?

(A) Patient A has persistent lower back pain with no radicular features, and no numbness, weakness, nor paresthesia; MRI reveals a disc herniation just abutting the thecal sac.
(B) Patient B is symptomatic with refractory back pain, but no signs of sensory or motor deficit; a large posterolateral herniation of L_5–S_1 is identified on MRI.
(C) Patient C has a 3-week history of lower back pain with right-leg sciatica, but no numbness, weakness, nor paresthesia; a straight-leg-raising test is positive on the right.
(D) Patient D has a 2-day history of severe, right-leg sciatica; patient notices progressive right-leg weakness with 3/5 right toe #1 dorsiflexion on exam; he has an MRI that reveals posterolateral disc herniation at L_4–L_5 impinging on the right L_5 nerve root.
(E) Patient E has an MRI (performed for evaluation of another condition) showing incidental disc herniation impinging on the thecal sac; this patient complains of lower back pain accompanied by no radicular features, numbness, weakness, nor paresthesia; the pain persists despite conservative management for 4 weeks.

DIRECTIONS (Items 14–15): Each of the numbered items or incomplete statements in this section is negatively phrased, as indicated by a capitalized word such as NOT, LEAST, or EXCEPT. Select the ONE lettered answer or completion that is BEST in each case.

14. A 20-year-old woman develops a flexed neck, rotated to one side, with a prominent sternocleidomastoid muscle. You learn that her head rests on several pillows during sleep. No blunt trauma has occurred to her head or neck; and no pain, numbness, or weakness radiates down her arms. She is afebrile. All of the following are appropriate in her management, EXCEPT

- (A) Cervical spine traction
- (B) Reassurance that the symptoms should resolve within 1 week
- (C) Application of moist heat
- (D) Nonsteroidal anti-inflammatory medication
- (E) Soft cervical collar for 2–3 days

15. Of various signs of radiculopathy which of the following is NOT consistent with an L_4 radiculopathy?

- (A) Numbness in anteromedial thigh
- (B) Decreased posterior tibial reflex
- (C) Quadriceps weakness
- (D) Pain radiation into the thigh
- (E) Decreased deep-tendon reflex at knee

ANSWERS AND EXPLANATIONS

1. The answer is E. Among the answer choices, motor vehicle accidents are associated with the greatest number of neck injury and neck pain cases. Most common among these is the "whiplash" injury. Playing football, dancing, practicing martial arts, and swimming produce a minority of cases.

2. The answer is A. Hyperextension of the neck is most commonly associated with a whiplash injury to the neck, typically produced when a victim is in a motor vehicle that is "rear ended" by another vehicle. In addition, hyperextension injuries may occur in contact sports (when the athlete is struck from the rear). "Passive" violent hyperextension carries the head and neck through an arc of extension that exceeds physiologic limits.

3. The answer is D. C_7 is the cervical root most affected in this patient's radiculopathy. Both C_6 and C_7 are the cervical nerve roots most commonly affected by cervical disc herniation and spondylosis.

4. The answer is A. Typically, atrophy of hand and arm muscles is seen in chronic cases of cervical radiculopathy. In acute compression radiculopathies, the EMG shows denervation changes only after 3 or 4 weeks; it shows no changes immediately. Patients do not usually report a history of recent blunt trauma to the neck; rather, they may report their symptoms began after activities that involve repetitive, lateral flexing and rotating of the cervical spine. If cervical radiculopathy is suspected, work-up should begin with cervical spine x-rays, not MRI. Spurling's neck compression test is highly specific, but poorly sensitive. The Spurling test consists of the application of external manual pressure downward on the patient's head with simultaneous turning of the head 30°–50° in the direction opposite to the symptoms and with dorsiflexion of 10°–15°. This applies increased pressure on the intervertebral foramina, on the symptomatic side. If symptoms, particularly radiating arm pain, are produced or worsened, the diagnosis of radiculopathy is confirmed.

5. The answer is E. Lower back pain is the leading cause of disability in patients younger than 50 years. It ranks second to heart disease as cause of disability in patients older than 50 years.

6. The answer is E. NSAIDs for 5–7 days should be recommended for this patient, whose presentation is consistent with lower back strain. An MRI is not used to confirm lower back strain. Prolonged bed rest is not beneficial, according to a recent study. Muscle relaxants are not indicated unless the patient is believed to be experiencing paravertebral muscle spasms. In the absence of controlled, double-blind studies, the effectiveness of physical therapy in this condition is not known.

7. The answer is D. L_4–L_5 and L_5–S_1 are the two levels at which more than 95% of all lumbar disc herniations occur. L_3–L_4 is the next most common level, and the incidence decreases at each higher lumbar level.

8. The answer is A. L_5–S_1 is the level at which this patient's disc herniation is present. The S_1 nerve root supplies motor enervation to plantar flexors that are needed for toe walking. An L_5–S_1 disc herniation affects the S_1 nerve root.

9. The answer is D. Bladder dysfunction is typical in a patient with cauda equina syndrome secondary to a centrally herniated lumbar disc. Being central, the herniated disc compresses the whole cauda (i.e., all the roots that exit at or below the herniation, rather than the usual herniation which compresses a root that exits at one side at a single level). Suspected cauda equina syndrome requires urgent orthopedic or neurosurgical assessment, because the compression of bilateral roots from a given level downward amounts to a cord transection, with all that implies. Patients will have a discrete sensory level on examination with saddle anesthesia, and will have anal sphincter weakness, bilateral lower leg and foot weakness, and bladder dysfunction. In addition to bladder and bowel dysfunction, cauda equina causes bilateral motor symptoms extending even to lower limb paralysis; thus dorsiflexion and ventriflexion would not be normal. Sciatica that involves one leg is typical of a unilateral, single-level herniation. Fever and weight loss are not sequelae of acute cauda equina syndrome.

10. The answer is B. A positive result of a contralateral straight-leg-raising (SLR) test is more specific for nerve-root compression on the contralateral side than on the ipsilateral side. A positive contralateral SLR test is poorly sensitive (approximately 25%), but highly specific for nerve root compression. Most patients with nerve root compression do not require surgery for their condition. A patient who is knowledgeable and motivated to malinger may be aware of the SLR test and simulate a positive response. The crossed-positive SLR is not a finding in sacroiliac (SI) strain. Radiating limb pain is not a symptom of SI strain nor the cauda equina syndrome.

11. The answer is E. Among patients with herniated discs, 95% experience spontaneous resorption of the nucleus pulposus material and resolution of their radicular pain. Only 5% require surgery.

12. The answer is C. Most patients with this condition (sacroiliac sprain syndrome) experience resolution of their symptoms in 4–6 weeks. Pregnancy often aggravates or precipitates this syndrome and other back problems (as a result of the displacement of the center of gravity forward, which places the posture muscles at mechanical disadvantage). Unlike patients with sacroiliitis, patients with sacroiliac sprain syndrome do not tend to be positive for HLA B-27. This condition is not amenable to surgery. Leaning forward is easier for a seated (rather than standing) patient. Reclining on the affected (rather than the unaffected) side increases the pain. Conservative treatment is with NSAIDS, moist heat, and rest; injection of corticosteroid is added if these measures result in no improvement.

13. The answer is D. Surgical intervention is indicated for "patient D" who has a 2-day history of right-leg sciatica, progressive right-weakness with 3/5 right toe #1 dorsiflexion on exam, and an MRI that reveals posterolateral disc herniation at L_4–L_5 impinging on the right L_5 nerve root. Surgical intervention should be considered only to correct radiculopathic causes of sensory or motor deficit, because postoperative surgical inflammation may result in more lower back pain than existed before the surgery. Cauda equina syndrome and progressive weakness are also indications for surgery. The MRI is so sensitive that herniations of no clinical significance may be found. Surgery is not indicated for patient E's asymptomatic disc herniation, found incidentally; and not indicated for patient A's back pain, for which herniation was unlikely to have been the cause. Patient B's herniation is more impressive anatomically, but more clinical evidence is necessary before surgery is considered. Patient C's case shows strong evidence for radiculopathy: The pain pat-

tern is that of sciatica (radiation down the lateral or posterior thigh), and the result of the straight-leg-raising test is positive. However, in the absence of neurologic deficit, conservative therapy can be tried: The patient is instructed to get adequate sleep and to assume the Williams position in bed, both during the night and during 2–3 daytime periods of bed rest of up to an hour each, daily. The Williams position consists of 20°–30° flexion at both the hips and knees, which results in opening the intervertebral spaces dorsally. Conservative therapy may be employed for 1–3 weeks. Electromyography (EMG) and a nerve-conduction velocity study may show evidence of motor unit denervation and slowing of nerve conduction before other evidence of neurologic deficit appears, strengthening the case for surgery for patients A and B. Thus, refractory and severe pain may ultimately be an indicator for surgery, but only when it is persistent for many weeks or months and the indication is supported not only by anatomical evidence (e.g., MRI), but by strong clinical and electrical evidence of radiculopathy.

14. The answer is A. Cervical spine traction is inappropriate treatment for this patient, whose history and physical examination are typical for torticollis. Neck traction, which can be useful in cervical radiculopathy that is caused by nerve root compression, is not useful in torticollis. Symptoms should resolve within 1 week. Reassurance, moist heat, nonsteroidal anti-inflammatory medication, and a soft cervical collar for a few days are all appropriate.

15. The answer is B. Decreased posterior tibial reflex is NOT seen in L_4 radiculopathy. It is seen in L_5 radiculopathy. Numbness in the anteromedial thigh, quadriceps weakness, pain radiation into the thigh, and decreased deep-tendon reflex at the knee are all consistent with an L_4 radiculopathy.

BIBLIOGRAPHY

Maropis CG: Musculoskeletal problems of the neck and back. In *Family Medicine* (House Officer Series). Edited by Rudy DR, Kurowski K. Baltimore, Williams & Wilkins, 1997, pp. 371–382.

Test 23

Common Problems of the Upper Extremities

DIRECTIONS (Items 1–15): Each of the numbered items or incomplete statements in this section is followed by answers or by completions of the statement. Select the ONE lettered answer or completion that is BEST in each case.

1. Which of the following is characteristic of impingement caused by rotator cuff tendinitis?

   (A) Pain is particularly increased by active abduction at the shoulder.
   (B) Flexing the arm to 90°, along with forced internal rotation, gives pain relief.
   (C) Calcium deposits in the rotator cuff tendon, seen on a radiograph, is very sensitive evidence of impingement.
   (D) The onset of pain is very abrupt.
   (E) The pain is localized to the anterior surface of the glenohumeral joint.

2. You examine a 20-year-old woman who fell on her abducted right arm. Her right acromion is prominent, and her right humeral head is palpated anterior to her acromion. Which of the following fractures is commonly associated with this dislocation?

   (A) Fracture of the distal third of the clavicle
   (B) Fracture of the posterior rim of the glenoid
   (C) Transverse fracture of the upper third of the humerus
   (D) Fracture of the posterolateral humeral head
   (E) Coracoid process fracture

3. You suspect a patient has a subluxation of the glenohumeral joint, and you want to see if you can elicit a positive apprehension sign. How must you position the patient's shoulder to produce this sign?

   (A) Adduction, internal rotation, flexion
   (B) Adduction, internal rotation, extension
   (C) Abduction, external rotation, extension
   (D) Abduction, internal rotation, extension
   (E) Abduction, external rotation, flexion

4. A 17-year-old high school student complains of pain in the area of the left shoulder since he used that shoulder to tackle a fellow student the day before. He is afebrile, with blood pressure of 120/80 and pulse of 78. He is holding his left arm with his right hand. The glenohumerus is not tender, and the range of motion is full. The left acromion seems prominent and is reduced by pulling down on the left clavicle. Tenderness and ecchymosis are present around the left acromioclavicular joint. Distal motion and sensory examinations are normal. The next step in management should be which of the following examinations?

   (A) Anteroposterior (AP) and lateral and modified axillary views of the left shoulder
   (B) Magnetic resonance imaging (MRI) of the left shoulder
   (C) Views of both acromioclavicular joints
   (D) An x-ray of the left clavicle
   (E) An arthrogram of the left acromioclavicular joint

5. A 40-year-old racquetball player complains of 3 weeks of right elbow pain, in the absence of any trauma. He denies any other joint pain or illness. Examination shows he has no fever and no elbow joint swelling; he has tenderness over the lateral epicondyle, but no erythema. Active extension of his wrist with his elbow held in extension produces pain. Your diagnosis is which of the following?

   (A) Olecranon bursitis
   (B) Rheumatoid arthritis of the elbow joint
   (C) Pitcher's elbow
   (D) Tennis elbow
   (E) Osteoarthritis of the elbow joint

6. Which of the following is a common initial treatment option for tennis elbow?

   (A) A tightening of the racquet strings
   (B) An elastic bandage on the elbow
   (C) A forearm splint
   (D) A course of medication with an oral corticosteroid
   (E) Daily exercises in which the wrist is flexed repetitively against resistance, while the elbow is held in extension.

7. Which of the following movements exacerbates medial epicondylitis?

(A) Wrist flexion
(B) Wrist extension
(C) Elbow flexion
(D) Elbow extension
(E) Forearm supination

8. A positive result to a Finkelstein's test is seen in which of the following conditions?

(A) Medial epicondylitis
(B) De Quervain's tenosynovitis
(C) Carpal tunnel syndrome
(D) Collateral ligament injury to the proximal interphalangeal joint
(E) Ulnar tunnel syndrome

9. You are examining a 15-year-old girl whose second finger was hit by a softball she was catching yesterday. You find tenderness and ecchymosis over the dorsal aspect of the distal interphalangeal (DIP) joint; the patient can flex the joint fully, but has lost 20° of extension of the joint. X-rays reveal no fracture. What is the appropriate treatment?

(A) Surgical repair of injured extensor mechanism
(B) Continuous splinting in extension for 6 weeks
(C) Continuous splinting in 20° of flexion for 6 weeks
(D) Continuous splinting in extension for 2 weeks
(E) A nonsteroidal anti-inflammatory drug (NSAID) alone

10. You are examining an 18-year-old male patient who has had pain in his third right finger since playing football yesterday. Tenderness and ecchymosis extend from the volar (ventral) aspect of the middle phalanx into the palm. The patient can extend the distal interphalangeal (DIP) joint fully, but he cannot flex the joint. X-rays are normal. Which of the following treatments should you recommend?

(A) Open surgical tendon reattachment in the next few days
(B) Continuous splinting in extension for 6 weeks
(C) Continuous splinting in 90° of flexion for 6 weeks
(D) Cast application from DIP joint to wrist
(E) Corticosteroid injection into the injured tendon

11. A 40-year-old man who sustained a sharp valgus stress to his left fifth finger yesterday (while playing football with his children) complains of pain in the proximal interphalangeal (PIP) joint area in the affected finger. Tenderness is present along the medial aspect of the fifth PIP. Ligament stress testing shows slight laxity of the medial collateral ligament. X-rays of the finger are normal. What is the appropriate treatment?

(A) Limit treatment to prescription of a nonsteroidal inflammatory drug.
(B) Splint the PIP joint in full extension for 6 weeks.
(C) "Buddy-tape" the fifth finger to the fourth finger for 6 weeks.
(D) Apply a cast from the wrist to the PIP joint, with the wrist and finger in full extension, for 6 weeks
(E) Refer the patient for open surgical ligament repair.

12. If not identified and treated appropriately, which of the following injuries can result in a boutonnière (buttonhole) deformity?

(A) Collateral ligament injury
(B) Volar plate tear
(C) Central slip tear
(D) Proximal interphalangeal (PIP) joint dislocation
(E) Rupture of flexor digitorum profundus tendon

13. Which of the following is the most appropriate management for most nonpathologic fractures of the proximal humerus that have 10° displacement?

(A) Open surgical reduction and internal fixation
(B) Immobilization with a shoulder sling for 6 weeks
(C) Hanging arm cast application for external fixation for 6 weeks
(D) Correction of displacement under regional or general anesthesia, followed by immobilization for 6 weeks.
(E) Immobilization with a sling, and the start of active range-of-motion exercises 1 week after the injury

14. You are examining a patient who has a fracture of the middle phalanx, extending into the distal interphalangeal joint, of left finger #4. You should consider referring the patient for open reduction and internal fixation if the percentage of the articular surface involved is greater than

    (A) 5%
    (B) 10%
    (C) 20%
    (D) 30%
    (E) 50%

15. You are examining a 50-year-old man who complains of a 3-month history of numbness and paresthesias in the ulnar portion of his hand and in his fourth and fifth fingers; the symptoms are worse when he flexes at the elbow. You do not notice any atrophy in the arm or fingers. No reproduction of symptoms is produced when his head is rotated to the side while downward compression is applied. Tinel's sign is negative over the volar aspect of the wrist, but positive over the medial posterior elbow. A slight weakness is present in the right fifth finger flexion. The patient can elevate his arm to shoulder level and keep it there for 2 minutes without pain. He has full-strength wrist flexion and extension. His biceps, triceps, and brachioradialis deep-tendon reflexes are all normal. Treatment is required for which of the following conditions?

    (A) Cubital tunnel syndrome
    (B) Carpal tunnel syndrome
    (C) Posterior interosseous nerve entrapment
    (D) Thoracic outlet syndrome
    (E) C-8 cervical radiculopathy

DIRECTIONS (Items 16–17): Each of the numbered items or incomplete statements in this section is negatively phrased, as indicated by a capitalized word such as NOT, LEAST, or EXCEPT. Select the ONE lettered answer or completion that is BEST in each case.

16. Which of the following muscle/tendon units is NOT part of the rotator cuff?

    (A) The supraspinatus
    (B) The infraspinatus
    (C) The teres major
    (D) The teres minor
    (E) The subscapularis

17. Which of the following is NOT recognized as a predisposing cause of carpal tunnel syndrome?

    (A) Pregnancy
    (B) Frequent, repetitive hand movements, performed in occupations such as tool and dye working
    (C) Diabetes mellitus
    (D) Hypothyroidism
    (E) Vitamin B_{12} deficiency

ANSWERS AND EXPLANATIONS

1. The answer is A. A particular increase in pain caused by active abduction at the shoulder is characteristic of impingement secondary to rotator cuff tendonitis. The pain of impingement is also aggravated by forced internal rotation with the arm in flexion. Radiographs are usually normal. Calcium deposits in the rotator-cuff tendon are specific evidence of chronic rotator-cuff tendinitis, a precursor of impingement; but such deposits are not sensitive for acute or subacute disease, either of which may lead to impingement. Magnetic resonance imaging (MRI) can reveal any swollen tendon that may be producing impingement and can identify tears in the rotator cuff. The pain of rotator cuff tendonitis usually has an insidious (not abrupt) onset, and it is poorly localized. Rotator cuff tendonitis occurs, with or without previous shoulder strain, in elderly patients whose tendons have undergone degeneration. It tends to occur in younger patients only if overhand lifting or throwing is a significant component of their work or sports activities. Conservative treatment includes nonsteroidal antiinflammatory drugs and cessation of the overhand activity. If these measures fail, subacromial injection with a corticosteroid may help.

2. The answer is D. A posterolateral humeral head fracture is commonly associated with a right anterior glenohumeral dislocation, the dislocation described in the question. When a patient with this condition falls on the outstretched arm, the humoral head can be forced through the weakest portion of the capsule, the anterior portion. Posterior dislocations are much rarer than anterior ones. Fractures of the posterolateral articular surface of the humerus (Hill-Sachs lesion) are seen frequently, particularly in cases of recurrent dislocations. The anterior rim of the glenoid can sometimes be fractured as the humerus herniates (dislocates) through the anterior capsule, but the posterior rim is not fractured with this type of injury. Fracture of the transverse humerus, coracoid process, and distal clavicle can result from a direct blow to the structure or from force transmitted through a fall onto an outstretched arm, but these fractures are not usually seen in association with anterior shoulder dislocations.

3. The answer is C. Abduction, external rotation, extension is the shoulder position in the patient that can elicit a positive apprehension sign. This position tends to pull the humeral head against the anterior aspect of the glenohumeral joint capsule and can produce subluxation if instability is present there. The maneuvers described in the other answer choices have no special significance.

4. The answer is C. Views of both acromioclavicular joints should be the next step in management. The high-riding left clavicle in this case suggests a grade III or IV sprain of the left acromioclavicular joint. A complete tear of these ligaments would cause an abnormally large separation at the acromioclavicular joint to be visible on the view of the affected side, which could be compared to the view of the contralateral side. Although weights (5–10 pounds) held in the patient's hands would accentuate the separation between the clavicle and acromion in the affected side and permit easier comparison with the contralateral side, this measure could also damage the ligaments further and cause the patient unnecessary discomfort. An MRI and an arthrogram are each capable of showing tears in the capsule, but these tests are more expensive than the other views, and unnecessary. Modified axillary views are most commonly obtained to assess for glenohumeral dislocation, not for acromioclavicular separation. A clavicle x-ray is indicated only if a clavicular fracture is also suspected.

5. The answer is D. This patient has tennis elbow (lateral epicondylitis). It is caused by excessive and repetitive supination, as in the tightening motion during right-handed use of a screw driver, or the isometric use of the same muscle (brachioradialis) in the hand-gripping motion of repetitive handshaking. Another example is repetitive extension at the wrist, as in an improper tennis backhand swing. (The backhand motion should be at the shoulder, with the elbow held rigidly in extension and the wrist in neutral position throughout the swing.) Golfer's (pitcher's) elbow is medial epicondylitis, caused by repetitive, forceful contraction of the forearm, wrist flexor, and pronator muscles that insert into the medial epicondyle. Olecranon bursitis (miner's elbow) is the condition of effusion into the olecranon bursa that results in a spongy "bag of fluid" overlying the extensor surface of the elbow. Both rheumatoid and osteoarthritis, by definition, involve the ulnohumeral (or true elbow) joint, not the lateral (nor medial) epicondyle.

6. The answer is C. Splinting the forearm is a common initial treatment for "tennis elbow" (lateral epicondylitis), the condition described in the preceding question. Although the wrist or forearm is splinted, the elbow itself is neither splinted nor wrapped. This is because the causative motion is forceful extension of the wrist, utilizing the brachioradialis muscle of the forearm. (The lateral epicondyle at the elbow is the point of insertion of the brachioradialis tendon and, therefore, the point of pain and tenderness.) The loosening (rather than tightening) of racquet strings and the increasing of racquet grip sizes for future playing have been found helpful. Ice is sometimes applied to the area within the first 48 hours; heat helps after 48 hours. Aggravating activities (e.g., racquetball) that produce extension of the wrist while the elbow is in extension are avoided until the inflammation subsides. Oral corticosteroid is not used for tennis elbow.

7. The answer is A. Wrist flexion exacerbates medial epicondylitis. Overuse of the flexor pronatus muscle group arising from the medial epicondyle produces the inflammation and pain.

8. The answer is B. A positive Finkelstein's test can be seen in De Quervain's tenosynovitis, an inflammation of the abductor longus pollicis and the extensor brevis tendons within the retinaculum. In this condition, the patient experiences pain in the region of the radial styloid, but usually the pain also radiates proximally as high as the elbow and distally into the thumb. Sometimes, palpable swellings and nodules are present within these tendon sheaths. In the Finkelstein's test, the patient clenches his or her thumb under the other fingers while forming a fist, and then places the wrist into ulnar deviation. The test is positive if it reproduces the patient's pain. A positive Finkelstein's test is not seen in medial epicondylitis, carpal tunnel syndrome, collateral ligament injury to the proximal interphalangeal joint, and ulnar tunnel syndrome.

9. The answer is B. Continuous splinting in extension for 6 weeks is appropriate treatment for the patient's mallet finger, a condition produced by a rupture of the terminal extensor tendon at its insertion into the distal phalanx. A mallet finger is caused by a forceful, abrupt hyperflexion of the distal interphalangeal (DIP) joint (i.e., impact on the tip of a finger that forces the DIP joint into flexion). Splinting in extension for 6–8 weeks is necessary for the extensor mechanism to heal. If treatment is delayed, the patient may become unable to extend the finger at the DIP joint without surgical intervention.

10. The answer is A. Open surgical tendon reattachment in the next few days is the appropriate treatment for this patient's jersey finger. A jersey finger is an avulsion of the flexor digitorum profundus tendon, caused by a violent hyperextension, such as the one that occurs when a hurtling football strikes a player's open hand near the distal interphalangeal (DIP) joint or strikes the digital phalanx of a single digit. The avulsed tendon tends to degenerate, so early reattachment is indicated.

11. The answer is C. "Buddy-taping" the affected fifth finger to the fourth finger for 6 weeks is the appropriate

treatment for this patient's mild, collateral ligament sprain of the finger. Buddy-taping permits better rotational alignment (alignment with respect to an axis drawn through the long axis of the bone) than does splinting in extension or flexion. Nonsteroidal anti-inflammatory drugs (NSAIDS), are for symptomatic relief, and would not provide the immobilization necessary for healing of the soft tissue injury. Splinting the PIP joint in extension would not guard against valgus stress during healing. Applying a cast to joints distal and proximal to the injury is the treatment approach for most fractures, but no fracture is present. Surgery is not indicated for a mild collateral ligament injury (no complete rupture).

12. The answer is C. A central slip tear, if not identified and treated appropriately, can result in a boutonnière deformity (also called a "buttonhole deformity"). A boutonnière deformity of a digit is a flexion deformity of the proximal interphalangeal (PIP) joint with the distal interphalangeal (DIP) joint in hyperextension. It develops weeks after an injury to the central slip, which is the extensor mechanism at, or proximal to, the PIP joint. A forced flexion of the PIP joint is the usual cause of tearing of the central slip; and laceration over the dorsal aspect of the PIP joint is another cause. Note how a boutonnière deformity differs from a swan-neck deformity: A swan-neck deformity is a hyperextension deformity of the PIP joint with flexion of the DIP joint; it results from disruptions to the volar plate structures on the volar aspect of the PIP joint. A forced hyperextension of the PIP joint could produce such an injury. In the presence of a rupture of the flexor digitorum profundus, the patient cannot flex the DIP joint, may have tenderness along the volar aspect of the finger, and may even have a palpable mass, representing the detached profundus tendon in the volar proximal finger or palm. Dislocation of the PIP joint usually damages the collateral ligaments, producing tenderness and variable amounts of laxity within these ligaments along the lateral aspect of the PIP joint line.

13. The answer is E. Immobilization with a shoulder sling, followed, at 1 week after the injury, by the start of active range-of-motion exercises is appropriate management for most nonpathologic fractures of the proximal humerus that have 10° displacement. The most common complication of these fractures, especially among the elderly, is not non-union of the fracture site, but a frozen shoulder. This complication can be forestalled in many cases by the early use of range-of-motion exercises and the discontinuance of the sling once local tenderness has subsided (usually within 2–3 weeks after the injury). Fractures with greater than 45° of displacement and fractures through pathologic bone usually require open reduction and fixation. Hanging arm casts are not used because they increase the incidence of non-union of the fragments.

14. The answer is D. If more than 30% of the articular surface is involved, you should consider open reduction and internal fixation. With closed treatment, a joint involved by this much of the fracture is likely to develop degenerative arthritic change.

15. The answer is A. This man's condition is cubital tunnel syndrome, in which the ulnar nerve is compressed in the groove behind the medial side of the elbow. Treatment consists of a nonsteroidal anti-inflammatory drug (NSAID) and elbow splinting. If the symptoms progress, surgical decompression is an option. Carpal tunnel syndrome (affecting the median nerve) involves only the other fingers of the hand and usually elicits a positive Tinel's sign (distal tingling on percussion) at the volar wrist. Posterior interosseous nerve entrapment primarily produces weakness in some of the wrist extensors. Thoracic outlet syndrome (involving the brachial plexus) usually produces pain as the primary symptom, although numbness and weakness in the neck and upper extremity may also be present. The pain is reproduced if the patient's arm is raised and kept at shoulder level for more than 1 minute. A C-8 cervical radiculopathy could produce the numbness in the ulnad fingers and hand, but would tend to be reproduced with rotation of the head and would not explain the positive Tinel's sign over the cubital tunnel area.

16. The answer is C. The teres major is NOT part of the rotator cuff of the shoulder. The rotator cuff is made up of the tendons of the supraspinatus, subscapularis, infraspinatus, and teres minor, all of which originate from the scapula and insert onto the lateral humeral head. Impingement can occur if the tendons are caught between the humeral head and the coracoacromial arch.

17. The answer is E. Vitamin B_{12} deficiency, well-recognized as a cause of combined systems degeneration, is NOT recognized as a predisposing cause of carpal tunnel syndrome (CTS) as a sole condition. CTS is a compressive irritation to the median nerve as it transverses the carpal canal. In any condition in which fluid overload occurs (e.g., renal failure, heart failure, the myxedema of hypothyroidism, or pregnancy, accumulated fluid in the carpal canal can compress the median nerve. In other conditions, growth of any of the other contents of the carpal canal can also produce this syndrome; examples include synovitis produced by rheumatoid arthritis, mechanical synovitis, and inflammation of the adjacent flexor tendons secondary to repetitive flexion of the wrist. The increased association between CTS and isolated peripheral nerve lesions, including median nerve neuropathy, believed to be secondary to inadequate arteriole perfusion, suggests that tissue ischemia may play a role as well. Any trauma (repetitive wrist movement constitutes trauma) to these nerves exacerbates any other tendency for swelling. Pregnancy and hypothyroidism are primary causes of edema of the carpal tunnel contents. Diabetes (chronic hyperglycemia) results in increased susceptibility of the peripheral nerves (e.g., the median) to causes of swelling.

BIBLIOGRAPHY

Myers A: Common problems of the upper extremities. In *Family Medicine* (House Officer Series). Edited by Rudy DR, Kurowski K. Baltimore, Williams & Wilkins, 1997, pp. 383–398.

Test 24

Mechanical Problems of the Lower Extremities

DIRECTIONS (Items 1–13): Each of the numbered items or incomplete statements in this section is followed by answers or by completions of the statement. Select the ONE lettered answer or completion that is BEST in each case.

1. A 17-year-old high school football player complains of hip pain after being tackled. The pain increases with rotation and lateral bending of the trunk. If this pain is secondary to a bony contusion, where is the most likely site of this contusion?

(A) Iliac crest
(B) Greater trochanter of the hip
(C) Lesser trochanter of the hip
(D) Acetabulum
(E) Pubic ramus

2. A 16-year-old girl, who is a high-school basketball player, complains of about 2 months of bilateral knee pain. She notices increased knee pain during repetitive jump shots and at the cinema when she is sitting with her knees flexed. She denies any trauma or twists to her knees. No effusions are visible or palpable above the knee, and no joint line or patellar area tenderness is present. Which of the following conditions is most consistent with this picture?

(A) Osgood-Schlätter disease
(B) Patellofemoral instability
(C) Prepatellar bursitis
(D) Patellar tendinitis
(E) Medial collateral ligament strain

3. A patient tore his anterior cruciate ligament 8 days ago. The swelling has decreased enough to permit adequate examination. Which of the following is likely to be found?

(A) A negative Lachman test
(B) A negative drawer test
(C) An absence of any knee effusion
(D) Tenderness over the anterior aspect of the knee
(E) An associated torn medial collateral ligament

4. You are examining a patient with a knee injury. You note a 10-millimeter opening when you apply valgus stress (a passive adduction of the lower leg with the knee fixed) with the patient's knee in 20° of flexion and an 8-mm opening when the knee is fully extended. No knee effusion is appreciated, but tenderness is present along the medial joint line. The Lachman test is normal. Which of the following is the likeliest lesion?

(A) Anterior cruciate ligament sprain and associated medial collateral ligament sprain
(B) Lateral collateral ligament sprain
(C) Patellofemoral instability
(D) Posterior cruciate ligament tear
(E) Medial collateral ligament tear with posterior capsule tear

5. With respect to tibial stress fractures, which of the following is correct?

(A) They are ruled out by normal x-rays.
(B) Limited running or jumping is permitted after 2 weeks of treatment.
(C) Amenorrhea is a risk factor.
(D) Cortical thickening is typically found on plain x-rays of early fractures.
(E) Swimming is forbidden for the first 4 weeks of treatment.

6. Which of the following is characteristic of medial tibial stress syndrome?

(A) Adults (as opposed to children in rapid growth) are at increased risk.
(B) Pain is brought on by activity and remains unrelieved for 1–2 days.
(C) Tenderness occurs along the anterior aspect of the distal tibia.
(D) Pes planus (a flattened arch) is a frequent aggravating factor.
(E) Heat application after activity is necessary in initial management.

7. You are examining an afebrile, 30-year-old athlete, who developed pain in the proximal posterior medial aspect of the right calf after long-distance running earlier in the day. He limps on his right leg and cannot "stand on his toes" on the right. Swelling, ecchymosis, and tenderness are present in an area approximately 5 centimeters in diameter in the proximal posterior medial aspect of the calf. Ecchymosis is also present in the lower leg and heel. Which of the following is the most likely diagnosis?

   (A) Achilles tendinitis
   (B) Achilles tendon rupture
   (C) Shin splints
   (D) Tibial stress fracture
   (E) Gastrocnemius tear

8. A 40-year-old athlete complains of posterior distal leg pain. With the patient supine and his knee flexed, you squeeze the mid-portion of his calf and observe no plantar flexion of the foot. Which of the following conditions is most strongly suggested by the result of this test?

   (A) Shin splints
   (B) Ruptured Baker's cyst
   (C) Deep venous thrombosis
   (D) Tibial stress fracture
   (E) Achilles tendon rupture

9. Which of the following ligaments in the ankle is the one most commonly sprained?

   (A) The anterior talofibular ligament
   (B) The anteromedial talofibular ligament
   (C) The calcaneofibular ligament
   (D) The deltoid ligament
   (E) The posterior talofibular ligament

10. On an anterior drawer test that assesses stability of a lateral ankle strain, where do you look for displacement?

   (A) The talus on the calcaneus
   (B) The talus on the navicular
   (C) The fibula on the talus
   (D) The talus on the tibia
   (E) The fibula on the calcaneus

11. You are examining a patient who sprained her right ankle 1 hour earlier. It is a lateral sprain, but, even with stress, no instability is present, and you suspect a second-degree sprain. X-rays reveal an intact ankle mortise and a small avulsion fracture of the lateral malleolus. If the patient has no contraindications to medication or procedures, which of the following treatments is most appropriate?

   (A) Immediate orthopedic consultation
   (B) Application of an ace wrap or soft-cast; decreased weight bearing on the right foot; and a 1-week prescription of an NSAID
   (C) Application of a short-leg walking cast
   (D) Arthroscopic surgery to remove a bone fragment
   (E) Open reduction and internal fixation of the bone fragment

12. For a patient who has a fracture of the posterior process of the talus, which of the following movements is particularly painful?

   (A) Ankle inversion
   (B) Ankle eversion
   (C) Plantar flexion
   (D) Dorsiflexion
   (E) Walking on the heels of the feet

13. The most aggressive management (including short-leg cast application, complete avoidance of weight-bearing, or open reduction and internal fixation) is necessary with respect to metatarsal stress fracture at which of the following sites?

   (A) First metatarsal
   (B) Second metatarsal
   (C) Third metatarsal
   (D) Fourth metatarsal
   (E) Fifth metatarsal

DIRECTIONS (Items 14–15): Each of the numbered items or incomplete statements in this section is negatively phrased, as indicated by a capitalized word such as NOT, LEAST, or EXCEPT. Select the ONE lettered answer or completion that is BEST in each case.

14. In the INITIAL management of a grade II muscle strain of the quadriceps, which of the following is NOT appropriate?

- (A) Stretching of the affected muscles to decrease shortening
- (B) Resistance training to rebuild muscle strength
- (C) Ice and compression with an elastic wrap
- (D) Use of a crutch until the patient can ambulate without limping
- (E) Avoidance of strenuous physical activity

15. Which of the following symptoms is NOT characteristic of a meniscal tear within the knee?

- (A) A "pop" or tearing sensation at the time of injury
- (B) Immediate, intense pain
- (C) A sensation that the knee is "locking"
- (D) An occasional sensation that the knee is "giving out"
- (E) The development of knee effusion

ANSWERS AND EXPLANATIONS

1. The answer is A. The iliac crest is the most likely site of the bony contusion causing this patient's pain. This bony contusion, called a "hip pointer," is usually produced by a direct blow to the iliac crest (e.g., the blow of a helmet during a football tackle). A blow to the greater trochanter (or overuse of the thigh abductor muscles at the insertion on the greater trochanter) produces pain and tenderness at the prominence of the trochanter. Sometimes trochanteric bursitis develops and produces pain radiating down the anterior thigh. The lesser trochanter of the hip, the acetabulum, and the pubic ramus are rarely involved in contusions in athletes.

2. The answer is B. Patellofemoral instability, which causes a great deal of pain during activities in which the knee is flexed (e.g., jumping during basketball, bicycle riding, running) is probably the cause of this patient's problem. Also called "chondromalacia patellae," patellofemoral instability represents an abnormal tracking of the patella through the normal range of motion of the knee. The pain is usually felt diffusely behind the patella. Osgood-Schlätter disease (traction apophysitis) occurs in adolescent boys during pubertal growth. It is caused by microtrauma to the anterior tibial tubercle. The pain is located in the tibial tubercle. Medial collateral ligament strain is caused by a forced valgus stress (such as that caused when a football player is tackled or blocked directly from the side). The pain is felt on the medial aspect of the knee. Prepatellar bursitis ("housemaid's knee") is caused by repeated kneeling on a hard surface. The pain is on the superficial inferior midline of the knee, just below the patella. Patellar tendinitis is not a clinical entity.

3. The answer is E. A torn medial collateral ligament is likely to be found in association with a torn anterior cruciate ligament of 8 days duration. In the Lachman test, the knee is flexed 10°–20°, and the lower thigh is grasped with one hand while the other hand pulls the tibia anteriorly. A positive result, the loss of the normal abrupt arrest of this movement and the ability to pull the tibia further forward than it can be pulled on the other leg, indicates that the anterior cruciate ligament has been torn. In the drawer test, a test that also looks for the absence of the normal abrupt halt to anterior translation, but that holds the knee in 90° of flexion, a positive result also indicates a torn anterior cruciate ligament. A large knee effusion is usually produced in these injuries, although it may be somewhat decreased after 8 days. The patient may have medial or lateral joint line tenderness, but no anterior aspect tenderness, secondary to menisci or collateral ligament injury.

4. The answer is E. A medial collateral ligament tear with posterior capsule tear are the expected lesions. Valgus is a turning out; valgus knee stress is an attempt to force the lower leg laterally, which stresses the medial collateral ligament. It is accomplished best when the knee is partially flexed. Varus is a turning in; varus knee stress involves the opposite stress and tests the lateral collateral ligaments. Even with a collateral ligament tear, if the knee is in full extension, components of the posterior capsule stabilize the knee during valgus and varus stress; therefore, an opening, even with full knee extension, indicates a posterior capsule tear also. Both anterior and posterior cruciate tears tend to produce abnormal Lachman tests, with no abrupt stop to tibial forward or backward displacement. Neither tears nor strains in these ligaments produce laxity when valgus and varus stressing is performed, unless other injuries are present as well. In patellofemoral instability, some laxity and apprehension may be present in patellar movement, but no abnormalities are seen on valgus, varus, or Lachman tests.

5. The answer is C. Amenorrhea is a risk factor for tibial stress fractures. Amenorrhea that results from an athlete's overly vigorous exercise program is a hypothalamic response to the weight loss produced by the exercise. More running produces more weight loss, which results in ovarian hypofunction and premature osteoporosis; repetitive running increases the chances for development of stress fractures. Plain x-rays do not always rule out stress fractures; bone scans may be necessary. Cortical thickening is a sign of advanced, not early, stress fractures. Running and jumping are forbidden for at least 6 weeks, but swimming is permitted, even during the healing period.

6. The answer is D. Pes planus ("flatfoot," "fallen arch") is a frequent aggravating factor of medial tibial stress syndrome (TSS). TSS is pain along the posterior medial edge of the tibia that occurs early in an athlete's running program or when the program is resumed after a period of inactivity. The pain usually dissipates within several hours. Pain that lasts longer than several hours after termination of exercise should be investigated for stress fracture. Rapid growth, pes planus, and hyperpronation are risk factors for TSS. The other answer choices are not characteristic of TSS

7. The answer is E. A gastrocnemius tear is the most likely cause of this athlete's pain. Ecchymosis distal to the injury site is typical. Tenderness and swelling are more proximal in gastrocnemius tears than in Achilles tendon tears. Achilles tendinitis manifests local tenderness (not involving the muscle), along with pain, upon the patient's attempt to stand or walk "on his toes." Achilles tendon rupture produces inability to toe-stand (as with gastrocnemius rupture), but pain is located in the tendon and a gap deformity is palpable and visible in the tendon. Swelling and ecchymosis are not typical in shin splints or tibial stress fractures, both of which produce anterior leg pain.

8. The answer is E. Achilles tendon rupture is the probable diagnosis in this case, as indicated by the absent plantar flexion in response to the Thompson test (test described in the question). An intact Achilles tendon would have produced plantar flexion. Achilles tendon rupture produces inability to toe-stand; pain is located in the tendon and a gap deformity is palpable and visible in the tendon. In shin splints, caused by overuse of the anterior leg muscles (ankle dorsiflexors) in unconditioned athletes, activity results in anterior to posterior medial leg pain; tenderness is not a prominent feature. In a tibial stress fracture, weight bearing produces pain in the bone. A Baker's cyst (popliteal cyst) is an evagination of the synovial joint lining of the knee. When it ruptures, it produces a painful swelling of the calf, but the Thompson test is negative, and the patient is able to toe-stand, albeit with pain. Thrombosis of deep calf veins results in calf tenderness and a positive Homan's sign. The Homan's test (poorly sensitive for deep venous thrombosis) involves forced dorsiflexion of the foot; the result is positive if the patient complains of calf pain. This test could be falsely positive in the presence of a ruptured Baker's cyst, therefore, venography and Dopler studies are needed to differentiate between the two.

9. The answer is A. The anterior talofibular ligament is the ligament in the ankle most likely to be sprained. Pain and tenderness are usually located just anterior and inferior to the lateral malleolus. Located laterally with the fibula, this ligament is vulnerable to the likeliest stress at the ankle, the inversion injury (foot turning inward as the body's center of gravity is carried laterally past the top of the joint). A mild sprain (pain with little swelling) is amenable to "walking it off." A moderate sprain manifests the "goose egg" swelling over the lateral malleolus. After 24 hours of cold packs and keeping the ankle from bearing weight, the patient can walk with a soft ankle-immobilizing splint or crutches, for as long as the pain dictates. After 2–3 days, extravasated (blue) subcutaneous blood appears; patients need assurance that this delayed appearance is normal. After 10 days, splinting

usually makes normal (nonathletic) activity possible. Healing is not complete for at least 3 weeks.

10. The answer is D. The talus on the tibia is where you look for displacement on an anterior drawer test. The tibia is stabilized and the calcaneus is pulled forward. Anterior displacement of the talus on the tibia signifies a positive test. As with the anterior drawer test of the knee, a positive test indicates loss of integrity of the ligament that prevents slipping of the lower half of the joint (talus) anteriorly with respect to the upper half (tibia and fibula as a block). A positive anterior drawer test indicates a more severe sprain. A VERY severe sprain is defined as the rupture of all three tendons (i.e., including the calcaneofibular and the posterior talofibular ligaments); such a strain may be suspected by the degree of movement on the anterior drawer test, but is confirmed by an x-ray showing tilt of the talus with stress. Consultation is necessary and surgery may be indicated.

11. The answer is B. Application of an ace wrap or soft cast, decreased weight-bearing on the right foot, and a 1-week prescription of an NSAID constitute appropriate treatment in this case. Treatment for an avulsion fracture is no different than for the sprain itself.

12. The answer is C. Plantar flexion is particularly painful for a patient who has a fracture of the posterior process of the talus. Rapid plantar flexing of the ankle (the bounce test) also produces pain in the posterior talus. Forced passive ankle inversion aggravates the pain of a lateral ankle sprain; forced passive ankle eversion aggravates the pain of a medial ankle sprain. Dorsiflexion causes pain in a ruptured, partially torn, or sprained Achilles tendon or plantar fasciitis (any injury or inflammation of a structure stretched by dorsiflexion). Walking on the heels of the feet involves volitional activation of the same tissues with the same results. Weakness or inability to heel-walk would occur with an Achilles rupture

13. The answer is E. A stress fracture at the fifth metatarsal site requires the most aggressive management. Metaphyseal fifth metatarsal stress fractures carry a higher risk than other metatarsal stress fractures of becoming complete fractures and failing to unite. Stress fractures at the first, second, third, and fourth metatarsal sites respond to conservative measures (e.g., cessation of offending activities for 6 weeks, along with a stiff-soled shoe for 3 weeks) without progressing to complete fracture.

14. The answer is B. Resistance training to rebuild muscle strength is NOT appropriate in the initial management of a grade II muscle strain of the quadriceps. Such exercises should not be initiated until swelling and pain have resolved and full range of motion has been restored. Generally, healing is complete within 3 weeks. Ice and compression with an elastic wrap is useful in the first 24 hours. Stretching of the affected muscles to decrease shortening, use of a crutch, and avoidance of strenuous activity are appropriate throughout the period of healing.

15. The answer is B. Immediate, intense pain is NOT characteristic of a meniscal tear within the knee. Pain is often minimal, especially immediately after the injury. A "pop" or tearing sensation at the time of injury, a sensation that the knee is "locking," an occasional sensation that the knee is "giving out," and the development of knee effusion are all typical with regard to a meniscal tear within the knee.

BIBLIOGRAPHY

Sickles RT: Mechanical problems of the lower extremities. In *Family Medicine* (House Officer Series). Edited by Rudy DR, Kurowski K. Baltimore, Williams & Wilkins, 1997, pp 399–412.

Test 25

Approach to the Patient with Rheumatic Disease

DIRECTIONS (Items 1–15): Each of the numbered items or incomplete statements in this section is followed by answers or by completions of the statement. Select the ONE lettered answer or completion that is BEST in each case.

1. A 35-year-old woman complains of numerous musculoskeletal aches, pains, "swelling," morning stiffness in several joints, and poor sleep quality of several months' duration. She thinks these problems may have begun some time after she miscarried a fetus 4 months ago. Examination is normal except for areas of tenderness. These are at bilateral matched points along the suboccipital ridge, left anterior cervical area at the C5–C6 interspace, bilateral second costochondral junctions, both lateral epicondyles, the medial fat pad of the left knee, and the right greater trochanter. No joint synovial swelling is present, even in areas in which the patient perceives swelling. Laboratory tests show normal sedimentation rate and complete blood count (CBC), as well as negative determinations for antinuclear antibody (ANA) and rheumatoid factor. This patient's condition is which of the following?

(A) Tennis elbow
(B) Trochanteric bursitis
(C) Cervical disc herniation
(D) Fibromyalgia
(E) Depression

2. A 60-year-old man complains that he lost right shoulder mobility after shoveling snow 6 months earlier. He denies any other joint complaint, any fall, and any blunt trauma to the shoulder or neck. He is afebrile, with strong radial pulses and normal results of motor and sensory examinations of the hands and arms. No tenderness is present in the cervical spine; and the patient can fully rotate, flex, and extend his cervical spine without reproducing the symptoms. He can actively abduct the shoulder to approximately 30°, but it can be moved passively to approximately 50°. No muscular bulging is evident with elbow flexion or extension, and no joint deformities or swelling is apparent. The most likely diagnosis is which of the following conditions?

(A) Injury to the rotator cuff
(B) Osteoarthritis (OA) of the glenohumeral joint
(C) OA of the acromioclavicular (AC) joint
(D) Biceps tendinitis
(E) Rupture of the long arm of the biceps tendon

3. With respect to patients with fibromyalgia (fibrositis), which statement is correct?

(A) They benefit from nonsteroidal anti-inflammatory drugs (NSAIDs).
(B) They complain of poor sleep quality.
(C) They have evidence of neuropathy consistent with the paresthesias they report.
(D) They have elevated sedimentation rates and C-reactive protein (CRP).
(E) They demonstrate diffuse joint effusion.

4. A 35-year-old man has a long history of arthralgias that previous physicians have been unable to explain. Physical examination demonstrates hyperextension at the knees, elbows, and fifth metacarpophalangeal (MCP) joints. Sedimentation rate is 10 mm/hr, blood count is normal, rheumatoid factor is negative, and uric acid is 3.2 mg/dl. The patient denies stiffness of the joints. The diagnosis is which of the following conditions?

(A) Generalized osteoarthritis (OA)
(B) Rheumatoid arthritis (RA)
(C) Generalized gout
(D) Ehlers-Danlos syndrome
(E) Patellar chondromalacia

5. A 60-year-old man who played halfback in football in high school and college complains of right groin pain radiating down his anterior thigh that has progressed during the last 5 years. In the mornings, as well as after periods of inactivity, he has noticed stiffness for approximately 5 minutes. Symptoms seem to worsen during the 12–24 hours before frontal weather systems. The patient denies recent falls or trauma. Examination shows he is afebrile and has no visible joint deformities, but he has poor, painful right hip abduction and slight pain on palpation. His sedimentation rate is normal. The likeliest diagnosis is which of the following conditions?

(A) Rheumatoid arthritis (RA)
(B) Gouty arthritis
(C) Trochanteric bursitis
(D) Contusion of the right iliac crest ("hip pointer")
(E) Osteoarthritis (OA)

6. Which of the following statements about osteoarthritis (OA) is correct?

(A) OA in women tends to involve a more limited number of joints than in men.
(B) Patients with OA typically complain of 1–2 hours of morning stiffness.
(C) OA is likelier to appear in a joint that has experienced significant trauma than in one that has not.
(D) Pain occurs only when the involved joint is experiencing active range of motion.
(E) OA is always symptomatic, with pain, crepitus, and stiffness.

7. You are planning on initiating pharmacologic therapy for a 65-year-old woman with early, minimal arthralgias from osteoarthritis (OA) who has no other health problems and no contraindications to any medication. Of the following agents, which is the most appropriate for this patient?

(A) Acetaminophen
(B) Ibuprofen
(C) Coated aspirin
(D) Oral prednisone
(E) Oral propoxyphene

8. Which of the following changes seen on x-rays would be most consistent with osteoarthritis (OA)?

(A) Joint erosions
(B) Osteoporosis of articulating bone
(C) Asymmetrical joint space narrowing
(D) Subperiosteal bone resorption
(E) Calcifications of the hyaline and fibrous cartilage

9. Which of the following is the most common mechanism for development of septic arthritis?

(A) Complication of intra-articular injection
(B) Contiguous spread of a cellulitis into the joint
(C) Hematogenous spread
(D) Contiguous spread of osteomyelitis into the joint
(E) Recent, closed trauma to the joint

10. A 22-year-old man who has had diffuse joint pains, a petechial rash on his fingers that resolved after 4 days, and an elevated temperature that also resolved, now complains of pain in his right knee. He has a right knee effusion. With respect to the most probable condition, which of the following statements is correct?

(A) Affected patients seldom seem very ill.
(B) Identification of the organism requires synovial, urethral, pharyngeal, or rectal cultures, or more than one of these.
(C) Septic effusions arc typically polyarticular.
(D) Parenteral penicillin is usually the treatment of choice.
(E) Systemic dissemination is common in patients infected with this organism.

11. A 60-year-old man complains of bouts of intense pain in his dorsal foot. Which of the following confirms (with certainty) a diagnosis of gouty arthritis?

(A) The patient complains of pain in the first metatarsophalangeal (MTP) joint.
(B) The patient has an elevated serum uric acid level.
(C) The patient has an erythematous, painful joint associated with fever and serum leukocytosis.
(D) A 24-hour urine uric acid is less than 800 mg/dl.
(E) Aspirated joint fluid viewed with a polarizing microscope shows negatively birefringent, needle-shaped crystals within white blood cells (WBCs).

12. With respect to calcium pyrophosphate deposition disease (CPDD, pseudogout), which of the following statements are correct?

(A) The incidence of CPDD increases with patient age.
(B) The crystals in CPDD are easier to detect than those in gout.
(C) CPDD may be associated with hypoparathyroidism.
(D) CPDD typically affects only the weight-bearing joints.
(E) CPDD attacks are always monoarticular.

13. An 8-year-old girl has had rheumatic fever (RF) and has developed murmurs of aortic and mitral regurgitation. You treated her with high-dose salicylates, bed rest, and penicillin for 10 days. She is now 6 weeks into the course, is no longer taking salicylates, and is asymptomatic. You clear her for returning to school. Which is the most appropriate treatment now?

(A) Low-dose, daily salicylates
(B) Oral corticosteroids
(C) Oral, low-dose, daily penicillin
(D) Monthly shots of intramuscular benzathine penicillin
(E) Penicillamine

14. Which of the following joints is commonly spared in patients with rheumatoid arthritis (RA)?

(A) Distal interphalangeal joint
(B) Metacarpophalangeal (MCP) joint
(C) Hip
(D) Wrist
(E) Cricoarytenoid joint

15. Among children who have arthritis, which of the following is most at risk for development of associated iritis?

(A) A child with rheumatic fever (RF)
(B) A child with Still's disease [systemic onset juvenile rheumatoid arthritis (JRA)]
(C) A child with polyarticular JRA
(D) A child with JRA that involves fewer than four joints within the first 6 months
(E) Any child with JRA and a positive rheumatoid factor

DIRECTIONS (Item 16): The numbered item in this section is negatively phrased, as indicated by the capitalized word NOT. Select the ONE lettered answer or completion that is BEST in this case.

---

16. Which of the following is NOT a treatment option for a patient with an acute gout attack?

(A) Ibuprofen 800 mg 4 times a day with food
(B) Aspirin 20 mg/kg/day
(C) Colchicine 0.5 mg every 8 hours until the attack resolves or nausea and emesis develop
(D) Intra-articular corticosteroid
(E) Intramuscular corticosteroid

ANSWERS AND EXPLANATIONS

1. The answer is D. This patient's condition is fibromyalgia, which is characterized by multiple aches and pains. For a diagnosis of fibromyalgia, at least 11 of 18 specific points (9 pairs of bilateral points) must be tender. Aside from the points found positive in this patient are the paired posterior superior iliac spine areas plus the paired areas of the supraspinatus and trapezius muscles. In addition, a precipitating traumatic event (physical or emotional) and sleep difficulties are common.

Fibromyalgia can be confused with rheumatoid arthritis (RA) because of a subjective sense of swelling (unconfirmed on examination) and morning stiffness. However, scrutiny reveals that the stiffness of fibromyalgia is caused by hypertonic musculature, rather than joint involvement. In RA, an elevated sedimentation rate is almost always present, and a positive rheumatoid factor occurs in 85% of cases. The antinuclear antibody (ANA) is an indicator of other autoimmune diseases. Neither tennis elbow nor trochanteric bursitis explains the clinical picture, despite tenderness in the appropriate areas. Although no particular finding rules out depression, the musculoskeletal complaints are not part of the clinical picture of depression.

2. The answer is A. A rotator cuff injury is the most likely cause of this patient's loss of shoulder mobility. The rotator cuff is composed of the tendons of the supraspinatus, infraspinatus, subscapularis, and teres major, as they merge and insert onto the lateral humeral head. Tears in the tendon can occur just before its insertion onto the humeral head, and these are called rotator cuff tears. Most rotator cuff tears are seen in the elderly, in whom the tendons have degenerated with age and are easily affected by minor strain or trauma. Such tears are unusual in young adults unless significant trauma has occurred to the shoulder (especially in the event of an anterior dislocation). Mild cases usually respond to rest, non-steroidal anti-inflammatory drugs (NSAIDs), and, when pain and inflammation are reduced, a course of range-of-motion exercises. Corticosteroid injections into the subacromial space can be added if symptoms persist. Surgical reanastomosis of the tendon (often in conjunction with acromioplasty) can be performed if conservative measures fail, if the tear is especially large, or if a younger patient is unwilling to accept any loss of shoulder function.

With respect to the other answer choices: Biceps tendinitis produces anterior, upper humeral area pain and tenderness, aggravated by elbow flexion. A rupture of the tendon of the long arm of the biceps, on flexion, results in a muscular mass (which eventually becomes painless) in the upper arm. Selective, symptomatic osteoarthritis (OA) of the shoulder joints is unusual relative to the more common rotator cuff injuries, which particularly affect abduction. More to the point, passive motion would aggravate OA of either the shoulder or the acromioclavicular (AC) joint.

3. The answer is B. Patients who have fibromyalgia (fibrositis) usually complain of poor sleep quality. This association is interesting, because sleep studies find decreased delta waves in most fibromyalgia patients and development of signs of fibromyalgia in some normal people whose delta sleep patterns are experimentally disturbed. Patients with fibromyalgia often have multiple tender points (see the explanation for question 1). Physical and laboratory evidence of joint inflammation is absent in these patients, as is documentable neuropathy, despite frequent complaints of paresthesias. Nonsteroidal anti-inflammatory drugs (NSAIDs) are useful only if patients have a superimposed osteoarthritis (OA) or other NSAID-responsive condition. Treatment, including a support group and a sedating antidepressant (e.g., amitriptyline), addresses factors (usually psychological) that disrupt the sleep cycle. Objective evidence of joint involvement and serologic evidence of inflammatory disease are absent.

4. The answer is D. The likeliest diagnosis is Ehlers-Danlos syndrome, a group of disorders whose most common manifestations include soft, hyperextensible skin; joint laxity; open, gaping wounds; and easy bruisability. To test for Ehlers-Danlos syndrome, the knee, elbow, and metacarpophalangeal (MCP) joint number five should be assessed for passive hyperextension. Most cases are inherited on an autosomal dominant basis and a few as autosomal recessives or X-linked recessives, but the hereditary pattern of each type is different. Most subtypes have no specific therapy (except for type VI, a lysyl hydroxylase deficiency, which is sometimes responsive to ascorbic acid oral supplementation), and most subtypes produce no loss in life expectancy. Ehlers-Danlos syndrome leads to arthralgias as a result of overuse aggravated by loose joint capsules. There are no osteophytic spurs [as in osteoarthritis (OA)], morning stiffness or gelling, or serologic abnormalities such as in rheumatoid arthritis (RA). Gout is seldom (if ever) generalized and usually manifests as hyperuricemia.

5. The answer is E. Osteoarthritis (OA) is the likeliest diagnosis because of the relationship to earlier trauma, the aggravation by frontal weather, and the brief period of morning stiffness. The location in the true groin, radiation down the anterior thigh, and aggravation by hip abduction are signs of involvement of the hip joint. Rheumatoid arthritis (RA) is unlikely for several reasons: RA remains monoarticular for as long as 5 years; its characteristic morning stiffness and postinactivity gelling last a minimum of 30 minutes, rather than a few minutes; and it is associated with an increased sedimentation rate. Gout is unlikely because, although it may occur in any joint, it seldom affects an isolated joint (or joints) chronically, attacks occur over time, and the disease eventually (well within 5 years) affects the great toe metatarsophalangeal (MTP) joint. Greater trochanter bursitis pain is unlikely because, although pain radiates down the anterior thigh, the pain is located at the trochanter (along with point tenderness) and is not aggravated by hip abduction or by frontal weather. A "hip pointer," as a contusion, commonly occurs in football players, but it causes acute (never chronic or recurrent) pain and tenderness at the iliac crest. It does not involve the hip joint and is not aggravated by hip abduction.

6. The answer is C. Osteoarthritis (OA) is more likely to occur in a joint that has experienced significant trauma than in one that has not. Women are likely to have more severe disease than men, with more numbers of involved joints and more deformity. Typical stiffness lasts for less than 30 minutes. Both passive and active range of motion produce pain in the involved joint. OA is frequently asymptomatic for years.

7. The answer is A. Acetaminophen is the first-line therapy for osteoarthritis (OA), especially in elderly patients or in those whose principal complaint is arthralgia. Nonsteroidal anti-inflammatory drugs (NSAIDs), including aspirin and ibuprofen, are associated with an increased risk of gastric ulcer and gastritis in elderly patients, and should be avoided except when acetaminophen fails to control symptoms. (Coated aspirin diminishes the risk, but does not eliminate it.) Elderly patients are more likely than others to experience acute gastrointestinal hemorrhage as their first side effect from NSAIDs, with no previous gastrointestinal warning symptoms. Oral or intramuscular corticosteroids are not used, but appropriately spaced intra-articular corticosteroid injections are sometimes used in the management of acute flairs of OA. Glucocorticoids have no place in the therapy of this noninflammatory condition. Narcotic analgesics (e.g., propoxyphene) are not used in the treatment of OA, except in some very elderly patients who cannot achieve pain control with acetaminophen and cannot tolerate NSAIDs, or in whom surgical approaches are contraindicated.

8. The answer is C. Asymmetrical joint space narrowing is a typical x-ray finding in osteoarthritis (OA). Bone spurs, joint space narrowing from loss of articular cartilage, and subchondral new bone formation are typical of OA. Although some inflammatory subcategories of OA are erosive, OA is generally not an erosive process. Osteoporosis (a loss of bone mass per unit volume) is most commonly seen as primary osteoporosis, especially in postmenopausal women; but secondary causes [including rheumatoid arthritis (RA)] are also seen. OA is not a cause of secondary osteoporosis. Subperiosteal bone resorption is relatively specific for hyperparathyroidism and not seen in OA; it is best seen in radiographs of the fingers where, on the radial surface of the phalanx, the cortex has undergone resorption, leaving the lacy, irregular edge of the underlying bone. Calcification of the hyaline and fibrous cartilage (chondrocalcinosis) is typical of calcium pyrophosphate deposition disease (CPDD) and is not seen in OA.

9. The answer is C. Hematogenous spread is the most common mechanism for the development of septic arthritis, although the mechanisms given in the other answer choices may also result in septic joint development. The bacteria that most commonly produce septic arthritis in adults are *Neisseria gonorrhoeae, Staphylococcus aureus, Streptococcus pyogenes,* and, rarely, gram-negative bacilli. The organisms most commonly responsible for postoperative cases and cases involving prosthetic joints include *Staphylococcus epidermidis, S. aureus,* and gram-negative bacilli. In addition, group B streptococci account for many cases in infants, and *Haemophilus influenzae* is found in many cases in children.

10. The answer is B. Synovial, urethral, pharyngeal, or rectal cultures, or more than one of these, are usually required for identification of the organism responsible for gonococcal arthritis, the condition to which this man's symptoms point. Patients with this condition usually present in a very ill state. Although a polyarthropathy may be present (apparently caused by a systemic immune response), septic effusions are typically monoarticular. Penicillin is not ideal for the treatment of gonorrhea, let alone gonococcal arthritis. The treatment of choice is intravenous ceftriaxone 1 g/day. Gonococcal arthritis is accompanied by systemic dissemination in only 2%–3% of cases.

11. The answer is E. Aspirated joint fluid that shows negatively birefringent, needle-shaped crystals within white blood cells (WBCs) when viewed with a polarizing microscope confirms gout. Pain in the first metatarsophalangeal (MTP) joint is classic, but not diagnostic [e.g., osteoarthritis (OA) may be a cause]. Patients may have hyperuricemia from overproduction or underexcretion and yet never have attacks of gouty arthritis. Septic joints are also erythematous with fever and serum leukocytosis. An interesting question concerns 24-hour urine uric acid. Obviously, a finding of less than 800 mg/dl in 24 hours is correlated with normality, but underexcretion with mild overproduction of uric acid may occur with gouty arthritis, and such patients excrete less than 800 mg/dl per 24 hours. These make up the great majority of cases. Only 10% of patients are primarily overproducers and excrete more than 1000 mg/dl in 24 hours.

12. The answer is A. The incidence of calcium pyrophosphate deposition disease (CPDD or pseudogout), especially in its idiopathic form, increases with patient age. CPDD can closely mimic gout, with similar potential joint involvement, including inflammation of the first metatarsophalangeal (MTP) joint and similar degrees of joint inflammation and pain. Both CPDD and gout can be exacerbated by trauma, surgery, or dehydration. However, CPDD is more likely than gout to involve the knee. Gout, but not CPDD, can be produced by thiazide diuretics, low-dose aspirin, and radiologic contrast dye. Gout, not CPDD, is accompanied by visible tophi on the extensor surfaces of the extremities or on the pinna of the ear. The only certain method of distinguishing between CPDD and gout is examination of aspirated joint fluid for crystals. A polarizing microscope shows either the needle-shaped, brightly negative, birefringent, monosodium urate crystals of gouty arthritis; the more rectangular, weakly positive, birefringent, calcium pyrophosphate crystals of pseudogout; or both, if the two conditions coexist. In addition, CPDD is associated with hyperparathyroidism (not hypoparathyroidism), gout, hypothyroidism, and hemochromatosis. It is more likely than gout to be polyarticular, and it is not limited to the weight-bearing joints.

13. The answer is D. The girl should receive monthly shots of intramuscular benzathine penicillin for 5 years in an effort to prevent further group A beta-hemolytic streptococcus infections that could lead to exacerbation of the rheumatic fever (RF) and further damage to the cardiac valves. RF is a syndrome of autoimmune inflammation of various tissues in response to infection with group A beta-hemolytic streptococcus. By definition, RF includes inflammation of the valvular endocardium but usually synovia of joints as well (if the latter occurs without valvulitis, RF cannot be diagnosed). In all but fewer than 10% of cases, the course of disease is self-limited (about 6 weeks). During this time, after treatment of the streptococcal infection with penicillin or other appropriate antibiotics, management consists of high-dose salicylates [e.g., nearly 1 grain (60 mg)/lb/day]. Corticosteroids have not been proven to be of value. Oral penicillin at a full therapeutic dosage is appropriate for the 10-day acute course but is impractical for long-term maintenance. Penicillamine is a third-tier treatment for RA.

14. The answer is A. In rheumatoid arthritis (RA), the distal interphalangeal joint is spared, in contrast to osteoarthritis (OA), in which the distal interphalangeal joints and weight-bearing joints are typically involved. Another condition that frequently attacks the distal interphalangeal joint is one of the patterns of arthritis seen in psoriatic arthritis. Patients with this condition often have prominent pitting and grooving in their fingernails. Rarely, psoriatic arthritis precedes for varying or even indefinite periods the typical skin lesions. Involvement of the cricoarytenoid joint in RA may cause patients to complain of laryngeal pain and swallowing difficulty. All other joints mentioned may be involved in RA.

15. The answer is D. A child whose juvenile rheumatoid arthritis (JRA) involves four or fewer joints within the first 6 months (called pauciarticular JRA) is the one most at risk for development of associated iritis. A positive antinuclear antibody (ANA) titer also increases the risk. Patients with pauciarticular JRA always test negative for rheumatoid factor, whereas those with polyarticular JRA and Still's disease (JRA with systemic onset) may or may not test positive. Patients with pauciarticular JRA require periodic slit-lamp examinations by an ophthalmologist. Children with Still's disease, a variant of JRA, appear acutely ill. They have fever, weight loss, rashes, and possibly pleural and pericardial effusion, hepatosplenomegaly, or adenopathy. In a few years, they often develop a severe polyarticular arthritis, but not iritis. Still's disease is initially treated with aspirin. Patients who have polyarticular JRA are often also ill with fevers, adenopathy, and hepatosplenomegaly, but they tend not to develop iritis. RF has no relationship to JRA, and coexistence of the two conditions would be a rare coincidence.

16. The answer is B. Aspirin is NOT a treatment option for a patient with an acute gout attack. Aspirin in low doses may actually exacerbate gout by decreasing renal excretion of uric acid. All other nonsteroidal anti-inflammatory drugs (NSAIDs), including ibuprofen, are excellent first-round choices for treatment of acute gout. Intra-articular and intramuscular corticosteroids may be useful, especially in patients who cannot tolerate NSAIDs. Colchicine is not popular for acute therapy because significant nausea, emesis, and diarrhea often develop before doses adequate to treat the gouty flare can be achieved; however, it remains a potentially effective agent for acute therapy.

BIBLIOGRAPHY

Seigel LB, Gall EP: Approach to the patient with rheumatic disease. In *Family Medicine* (House Officer Series). Edited by Rudy DR, Kurowski K. Baltimore, Williams & Wilkins, 1997, pp 413–438.

Test 26

Musculoskeletal Problems in Children

DIRECTIONS (Items 1–7): Each of the numbered items or incomplete statements in this section is followed by answers or by completions of the statement. Select the ONE lettered answer or completion that is BEST in each case.

1. You are examining a newborn. With the baby's hips abducted 90°, you place your long fingers on the greater trochanters. As you press the trochanters anteriorly, you feel the distinct sensation on the left of the trochanter moving anteriorly and medially. With regard to this condition, which of the following statements is correct?

(A) The procedure described in the Barlow maneuver.
(B) Presence of symmetrical hip creases is a highly sensitive but not highly specific sign.
(C) Universal sonographic screening of newborns is recommended.
(D) Delayed diagnosis may lead to avascular necrosis of the hip.
(E) Family history is positive in 80% of cases.

2. Which of the following combinations of characteristics entirely applies to the condition that affects the patient in question 1?

(A) Males are affected more than females; the majority of affected patients have a positive family history.
(B) Males are affected more than females; the left hip is affected more than the right hip.
(C) Females are affected more than males; the right hip is affected more than the left hip.
(D) Females are affected more than males; the left hip is affected more than the right hip.
(E) The presence of intoeing effectively rules out the condition.

3. A 6-year-old boy who developed a limp without pain within the last 2 weeks has Legg-Calvé-Perthes disease. This disease is characterized by which of the following conditions?

(A) Periarticular purulence and joint capsule effusion of the hip
(B) Leukocytosis and increased sedimentation rate
(C) Slipping of the femoral head from the femoral neck
(D) Traction apophysitis of the tibial tubercle, as a result of recurring microtrauma
(E) Avascular necrosis of the femoral head

4. Which of the following is the most significant risk factor for contracting postchlamydial infectious arthritis?

(A) History of rheumatic fever
(B) Multiple sex partners
(C) Recent diarrhea
(D) Recent clinical diagnosis of fifth disease (parvovirus B19)
(E) HIV infection

5. A 7-year-old boy has developed pain in the right knee gradually, over the past 3 weeks. He says that the pain increases during athletic play and when he kneels on a hard surface. You find a hard, tender swelling inferior to the patella. The boy has which of the following diseases?

(A) Prepatellar bursitis
(B) Osgood-Schlätter disease
(C) Juvenile rheumatoid arthritis (JRA)
(D) Poststreptococcal reactive arthritis
(E) Referred hip pain caused by slipped femoral capital epiphysis (SFCE)

6. With respect to Osgood-Schlätter disease, which of the following statements is correct?

    (A) Quadriceps exercises are a mainstay of treatment during the acute phase.

    (B) Knee joint effusion is usually associated.

    (C) It is an expression of juvenile rheumatoid arthritis (JRA).

    (D) It usually remits after fusion of the tibial tubercle with the diaphysis.

    (E) It is caused by premature closure of the tibial tubercle with the diaphysis.

7. A 10-year-old boy has been limping for the past 3 days and has cried because of pain in the right inguinal region. He has had no previous urinary tract infections (URIs). His temperature is 100.5°F (38.5°C). Physical examination indicates that pain in the right groin area is aggravated by both inversion and abduction of the right hip joint. The genitalia are normal to examination. No other joints are involved. Laboratory tests reveal a white blood cell (WBC) count of 15,500 cells/mm^3, with 75% neutrophils and 15% band forms, and a sedimentation rate of 35 mm/hr. Streptococcal throat screen of the throat is negative. What is the most likely diagnosis?

    (A) Toxic synovitis of the hip

    (B) Septic arthritis of the hip

    (C) Legg-Calvé-Perthes disease

    (D) Slipped femoral capital epiphysis (SFCE)

    (E) Inguinal hernia

DIRECTIONS (Item 8): Each of the numbered items or incomplete statements in this section is negatively phrased, as indicated by a capitalized word such as NOT, LEAST, or EXCEPT. Select the ONE lettered answer or completion that is BEST in each case.

8. Which of the following statements regarding intoeing is NOT true?

    (A) Metatarsus adductus (MA) may be the cause.

    (B) Internal tibial torsion (IIT) may be the cause.

    (C) Excessive femoral anteversion (EFA) may be the cause.

    (D) The vast majority of cases resolve spontaneously.

    (E) Surgical correction is required in most cases that have not resolved by the age of 8 years.

ANSWERS AND EXPLANATIONS

1. The answer is D. Delayed diagnosis of dislocated (as opposed to "dislocatable") developmental dysplasia of the hip [developmental dislocation of the hip (DDH), congenital dislocation of the hip] may have critical implications, including permanent joint changes that result in a waddling gait, osteoarthritis (OA), and cosmetic deformity. Before the age of 6 months, DDH can generally be corrected without surgery, but management is not as easy without bracing during the first few months of life.

The procedure described in the question is the Ortolani maneuver, which is positive for DDH. The trochanter movement palpated on the left is the classic, notorious "click," which represents the palpable reduction (i.e., reentry of the femoral head into the acetabulum). The Barlow maneuver is positive when a reduced hip joint is dislocated with a palpable "click" on 90-degree abduction of the hips while medial pressure is applied to the femoral heads posteriorly by the thumbs of the examiner (placed high in the medial thighs)—the opposite movement of that in the Ortolani maneuver. Diagnosis of irreducible dislocation involves Allis' sign. To elicit this sign, both hips and knees are flexed 90°; the knees on the dislocated side manifest a lower position. Universal sonographic screening of newborns is not recommended unless family history for DDH is positive, which occurs in 20% of cases.

2. The answer is D. Females are affected more than males. In addition, the left hip is affected alone 60% of the time, and the affliction is bilateral 20% of the time. The right hip is affected alone in 20% of cases. A positive family history exists in 20% of cases. Intoeing as a diagnosis of gait disturbance does not necessarily rule out developmental dislocation of the hip (DDH). Metatarsus adductus (MA), a cause of intoeing, may be associated with DDH.

3. The answer is E. Avascular necrosis of the femoral head characterizes Legg-Calvé-Perthes disease, a disease that affects the hip joint in males more than females by a ratio of 5:1. Purulent joint capsule effusion of the hip describes septic arthritis. This condition, not avascular necrosis, results in leukocytosis and increased sedimentation rate. Slipping of the femoral head from the femoral neck, secondary to shearing forces, and occurring before epiphyseal closure, describes slipped femoral capital epiphysis (SFCE). Traction apophysitis of the tibial tubercle as a result of recurring microtrauma is the pathologic process of Osgood-Schlätter disease.

4. The answer is B. A history of multiple sex partners is the most significant risk factor for postchlamydial infectious arthritis. All the other factors are more likely (than by chance) to be followed by postinfectious arthritis as well, but chlamydia is not implicated as the primary or secondary sensitizing organism in those cases.

5. The answer is B. This boy has Osgood-Schlätter disease. It is caused by traction apophysitis of the tibial tubercle, which becomes an enlarged apophysis in preadolescent boys (more often in boys than girls), and the unclosed connection to the diaphysis becomes inflamed as a result of microtrauma and traction on the tubercle by the quadriceps apparatus at its attachment. The condition is called a "traction apophysitis." Prepatellar bursitis, once called housemaid's knee, causes pain on repeated kneeling by serial trauma to the bursa, resulting in a palpable spongy area corresponding to the prepatellar bursa between the patella and the tibial tuberosity. From the preceding discussion, it is clear that the knee joint is not involved; therefore, the condition cannot be juvenile rheumatoid arthritis (JRA) or poststreptococcal reactive arthritis. By definition of local tenderness, the knee pain cannot be referred from the hip, as in slipped femoral capital epiphysis (SFCE).

6. The answer is D. Osgood-Schlätter disease usually remits when the tubercle fuses with the diaphysis, generally when the child is between the ages of 9 and 15 years. Quadriceps exercises, which would probably aggravate the condition in the acute phase, are not a treatment. (In general, activity level is guided by the symptoms; activities that aggravate the condition are curtailed.) Joint effusion is not associated, because the knee joint is not involved. Osgood-Schlätter disease is not related to juvenile rheumatoid arthritis (JRA). Because Osgood-Schlätter disease is a result of trauma to an unclosed ossification system, it cannot be a sequela of a premature closure of tubercle with diaphysis.

7. The answer is B. This boy most likely has septic arthritis of the hip. The best evidence given is the significant leukocytosis and elevated sedimentation rate. The primary confounding condition is toxic synovitis of the hip, which occurs in the same age-group, is usually monoarticular, and causes a limp. However, whereas septic arthritis is a medical (and sometimes surgical) emergency, toxic synovitis has a self-limited course of 7 days or less. Septic arthritis causes a much greater picture of illness but may be confounding early in the course. In toxic synovitis, the white blood cell (WBC) count and the sedimentation rate are not significantly elevated.

The results of joint aspiration are considered the definitive and only reliable means of distinguishing between the two diseases. In septic arthritis, Gram stain guides identity of the organism in 30%–50% of cases, but culture of joint fluid is also generally necessary. *Staphylococcus aureus* and *Streptococcus pyogenes* cause the vast majority of cases of infectious arthritis, which is monoarticular in 90% of cases. In toxic synovitis, aspiration yields only yellow fluid. In addition, limitation of motion typically involves internal rotation more than other movements.

Serial x-rays are important to detect the few cases that may be harbingers of aseptic necrosis of the femoral head (Legg-Calvé-Perthes disease). Legg-Calvé-Perthes or slipped femoral capital epiphysis (SFCE) is possible in this situation, because neither condition results in leukocytosis nor an elevated sedimentation rate.

8. The answer is E. The vast majority (95%) of cases of intoeing resolve spontaneously before children reach the age of 8 years, leaving no cosmetic or gait abnormalities. Surgical correction is required in most cases that have not resolved by this time. The most common cause of intoeing is excessive femoral anteversion (EFA), which has its onset in early childhood. It causes cosmetic, and sometimes functional, gait changes and may lead to osteoarthritis (OA). Intoeing is associated with inturning of the patellae as well, because the problem exists at the hips. The femurs and tibiae themselves are normally formed in EFA. Cases that have not resolved by age eight, except for very severe cases, are best accepted in the patient's state of accommodation, because osteotomy, the only treatment, carries dangers of serious complications. Metatarsus adductus (MA), which also causes intoeing, is recognized by the C-shaped curve of the lateral aspect of the foot. Approximately 85%–90% of cases resolve spontaneously by the age of 1 year. In internal tibial torsion (ITT), another cause of intoeing, the bones are oriented in the normal anterior position, and the foot curvature is normal. However, the tibia is twisted internally.

BIBLIOGRAPHY

Wenacur R, Tucker JB: Musculoskeletal problems in children. In *Family Medicine* (House Officer Series). Edited by Rudy DR, Kurowski K. Baltimore, Williams & Wilkins, 1997, pp 439–446.

Test 27

Approach to the Connective Tissue Diseases

DIRECTIONS (Items 1–9): Each of the numbered items or incomplete statements in this section is followed by answers or by completions of the statement. Select the ONE lettered answer or completion that is BEST in each case.

1. Which of the following patterns of antinuclear antibody (ANA) is most specific (rather than most sensitive) to systemic lupus erythematosus (SLE)?

(A) Rim or peripheral pattern
(B) Homogeneous pattern
(C) Speckled pattern
(D) Nucleolar pattern
(E) Diffuse pattern

2. The presence of which of the following is most commonly associated with neonatal lupus?

(A) Anti-Smith (anti-Sm) antibody
(B) Soluble ribonucleoprotein (S-RNP)
(C) Positive LE cell preparation
(D) Anti–SS-A (anti-Ro) antibody
(E) Anti–SS-B (anti-La) antibody

3. In a patient who is taking no other medication, treatment with oral or parenteral corticosteroids is most likely to be required in the presence of which of the following manifestations of systemic lupus erythematosus (SLE)?

(A) Malar rash
(B) Thrombocytopenia of 40,000/mm³
(C) Tenderness and swelling of three peripheral joints
(D) Pleuritis without effusion
(E) Photosensitive rash on the arms

4. In limited systemic sclerosis (LSS), which of the following is a characteristic clinical feature?

(A) Pulmonary hypertension
(B) Obstructive pulmonary disease
(C) Intestinal malabsorption
(D) Indurated skin on trunk
(E) Proximal muscle weakness

5. Which of the following correlates most specifically with limited systemic sclerosis (LSS)?

(A) Anticentromere antibodies
(B) Anti–double-stranded DNA (anti-dsDNA) antibodies
(C) A peripheral or rim pattern on antinuclear antibody (ANA) tests
(D) Anti-Smith (anti-Sm) antibodies
(E) Antimitochondrial antibodies

6. A 60-year-old woman has found climbing stairs, getting in and out of her car, and combing her hair difficult for the last 3 weeks. You note violaceous plaques on the dorsal aspect of her interphalangeal joints, as well as edema and violaceous coloring of her upper eyelids. Which of the following malignancies is most commonly associated with her condition?

(A) Colorectal carcinoma
(B) Osteogenic sarcoma
(C) Lung carcinoma
(D) Endometrial carcinoma
(E) Malignant melanoma

7. The definitive diagnosis of a polymyositis is established by which of the following?

(A) Elevated sedimentation rate
(B) Elevation of creatine phosphokinase (CPK)
(C) Elevation of aspartate aminotransferase (SGOT) and lactate dehydrogenase (LDH)
(D) Open surgical muscle biopsy
(E) Needle muscle biopsy

8. Which of the following laboratory results would be most consistent with, and specific for, Sjögren's syndrome (SjS)?

(A) Positive antinuclear antibody (ANA) in a homogeneous pattern
(B) Positive anti-Smith (anti-Sm) antibodies
(C) Positive anti–SS-A (anti-Ro) and anti–SS-B (anti-La) cytoplasmic antibodies
(D) Positive anticentromere antibodies
(E) None of the above (all would be negative)

9. In addition to the clinical features of two or more connective tissue diseases (CTDs), elevations of which of the following antibody titers is necessary for a diagnosis of mixed CTD?

(A) Anti–SS-A (anti-Ro) and anti–SS-B (anti-La)
(B) Anti-Smith (anti-Sm)
(C) Anti–double-stranded DNA (anti-dsDNA)
(D) Antiribonucleic protein (anti-RNP)
(E) Anti–SCL-70

DIRECTIONS (Items 10–11): Each of the numbered items or incomplete statements in this section is negatively phrased, as indicated by a capitalized word, such as NOT, LEAST, or EXCEPT. Select the ONE lettered answer or completion that is BEST in each case.

---

10. Which of the following is NOT one of the established criteria for the diagnosis of systemic lupus erythematosus (SLE)?

(A) Painless oral ulcer
(B) Seizure without other known causative etiology
(C) Erosive arthritis of the lumbar spine
(D) Pleuritis
(E) White blood cell (WBC) count of 2900/mm^3 and 2600/mm^3 on respective occasions within 2 weeks

11. A 60-year-old woman has had a dry mouth and gritty, irritated eyes for years. She sips water frequently and uses artificial tears regularly. A Schirmer test 2 years ago showed decreased tear flow. A slit-lamp examination 6 months ago showed no corneal damage. She has no clinical features of any other autoimmune disease. She is at increased risk of developing all of the following conditions EXCEPT

(A) chronic lymphocytic leukemia
(B) vasculitis
(C) interstitial lung disease
(D) renal tubular acidosis
(E) interstitial nephritis

DIRECTIONS (Items 12–15): For each numbered clinical vignette containing symptoms or demographic data, select the letter of the best matching clinical syndrome or disease. Each lettered option may be selected once, more than once, or not at all.

(A) Takayasu's arteritis
(B) Polymyalgia rheumatica (PMR)
(C) Wegener's granulomatosis (WG)
(D) Henoch-Schönlein purpura (HSP)
(E) Behçet's syndrome

12. A 3-year-old girl presents with a fever, general malaise, abdominal pains, and a petechial rash. Her stool contains no melena or bright red blood, but it is guaiac-positive. Neither she nor her parent has noted dysuria or hematuria, but a urine analysis is positive for small amounts of protein and blood. The child has palpable, purpuric lesions on her legs.

13. A 65-year-old woman complains of a 3-week history of pain and a sense of weakness in her neck, shoulders, and hip. She has a low-grade fever. Otherwise, she feels well and has no other symptoms. Her eyelids and hands appear normal; she has no rashes. Her neck, shoulder, and hips have full range of motion, and she has normal strength. Her sedimentation rate is markedly elevated, but her creatine phosphokinase (CPK) is normal.

14. A 30-year-old Chinese woman complains of 1 year of painful, aphthous ulcers in her mouth and similar lesions in her vagina. They heal after about 1 week, but they recur. An ophthalmologist treated the woman for iritis about 6 months ago.

15. A 40-year-old Caucasian man complains of a runny nose, cough, low-grade fever, and hemoptysis. He has noted some diffuse muscle pains. A small amount of blood and protein are appreciated on urine analysis.

ANSWERS AND EXPLANATIONS

1. The answer is A. The rim or peripheral pattern is most specific for systemic lupus erythematosus (SLE). This type of appearance also correlates with greater degrees of renal and central nervous system involvement. Although the homogeneous pattern is the most common pattern seen in patients with SLE, it is not specific. This pattern is also characteristic of and sensitive for drug-induced lupus [e.g., with hydralazine and isoniazid (INH)] and certain chronic infections (e.g., tuberculosis and histoplasmosis).

2. The answer is D. Anti–SS-A (Anti-Ro) antibody is most commonly associated with neonatal lupus. This cytoplasmic antibody crosses the placenta and can produce neonatal lupus with congenital heart block.

3. The answer is B. Thrombocytopenia of 40,000/mm³ is the manifestation of systemic lupus erythematosus (SLE) most likely to require treatment with oral or parenteral corticosteroids because the condition is potentially life threatening. Such treatment is also considered for hematologic lupus, lupus nephritis, CNS lupus, or severe lupus pericarditis. Although each of the other choices may be present (or in the case of malar rash, sterotypical of SLE), none constitutes an indication for glucocorticoid treatment.

4. The answer is A. Pulmonary hypertension is a characteristic clinical feature accompanying limited systemic sclerosis (LSS), which is a more slowly progressive form of systemic sclerosis (SS). Although pulmonary hypertension may occur with any of the connective tissue diseases (CTDs), pulmonary hypertension may supervene early (i.e., before other symptoms of LSS are prominent). Lung involvement of SS exists as well, but it is characterized by a restrictive pattern with decreased diffusion capacity. In contrast to the features in progressive systemic sclerosis (PSS), however, skin changes do not extend proximal to wrists and ankles, and malabsorption does not occur. Obstructive pulmonary disease is not a particular characteristic of either PSS or LSS. However, either condition may ultimately lead to restrictive lung disease, which may be termed pseudo-obstructive lung disease. Proximal muscle weakness is a hallmark of myopathy, not SS.

5. The answer is A. Anticentromere antibodies correlate most specifically with limited systemic sclerosis (LSS). A nucleolar (not rim) pattern is most commonly seen with both kinds of systemic sclerosis (SS), progres-

sive and limited. Anti-dsDNA, anti-Smith (anti-Sm) antibodies, and rim patterns on antinuclear antibody (ANA) are more specific markers for SLE. Antimitochondrial antibodies are commonly seen in patients with primary biliary cirrhosis, not SS.

6. The answer is C. Lung carcinoma is most commonly associated with dermatomyositis, the disease to which this classical presentation points. Dermatomyositis is an autoimmune inflammatory disease involving skin and muscle. The purplish rash about the eyes has been compared to the heliotrope flower. Breast, ovary, and stomach carcinomas are also commonly associated with lung carcinoma. The autoimmune development is apparently triggered by the DNA mutations that occur in association with this syndrome.

7. The answer is D. Open surgical muscle biopsy establishes the definitive diagnosis of a polymyositis, although sedimentation rate, creatine phosphokinase (CPK), aspartate aminotransferase (SGOT), and lactate dehydrogenase (LDH) are usually elevated in this disorder, and should be obtained if polymyositis is suspected. Needle insertion can damage muscle tissue and produce localized inflammation, which confuses pathologic diagnosis. For the same reason, electromyographic (EMG) studies are avoided on the side where the muscle biopsy is to be taken.

8. The answer is C. Positive anti–SS-A (anti-Ro) and anti–SS-B (anti-La) cytoplasmic antibodies are most consistent and specific for Sjögren's syndrome (SjS), although patients with SjS may demonstrate positive antinuclear antibody (ANA) [usually in the nucleolar pattern] and may have positive rheumatoid factor. SjS, an autoimmune inflammatory process that involves exocrine glands, in particular the salivary and lacrimal glands, causes reduced function (i.e., dry mouth and eyes).

9. The answer is D. Besides clinical evidence of two or more connective tissue diseases (CTDs), elevation of antiribonucleoprotein (anti-RNP) antibody titer is necessary for a diagnosis of mixed CTD. Anti-Smith (anti-Sm) antibody and anti–double-stranded DNA (anti-dsDNA) are more specific for SLE. Anti-SCL-70 is seen in progressive systemic sclerosis (PSS).

10. The answer is C. Erosive arthritis of the lumbar spine is NOT one of the established criteria for the diagnosis of systemic lupus erythematosus (SLE), a multisystemic disease, due in large part to autoimmune involvement of small vessels. Four of nine findings must be present for a diagnosis of SLE. To satisfy the criteria, an arthritis must be nonerosive and must involve two or more peripheral joints. Hematologic manifestations of SLE include hemolytic anemia, thrombocytopenia, and leukopenia. Additional criteria include the presence of pleuritis, pericarditis (or other serositis), and a malar or photosensitive rash, nonhealing oral ulcers (presumably due to microvasculitis and resultant ischemia), discoid rash, renal disease, and neurologic disorders. Seizures and psychosis can be manifestations of CNS lupus.

11. The answer is A. Chronic lymphocytic leukemia is NOT one of the conditions for which this woman is at increased risk because of primary Sjögren's syndrome (SjS). An autoimmune inflammatory process, SjS involves exocrine glands, in particular, salivary and lacrimal and causes reduced function (i.e., dry mouth and eyes). In this case, the symptoms point to SjS, which carries a higher than expected risk of extraglandular involvement and puts the patient at increased risk for lymphomas but not chronic lymphocytic leukemia. As an autoimmune disease, SjS not surprisingly overlaps with other connective tissue diseases (CTDs) [another term for autoimmune diseases]. SjS carries a higher-than-expected risk for vasculitis, interstitial lung disease, renal tubercular acidosis, and interstitial nephritis.

12. The answer is D. Henoch-Schönlein purpura (HSP), a self-limited autoimmune vasculitis, is the most likely diagnosis of this child's disease. In HSP, as in rheumatic fever (RF), an autoimmune response is triggered by a respiratory infection—a virus as opposed to a streptococcal infection. Vasculitides lead to capillary and arteriolar permeability, resulting in bleeding from various sites. Polyarteritis nodosa, which can produce a similar constellation of symptoms, is most commonly seen in adults of 50–70 years but sometimes occurs in children. Polyarteritis is a chronic disease that leads to pulmonary hypertension, renal failure, coronary insufficiency, and other multisystemic involvements, whereas HSP has none of those findings and has run its course in a few weeks (i.e., usually ≤ 3). Takayasu's arteritis is large-vessel, occlusive disease involving young females. Diagnosis is confirmed by arteriograms of affected organs and seldom requires biopsy for confirmation.

13. The answer is B. This patient has polymyalgia rheumatica (PMR), an inflammatory disease of unknown etiology, which is seen in patients older than 50 years (especially women). This condition is characterized by pain in the neck as well as in the shoulder or hip girdle (or both). Patients subjectively sense weakness in these muscles, but objective testing shows normal strength.

The lack of rashes on the eyelids, face, or hands excludes dermatomyositis, an autoimmune inflammatory disease involving skin and muscle. The normal muscle strength and creatine phosphokinase (CPK) exclude polymyositis and dermatomyositis. The woman's age excludes Henoch-Schönlein purpura (HSP), which is principally a disease of children, sometimes seen in young adults, but not seen in the elderly. Takayasu's arteritis, a large-vessel, occlusive disease that affects young women, produces claudication, angina, and cold in the extremities, but not shoulder and hip pain.

Although PMR is self-limited, it has a longer course (6–9 months) than other self-limited connective tissue diseases (CTDs). Treatment consists of oral glucocorticoid maintenance at modest levels (e.g., prednisone 15 mg daily). The most significant aspect of PMR is its association with temporal arthritis, which causes vascular headaches centered on a tender and enlarged temporal artery. Temporal arthritis can lead to sudden blindness and responds dramatically to glucocorticoids but at higher dosages than those used in uncomplicated PMR. This also removes the risk of blindness.

14. The answer is E. This woman has Behçet's syndrome, a disease common in Asian populations. Almost all affected patients have recurrent aphthous ulcers, and over 90% have ocular manifestations consisting of uveitis, either anterior or posterior.

15. The answer is C. This man's problem is Wegener's granulomatosis (WG). Unlike polymyalgia rheumatica (PMR), which is rare before age 50 and more common in females than in males, WG is more common in males and has a peak incidence in middle age. The "triad" of WG includes clinical disease in the upper respiratory tract, lower respiratory tract, and kidneys. Upper respiratory tract involvement includes the mucosae of the nose and sinuses, which bleed regularly and predispose the patient to secondary sinusitides. Pulmonary involvement results in hemoptysis. It is now known that the disease is multisystemic, and symptoms include bouts of fever, arthralgias, and episcleritis. The differences between this connective tissue disease (CTD) and systemic lupus erythematosus (SLE) result in part from the histologic forms of vasculitis, manifesting granulomatous vascular proliferation and SLE intimal changes of a more proliferative nature. As with all chronic CTDs, treatment is symptomatic or aimed at intercurrent infections. Glucocorticoids are used only in life-threatening situations.

BIBLIOGRAPHY

Seigel L, Gall EP: Approach to the connective tissue diseases. In *Family Medicine* (House Officer Series). Edited by Rudy DR, Kurowski K. Baltimore, Williams & Wilkins, 1997, pp 447–466.

SECTION X

Sports Medicine

Test 28

Sports Medicine

DIRECTIONS (Items 1–3): Each of the numbered items or incomplete statements in this section is followed by answers or by completions of the statement. Select the ONE lettered answer or completion that is BEST in each case.

1. With regard to athletics, what is the main objective of the preparticipation medical evaluation?

   (A) To diagnose hypertrophic subaortic stenosis in a candidate for high energy output athletics
   (B) To diagnose exercise-induced asthma and significant cardiac conditions that pose a threat to an exertional athlete or an athlete in a high-contact sport
   (C) To identify medical threats to an exertional athlete and to recommend techniques of training that tend to maximize success in athletics
   (D) To identify conditions that place the athlete at risk for exacerbating an existing illness or injury or incurring a new problem
   (E) To protect a practitioner against liability after approval for athletic participation of an athlete with a condition that might lead to sudden death

2. The 13-point examination is an example of which type of physical examination?

   (A) Complete general medical examination
   (B) Sport-specific examination
   (C) Limited musculoskeletal examination
   (D) Complete musculoskeletal examination
   (E) An examination to maximize cardiovascular security within the constraints of office primary care practice

3. A high school football player is lying on the field after performing an illegal spear block (the blocker has struck his targeted defender straight on with his head instead of a shoulder or the broad side of this body). He is conscious and alert, complaining of neck pain, and his teammates have prevented him from moving. Which of the following is the most appropriate next step?

   (A) Pull upward on his waist belt to help him regain his "wind."
   (B) Check for range of motion at the neck.
   (C) Keep his neck immobilized in a neutral position.
   (D) Check his pupils for reactivity.
   (E) Test his upper extremities for deep tendon reflex reactivity and symmetry.

DIRECTIONS (Items 4–6): Each of the numbered items or incomplete statements in this section is negatively phrased, as indicated by a capitalized word such as NOT, LEAST, or EXCEPT. Select the ONE lettered answer or completion that is BEST in each case.

4. High-contact sports are NOT contraindicated by which one of the following conditions?

   (A) Atlantoaxial instability
   (B) Absence of one kidney
   (C) Hepatomegaly
   (D) Hypertension
   (E) Poorly controlled convulsive disorder

5. Limited-contact sports are NOT contraindicated by which one of the following conditions?

   (A) Atlantoaxial instability
   (B) Absence of one kidney
   (C) Hepatomegaly
   (D) Enlarged spleen
   (E) Poorly controlled convulsive disorder

6. In the prevention of heat injury, which of the following measures is NOT appropriate?

   (A) Adjusting activities to avoid days on which heat and humidity are highest
   (B) Scheduling regular breaks for fluid and rest
   (C) Administering salt tablets with each water break
   (D) Advocating the use of light-colored, loose-fitting clothing

DIRECTIONS (Items 7–9): For each numbered grade of concussion in these matching questions, select the letter of the defined clinical picture. Each lettered option may be selected once, more than once, or not at all.

(A) Dazed without other symptoms
(B) Confusion without amnesia
(C) Confusion with amnesia
(D) Confusion with pupil changes
(E) Loss of consciousness

7. Grade I concussion

8. Grade II concussion

9. Grade III concussion

DIRECTIONS (Items 10–12): For each numbered grade of first concussion in these matching questions, select the letter of the guideline for when to return the athlete to play. Each lettered option may be selected once, more than once, or not at all.

(A) Terminate the athlete's play and practice; permit the athlete to return to play if symptoms are absent for at least 1 week.
(B) Permit the athlete to return to play if symptoms are absent for at least 20 minutes.
(C) Terminate the athlete's play and practice for the season; permit the athlete to return next season if symptoms are absent for the remainder of this season.
(D) Terminate the athlete's contest or practice; transport him or her to the hospital; permit the athlete to return to play 1 month after 2 consecutive asymptomatic weeks; permit conditioning after 1 asymptomatic week.
(E) Terminate the athlete's play and practice for the season; strongly discourage the athlete from returning to contact sports.

10. Grade I concussion

11. Grade II concussion

12. Grade III concussion

ANSWERS AND EXPLANATIONS

1. The answer is D. The primary goal is the identification of conditions that place the athlete at risk for exacerbation of an existing illness or injury or incurring a new problem. All other objectives listed are worthy, including medicolegal mindfulness, but they are overshadowed by the goal of protection of the athlete from harm by participating in an event with a potentially dangerous condition.

2. The answer is C. The 13-point examination is a limited musculoskeletal examination that is acceptable for preparticipation sports clearance, provided the athlete is certifiably healthy, preferably by having had a negative complete history and physical examination within a "medically uneventful" year. [See Table 28.3, in *Family Medicine* (House Officer Series).] A sports-specific examination is warranted for this same athlete later in the season if reevaluation is required for certain eventualities. An example would be an abdominal examination to rule out splenomegaly in an athlete who participates in a contact sport and who has convalesced from infectious mononucleosis within the previous 3 months.

3. The answer is C. The protocol for trauma life support should be followed by keeping the athlete's neck immobile in the neutral position. Thus, checking the range of motion of the neck, the pupils, and reflexes is not appropriate. The belt pull-up is helpful in an athlete who needs to "regain his wind." However, this patient exhibits no respiratory difficulty, and, in any case, neck injury assessment and management is the first priority. [Mouth-to-mouth insufflation (without neck extension) would be more appropriate to restore respiration than the belt-lift.]

4. The answer is D. Hypertension does NOT contraindicate participation in a high-contact sport. A challenge of sports medicine is to detect medical problems that pose risks to athletes who wish to participate in contact sports. Contact sports have been subdivided into high-contact and limited-contact categories. [For definitions of high-contact, limited-contact, and noncontact sports, see Table 28.2 in *Family Medicine* (House Officer Series).] Atlantoaxial instability, absence of one kidney, hepatomegaly, and poorly controlled convulsive disorder (among other conditions) contraindicate participation in a high-contact sport. [For further recommendations with respect to participation in competitive sports, see Table 28.1 in *Family Medicine*.]

5. The answer is B. The absence of one kidney does NOT contraindicate participation in limited-contact sports (e.g., basketball, baseball), although it DOES forbid participation in high-contact sports. Atlantoaxial instability, hepatomegaly, enlarged spleen, and poorly controlled convulsive disorder DO contraindicate participation in limited-contact sports. [For further recommendations with respect to participation in competitive sports, see Table 28.1 in *Family Medicine*.]

6. The answer is C. The administration of salt tablets is NOT an appropriate measure in the prevention of heat injury. In the past, salt tablets were given routinely, along with water, during summer football practice, but research shows that intake of generous amounts of water alone is superior for prevention of heat injury (e.g., heat exhaustion). The danger of hypernatremia associated with dehydration is greater than that of salt depletion and hypovolemia.

7. The answer is B. A grade I concussion produces confusion without amnesia.

8. The answer is C. A grade II concussion produces confusion with amnesia.

9. The answer is E. A grade III concussion produces loss of consciousness.

10. The answer is B. An athlete with a grade I concussion (first occurrence) may return to play if symptoms are absent for at least 20 minutes.

11. The answer is A. An athlete with a grade II concussion (first occurrence) should terminate play or practice, and may return to play if symptoms are absent for at least 1 week.

12. The answer is D. An athlete with a grade III concussion (first occurrence) should terminate play or practice and be transported to the hospital; the athlete may return to conditioning after one asymptomatic week, and may return to play 1 month after two consecutive asymptomatic weeks. [See Table 28.4, Grading Concussions in Sports and Guidelines for Return to Play, in *Family Medicine* (House Officer Series). Guidelines differ according to whether the concussion is the first, second, or third occurrence.]

BIBLIOGRAPHY

Lombardo JA: Sports medicine. In *Family Medicine* (House Officer Series). Edited by Rudy DR, Kurowski K. Baltimore, Williams & Wilkins, 1997, pp 467–480.

SECTION XI

Other Infectious Diseases Encountered in Primary Care

Test 29

Adult Acquired Immune Deficiency Syndrome

DIRECTIONS (Items 1–16): Each of the numbered items or incomplete statements in this section is followed by answers or by completions of the statement. Select the ONE lettered answer or completion that is BEST in each case.

1. A 26-year-old male intravenous drug abuser has been diagnosed with HIV by positive enzyme-linked immunosorbent assay (ELISA) and Western blot tests. His CD4 count was originally 440 cells/mm^3. He has been taking zidovudine (AZT) and didanosine (ddI) for 6 months. He has received treatment for oral candidiasis on two occasions. Otherwise, he has felt well except for increased incidence of seborrhea and has continued to work as a buyer for a large department store.

Two months ago, he noticed 10 to 15 multilocular button-like lesions that were 2–3 mm in diameter on the lower abdominal wall. The lesions, which contained a thick, gelatinous substance, popped off easily with a curette. After the lesions had completely disappeared for 6 weeks, they recurred. Which of the following is the likely diagnosis?

(A) Folliculitis
(B) Smallpox
(C) Varicella
(D) Epidermoid cysts
(E) Molluscum contagiosum

2. Considering the diagnosis of the rash in the HIV-infected patient in question 1, what would now be the predicted CD4 count?

(A) < 200 cells/mm^3
(B) 200–500 cells/mm^3
(C) 500–1000 cells/mm^3
(D) ≥ 1000 cells/mm^3

3. Given the change in status of the HIV-infected patient described in questions 1 and 2, which of the following statements concerning overall management is reasonable?

(A) Continue the regimen consisting of AZT and ddI.
(B) Discontinue ddI and add lamivudine (3TC).
(C) Discontinue ddI and add zalcitabine (ddC).
(D) Discontinue ddI and add 3TC and ritonavir (RIT).
(E) Discontinue AZT and add stavudine (d4T).

4. What percentage of adults infected for 10 years with the HIV virus have no clinical evidence of AIDS and have normal CD4 lymphocyte counts even without treatment?

(A) 1%–2%
(B) 5%–10%
(C) 25%–30%
(D) 40%–50%
(E) 60%–75%

5. In patients experiencing an acute, initial infection with HIV, which of the following is typical?

(A) Folliculitis
(B) Hairy leukoplakia
(C) Diarrhea
(D) Lymphadenopathy
(E) *Pneumocystis carinii* pneumonia

6. Which of the following body fluids is believed to carry the most significant amount of the virus in patients with HIV infection?

(A) Saliva
(B) Synovial fluid
(C) Urine
(D) Vomitus
(E) Nasal secretions

7. In asymptomatic patients with no previous history of the disease, prophylaxis for *Pneumocystis carinii* pneumonia is indicated beginning at which CD4 count?

(A) < 500 cells/mm^3
(B) < 200 cells/mm^3
(C) < 100 cells/mm^3
(D) < 50–75 cells/mm^3
(E) < 25 cells/mm^3

8. The patient group likeliest to develop Kaposi's sarcoma as a manifestation of AIDS is which of the following?

(A) Homosexual men
(B) Intravenous drug abusers of either sex
(C) Heterosexual women
(D) Hemophiliacs
(E) Medical personnel who acquired the infection through needle sticks

9. In treatment of HIV-infected patients with antiretroviral therapy, which of the following should be avoided?

(A) Change of two drugs at once when changing regimens

(B) Use of full-dose therapy after graduated dosage increase

(C) Two-drug therapy with the nucleoside reverse transcriptase inhibitors zidovudine (AZT) and stavudine (d4T)

(D) Therapy combining nucleoside reverse transcriptase inhibitors with non-nucleoside reverse transcriptase inhibitors

(E) Belief that the treatment regimen failed in the absence of at least a 3-log drop in HIV RNA titers within 1 month of therapy.

10. You are considering starting antiretroviral therapy in a 30-year-old man who is positive for HIV. Which of the following clinical situations most warrants initiating such treatment?

(A) Patient is asymptomatic; CD4 = 740 cells/mm^3; viral load is undetectable

(B) Patient is asymptomatic; CD4 = 1000 cells/mm^3; viral load = 100 copies/ml

(C) Patient is asymptomatic; CD4 = 600 cells/mm^3; but was 700/mm^3 6 months earlier; viral load = 30 copies/ml

(D) HIV infection is acute, CD4 = 1200 cells/mm^3; viral load > 5000 copies/ml

(E) CD4 count = 1000/mm^3; patient has a positive ELISA and Western blot confirmatory test

11. Which of the following medications is most likely to produce pancreatitis as a side effect?

(A) Lamivudine (3TC)

(B) Didanosine (ddI)

(C) Stavudine (d4T)

(D) Zidovudine (AZT)

(E) Zalcitabine (ddC)

12. You are treating a symptomatic HIV patient with zidovudine (AZT) and lamivudine (3TC). Besides CD4 counts and viral loads, which of the following should be monitored periodically because of the side-effect profile of these medications?

(A) Complete blood counts (CBCs)

(B) Serum electrolytes

(C) Liver function

(D) Serum creatinine

(E) Thyroid function

13. An asymptomatic, HIV-infected man with a CD4 count of 450 cells/mm^3 has no known exposure to tuberculosis and has normal results on chest x-ray. You are considering prophylaxis with isoniazid (INH) 300 mg/day. What diameter of induration is required on the purified protein derivative (PPD) reading to warrant prophylaxis?

(A) ≥ 2 mm

(B) ≥ 5 mm

(C) ≥ 10 mm

(D) ≥ 15 mm

(E) ≥ 20 mm

14. With respect to the HIV-positive patient described in question 13, how long should isoniazid (INH) therapy be given?

(A) 2 months

(B) 6 months

(C) 1 year

(D) 2 years

(E) Indefinitely

15. A 34-year-old man with AIDS, whose CD4 count 2 months ago was 40 cells/mm^3, complains of a 2-day history of fever, occipital headache, and general malaise. No seizures are reported. The patient's temperature is 101°F (38.3°C), his blood pressure is 140/80 mm Hg, and his pulse is 100 beats/min and regular. His pupils are normal and reactive, extraocular movements are normal, and there is no papilledema. The patient appears ill but in no acute distress. He is alert and oriented to time, person, and place. Motor and sensory examinations are normal. Deep tendon reflexes are normal and symmetrical. Which of the following organisms is most likely responsible for his symptoms?

(A) *Cryptococcus neoformans*

(B) *Toxoplasma gondii*

(C) *Mycobacterium avium* complex

(D) Cytomegalovirus (CMV)

(E) HIV

16. In the spring of the year, you are treating a 40-year-old woman with HIV with a CD4 count of 400 cells/mm^3. She has a history of intravenous drug abuse, and she is positive for hepatitis B surface antigen. Her childhood immunizations were all completed, and she received a diphtheria–tetanus booster 2 years ago. Which of the following immunizations is indicated?

(A) Hepatitis B vaccination series

(B) Oral polio booster

(C) Measles–mumps–rubella booster

(D) Varicella vaccination

(E) Pneumococcal vaccine

DIRECTIONS (Items 17–18): Each of the numbered items or incomplete statements in this section is negatively phrased, as indicated by a capitalized word such as NOT, LEAST, or EXCEPT. Select the ONE lettered answer or completion that is BEST in each case.

17. Until CD4 counts in HIV-infected patients have dropped to below 200/mm^3, which of the following is NOT usually seen?

    (A) Cytomegalovirus (CMV) retinitis

    (B) Oral thrush

    (C) Seborrhea

    (D) Hairy leukoplakia

    (E) Persistent diarrhea

18. With respect to the use of viral load determinations in assessing HIV-infected patients, all of the following statements are true EXCEPT

    (A) A doubling of the viral load in 6 months (between checks) is a poor prognostic sign.

    (B) Viral load and CD4 counts should be obtained every 6 months in asymptomatic patients who have CD4 counts greater than 500/mm^3.

    (C) Viral load determinations can be used to monitor the progression of HIV disease.

    (D) Viral load determinations can be used to monitor response to antiviral therapy.

    (E) Viral load determinations are useful in assessing prognosis.

ANSWERS AND EXPLANATIONS

1. The answer is E. Molluscum contagiosum is a benign infection caused by a member of the parapoxvirus group of the Poxviridae. Although this condition may occur in healthy individuals, its recurrence signifies a connection with the HIV infection. Folliculitis is a pustular rash reminiscent of acne. Although it could occur in the patient described at a higher-than-expected rate, considering all known information (namely positive HIV status with CD4 count < 500/mm³), it does not fit the given description. Because smallpox no longer exists in the world, its presence is highly unlikely in this case. In any event, smallpox appears as a centrifugally distributed rash of unilocular vesicles that is much more generalized, and it results in severe systemic febrile illness. Varicella, or chickenpox, which is caused by a member of the Herpesviridae, is a systemic illness. It is a centripetally distributed rash of many more lesions, consisting of multilocular vesicles (not fitting the description of the lesions in the present case). Finally, epidermoid "cysts" are subcutaneous collections of invaginated keratin from the cornified layer of skin, which are normally sloughed off in bathing. A telltale punctum marking the location of each "cyst" represents the point of submergent invagination. The material is contained in semimobile pseudocapsules (merely impacted layered keratin; hence the proper generic category, pseudocyst). The removal of such cysts, which are common in healthy individuals, are the subject of many minor office procedures.

2. The answer is A. In HIV-positive patients whose CD4 counts go below 200 cells/mm³, there is increased susceptibility to molluscum contagiosum [see Figure 29.1 in *Family Medicine* (House Officer Series)]. Significantly, a CD4 count of less than 200 cells/mm³ constitutes the official definition of AIDS, with different criteria for follow-up. With CD4 counts of 200–500 cells/mm³, HIV-positive patients are more likely to contract thrush (candidiasis), hairy leukoplakia of the oral mucosa, persistent diarrhea, and weight loss, but they are not more susceptible to the other conditions mentioned above. With CD4 counts of 500–1000 cells/mm³, folliculitis and seborrhea, two conditions encountered in normal individuals, are more likely than expected to occur. However, in this range, individuals are not more than normally susceptible to hairy leukoplakia, persistent diarrhea, or weight loss.

3. The answer is D. 3TC and RIT should be used. Two main points must be made here. The patient has entered a new phase, now meeting a criterion for AIDS and is at risk for rapid progression of disease. Therefore, a regimen with three drugs is more appropriate than one with just two, especially when the two drugs include one that the patient has already been taking [note that zidovudine (AZT) has been retained]. As in treating tuberculosis, a single drug should never be used except in unusual circumstances, and a single drug change in regimen should not be made. Thus, all the choices in which one drug is retained, one discontinued, and one added are incorrect. Stavudine (d4T) works well with ddI even in patients who are at risk for rapid progression (choice E, in which ddI is retained while AZT is discontinued) but is incorrect in that in this instance only a single drug would have been affected.

4. The answer is B. Between 5% and 10% of patients infected with HIV virus for 10 years have no clinical evidence of AIDS and have normal CD4 lymphocyte counts even without treatment. Most patients, however, develop low CD4 counts or clinical AIDS within this 10-year period if no treatment is given.

5. The answer is D. Lymphadenopathy, as well as fever, sore throat, rash, and headache are typical symptoms of an acute, initial infection with HIV. Folliculitis, hairy leukoplakia, diarrhea, chronic lymphadenopathy, and *Pneumocystis carinii* pneumonia are seen in later stages of the disease.

6. The answer is B. Synovial fluid, blood, semen, vaginal secretions, as well as pleural, peritoneal, and cerebrospinal fluids are all believed to contain significant amounts of the virus. Except for vaginal secretions, all of these normally do not interface with the extracorporeal environment. All other choices represent fluids that are normally excreted (i.e., they are found outside the body without the required invasion or injury), and they do not contain significant HIV virus in infected individuals.

7. The answer is B. A CD4 count less than 200 cells/mm³ is the level at which prophylaxis for *Pneumocystis carinii* pneumonia begins to be indicated. CD4 counts less than 500 cells/mm³ warrant checks of CD4 count and viral load every 3 months but do not warrant prophylaxis. When the CD4 count falls below 50–75 cells/mm³, prophylaxis is added (with clarithromycin, azithromycin, or rifampin) against *Mycobacterium avium* complex.

8. The answer is A. Homosexual men are more likely than other patient groups to develop Kaposi's sarcoma as a manifestation of AIDS. Treatment does not improve patients' chances of survival, but may diminish the size of lesions for cosmetic reasons. The more frequent occurrence of Kaposi's sarcoma in homosexuals may relate to its possible initiation by a herpes virus, which may be transmitted during homosexual activity but not through needles or heterosexual relations. All other groups mentioned are at risk for AIDS.

9. The answer is C. Two-drug therapy with the nucleoside reverse transcriptase inhibitors zidovudine (AZT) and stavudine (d4T) should be avoided in treating HIV-infected patients who are receiving antiretroviral therapy because of potential antagonistic action of the two agents. Other kinds of two-drug therapy with nucleoside reverse transcriptase inhibitors and three-drug therapy with either a protease inhibitor or a non-nucleoside reverse transcriptase inhibitor are used. At least two drugs should be changed whenever treatment is changed. Lower graduated doses are avoided because they may encourage development of resistance. Initial therapy is judged a failure only in the face of a persistent decline in CD4 counts or less than a 1-log decline in HIV RNA titers.

10. The answer is D. The clinical situation in which the HIV infection is acute, CD4 = 1200/mm^3, and viral load = 5000 copies/ml would most warrant initiation of anti-retroviral therapy. Following acute retroviral syndrome, treatment with nucleoside reverse transcriptase inhibitors combined with protease inhibitors for at least 2 years is believed to slow later progression of the disease. Chronic infections are treated if the patient has symptomatic AIDS or even symptomatic HIV disease (e.g., recurrent candidiasis, oral hairy leukoplakia, chronic fever, or weight loss). Treatment is also indicated in asymptomatic chronic infections if the CD4 count is less than 500/mm^3, or if the viral load is more than 500 copies/ml and, with increasing agreement among clinicians, especially if it is greater than 5000 copies/ml. The Western blot test is a more expensive, more specific test that is used to confirm HIV infection in patients who are positive on the ELISA screen, but this test cannot assist in establishing stage, prognosis, or treatment of the disease.

11. The answer is B. Didanosine (ddI) produces pancreatitis as a side effect in approximately 5%–9% of cases. Zalcitabine (ddC) produces pancreatitis less commonly (1%). None of the other drugs mentioned here have pancreatitis as a side effect. [See Table 29.7 in *Family Medicine* (House Officer Series).]

12. The answer is A. Complete blood counts (CBCs) should be obtained periodically because zidovudine (AZT) and lamivudine (3TC) can produce neutropenia and anemia. Liver function should be monitored in patients who are taking didanosine (ddI), zalcitabine (ddC), and most of the protease inhibitors. Electrolytes, renal function, and thyroid function need to be monitored during periods of administration of any of the drugs currently in use to control HIV infection.

13. The answer is B. An induration diameter of 5 mm or more on the purified protein derivative (PPD) reading is required to warrant prophylaxis in this case. In contrast, for adults who are not HIV infected and who are free of risk factors (e.g., prison incarceration, intravenous drug use), a diameter of 15 mm or more is required.

14. The answer is C. The patient in question 13 should be given isoniazid (INH) therapy for 1 year. In contrast, individuals who are not HIV infected should be given this treatment for only 6 months.

15. The answer is A. *Cryptococcus neoformans* is the organism most likely responsible for the 2-day history of fever, occipital headache, and malaise in this patient with AIDS. HIV, too, also produces this picture, but it does so less commonly than *C. neoformans*. Toxoplasmosis, the most common opportunistic central nervous system infection in AIDS patients, usually results in a space-occupying lesion with focal neurologic deficits. Cytomegalovirus (CMV) most often causes retinitis characterized by serious visual disturbance. Less often it leads to esophagitis, enteritis, colitis, hepatitis, transverse myelitis, or radiculitis. *Mycobacterium avium* complex most likely causes pulmonary symptoms similar to classic tuberculosis.

16. The answer is E. Pneumococcal vaccine is indicated in this patient. If she did not already test positive for the hepatitis B antigen, she would be a candidate for hepatitis B vaccination. Live attenuated viral vaccines, including oral polio and varicella, are contraindicated in HIV patients. The measles–mumps–rubella booster is also a live attenuated virus vaccine, but if patients have no immune experience with rubeola, the risk of measles is believed to outweigh the risks of the vaccine in patients with asymptomatic HIV disease who are less than 21 years of age.

17. The answer is A. Cytomegalovirus (CMV) retinitis, as well as pneumocystis pneumonia and Kaposi's sarcoma, is NOT usually seen in HIV-infected patients until their CD4 counts have dropped to 200/mm^3 or less. Oral thrush, diarrhea, seborrhea, folliculitis, and hairy leukoplakia all occur when CD4 counts are well above 200/mm^3.

18. The answer is A. A doubling of the viral load in 6 months (between checks) is NOT necessarily a poor prognostic sign. Viral load measurements vary widely and only differences greater than at least 0.5-log are significant. All of the statements in the other answer choices are correct.

BIBLIOGRAPHY

Weinstock MB, Crane R: Adult acquired immune deficiency syndrome. In *Family Medicine* (House Officer Series). Edited by Rudy DR, Kurowski K. Baltimore, Williams & Wilkins, 1997, pp 481–500.

Test 30

Less Common Infectious Diseases in Primary Care

DIRECTIONS (Items 1–14): Each of the numbered items or incomplete statements in this section is followed by answers or by completions of the statement. Select the ONE lettered answer or completion that is BEST in each case.

1. Which of the following is the natural habitat for *Legionella pneumophila?*

   (A) Human respiratory tract
   (B) Soil
   (C) Grains and cereals
   (D) Bodies of water
   (E) Fomites

2. Which of the following is a major risk factor for the development of legionnaires' disease?

   (A) Age of 30–50 years
   (B) Chronic obstructive pulmonary disease
   (C) Congestive heart failure
   (D) Obesity
   (E) African-American ethnicity

3. A 57-year-old woman with a 40-year history of smoking two packs of cigarettes a day has developed fever, headache, cough, and anorexia after long sessions in a new gambling casino. Which of the following would serve as additional evidence to support the most likely diagnosis in this patient?

   (A) A Gram stain of sputum that reveals more bacteria than neutrophils
   (B) An incubation period of 2–4 weeks
   (C) Ear pain
   (D) Constipation
   (E) Elevated serum creatine kinase

4. Which of the following is the recommended initial treatment for patients with legionnaires' disease?

   (A) Any first-generation cephalosporin
   (B) Amoxicillin with clavulanic acid
   (C) Erythromycin with rifampin
   (D) Gentamicin
   (E) Sulfamethoxazole

5. You are evaluating a 34-year-old woman who removed a deer tick from her skin on awakening one morning during a camping vacation. Within 6 days she noted an expanding, nonpruritic, blanching, raised, red lesion around the site of removal. She is not ill. What is the diagnosis?

   (A) Rocky Mountain spotted fever (RMSF)
   (B) Meningococcemia
   (C) Lyme disease
   (D) Discoid lupus erythematosus
   (E) Urticaria

6. In which of the following regions is the deer tick population most likely to be a reservoir for Lyme disease?

   (A) Northern California
   (B) Montana
   (C) Indiana
   (D) Kentucky
   (E) South Dakota

7. What is the peak time of the year for Lyme disease?

   (A) Spring
   (B) Winter
   (C) Autumn
   (D) Summer
   (E) Any season

8. Which of the following is a frequent manifestation of stage 3 Lyme disease?

   (A) Annular red lesions on chest and back
   (B) Facial palsy
   (C) Joint swelling
   (D) Myalgia
   (E) First-degree atrioventricular heart block

9. What is the causative agent of Lyme disease?

   (A) A spirochete bacterium
   (B) A virus
   (C) A rickettsia
   (D) A mycobacterium
   (E) A tick of the *Ixodes* genus

10. A 50-year-old woman, who has no allergies and is taking no medication, develops erythema chronicum migrans as well as head and muscle aches after camping in Vermont a week earlier. Her last menstrual period was 3 years ago. Her temperature is 99.9°F (37.7°C), and her blood pressure is 120/75 mm Hg. She is fully alert and oriented to time, person, and place. Motor and sensory examinations are within normal limits, as are deep tendon reflexes and cranial nerves. Her neck is supple, and her lungs are clear. Cardiovascular examination reveals a regular rhythm and no friction rubs or murmurs. Which of the following treatments or tests do you recommend next?

(A) Empiric treatment with amoxicillin 500 mg by mouth 3 times a day for 30 days

(B) Empiric treatment with doxycycline 100 mg by mouth 2 times a day for 10 days

(C) A lumbar puncture for examination of cerebrospinal fluid

(D) An enzyme-linked immunosorbent assay (ELISA) test for Lyme disease

(E) An antibody-capture immunoassay serologic test for Lyme disease

11. The greatest risk of tuberculosis exists in which of the following populations?

(A) Migrant workers

(B) Prisoners

(C) Middle-aged smokers

(D) Intravenous drug users

(E) Alcoholics

12. You are treating a 54-year-old man with AIDS. Four weeks ago his CD4 count was 20 cells/mm³. He has been having chills, fever, and an occasional cough. You apply a single intracutaneous skin test—5 tuberculin units of purified protein derivative (PPD). Three days later you appreciate no induration at the injection site. Which of the following statements is correct?

(A) The lack of at least 5 mm of induration precludes a diagnosis of tuberculosis.

(B) The lack of at least 15 mm of induration precludes a diagnosis of tuberculosis.

(C) A chest x-ray can confirm a diagnosis of tuberculosis if it shows upper lobe cavities, infiltrate, or hilar adenopathy.

(D) Tuberculosis cannot be excluded in this situation.

(E) Prophylaxis with isoniazid (INH) for 12 months is indicated.

13. You are assessing a 60-year-old woman who immigrated to the United States from eastern Europe 5 years ago. She feels well and denies cough, fever, or chills, and she also denies high-risk activity for HIV, a history of diabetes, immunocompromise, or liver dysfunction. She does not know her vaccination history and is taking no medication. She is afebrile, with lungs clear to auscultation and percussion, and she has no cervical or supraclavicular adenopathy. Her tuberculin skin test shows 18 mm of induration. Her chest x-ray reveals a few scattered, calcified granulomas. How should you proceed?

(A) Obtain three morning sputum samples for acid-fast bacillus and tuberculosis cultures.

(B) Obtain gastric aspirate for acid-fast bacillus and tuberculosis cultures.

(C) Prescribe isoniazid (INH) 300 mg by mouth each day for 6 months.

(D) Prescribe isoniazid (INH) 300 mg by mouth each day, plus rifampin 600 mg by mouth each day, for 9 months.

(E) Obtain no smears or cultures, and prescribe no treatment.

14. A 32-year-old woman with AIDS, who says she feels well and denies any fever or cough, has 8 mm of induration on a tuberculin skin test. Her last menstrual period was 1 week ago. Her chest x-ray is normal. She is taking zidovudine (AZT) and lamivudine (3TC). How should you manage this patient?

(A) Refrain from treating.

(B) Prescribe isoniazid (INH) 300 mg by mouth each day for 1 year.

(C) Prescribe ethambutol 25 mg/kg each day for 9 months.

(D) Prescribe isoniazid (INH) 300 mg each day and rifampin 600 mg each day for 6 months.

(E) Repeat the tuberculin skin test to see if there is a booster effect.

15. A 21-year-old college student develops a fever after taking a camping trip to the southern Appalachian Mountains. Four days later the student develops a severe headache and an erythematous, nonpruritic, blanching rash consisting of red macules about the wrists and ankles. Two days later the macules enlarge to ½–1 cm in diameter and manifest central nonblanching areas. What is the diagnosis?

(A) Meningococcemia

(B) Lyme disease

(C) Rocky Mountain spotted fever (RMSF)

(D) Rubeola

(E) Urticaria

DIRECTIONS (Item 16): Each of the numbered items or incomplete statements in this section is negatively phrased, as indicated by a capitalized word such as NOT, LEAST, or EXCEPT. Select the ONE lettered answer or completion that is BEST in each case.

16. A 28-year-old female Korean immigrant complains of a 6-week history of cough and fever. Sputum culture grows acid-fast bacilli in 6 weeks. Which of the following symptoms is NOT typical of her condition?

(A) Wheezing
(B) Weight loss
(C) Anorexia
(D) Night sweats
(E) Fatigue

ANSWERS AND EXPLANATIONS

1. The answer is D. Bodies of water, mostly from man-made sources, are the natural habitat for *Legionella pneumophila*. Humans may inhale aerosols from cooling towers or condensers. Humans do not pass *L. pneumophila* from person to person; thus, the human respiratory tract is not the source. Soil, particularly around construction sites, once thought to be a habitat, has not proven to be a source of legionnaires' disease. Grains, cereals, and fomites are not sources.

2. The answer is B. Chronic obstructive pulmonary disease is a major risk factor for legionnaires' disease. Other risk factors include advanced age (> 65 years), immunosuppression, and smoking, especially when combined with excessive alcohol intake. Legionnaires' disease is now thought to be more common in patients with excessive alcohol consumption. Congestive heart failure, obesity, and African-American ethnicity are not known risk factors.

3. The answer is E. The presentation in this patient is typical of legionnaires' disease. According to a recent review of literature, an elevated creatine kinase distinguishes the other pneumonitides from legionnaires' disease. A cough may be nonexistent or mild compared to the remaining clinical picture, including chest x-ray. Legionnaires' disease is one of the "atypical" pneumonitides; the term "atypical" was originally defined as manifesting x-ray findings out of proportion to historical and physical findings. Anorexia, myalgias, and hyponatremia frequently occur. On Gram stain, many more neutrophils than bacteria are usually present, perhaps because of the small dose of organism required to produce disease and, conversely, the virulence of the organism. The incubation period is 2–10 days, and diarrhea, rather than constipation, is an associated finding. Ear pain from an associated otitis media can be seen with *Mycoplasma pneumoniae* and some streptococcal infections, but not typically with legionnaires' disease.

4. The answer is C. Erythromycin with rifampin is the recommended initial treatment for legionnaires' disease. Erythromycin alone can be used with milder cases. (Rifampin, to which resistance develops rapidly, should not be used alone.) Other macrolides are also alternatives. Sulfamethoxazole is sometimes effective but is not the first-line agent. *Legionella* is not sensitive to penicillin, cephalosporins, or aminoglycosides.

5. The answer is C. The patient has Lyme disease. Discovered in the morning, the tick could have been attached for 24 hours, the minimum exposure time thought to be necessary for transmission of Lyme disease. The patient's rash, erythema chronicum migrans, constitutes stage 1 of the disease. This stage is present in 80% of cases after an incubation period of approximately 7 days (most often). Stage 2, characterized by dermal, central nervous, or musculoskeletal systemic symptoms, usually begins approximately 30 days after exposure, but may overlap with stage 1 as early as the first week.

Rocky Mountain spotted fever (RMSF) causes an acute, toxic systemic picture. Generalized 1–3-mm red macules, which blanch early, then become nonblanching with pressure and evolve into petechiae. Meningococcemia produces still more critically ill patients who have purpuric lesions that enlarge to several centimeters and coalesce with one another. Discoid lupus erythematosus produces large papules such as those described, some of which may become annular, but occurrence of a single such lesion around an insect bite would be sheer coincidence. Finally, by definition, urticaria is a rash of pruritic and evanescent wheals (appearing de novo in some areas while subsiding in others). Urticaria is an acute, systemic allergic condition.

6. The answer is A. Most cases of Lyme disease are seen in New England, Minnesota, Wisconsin, California, and Oregon. The disease also occurs in New Jersey and Pennsylvania.

7. The answer is D. In general, Lyme disease peaks during the summer months, but it also occurs as early as May and as late as November.

8. The answer is E. First-degree atrioventricular heart block is a manifestation of stage 3 Lyme disease. Facial palsy, joint swelling, and myalgia, as well as annular red lesions on the chest and back (days after development of erythema with central clearing around a tick bite), are characteristic of stage 2 disease. However, after a period of months to years in approximately 60% of cases, stage 3 disease may occur with further manifestations of musculoskeletal symptoms, including arthritis and synovitis (i.e., recrudescence of stage 2 manifestations), as well as subacute encephalopathy and polyneuropathy and a late dermopathy, acrodermatitis chronicum atrophicans. The latter is a purplish discoloration, with associated swelling, of a distal extremity.

9. The answer is A. A spirochete bacterium, *Borrelia burgdorferi,* causes Lyme disease. Ticks of *Ixodes* species (*Ixodes dammini, Ixodes pacificus*) [deer ticks] are the vector, but not the causative agent.

10. The answer is B. Empiric treatment with doxycycline 100 mg by mouth 2 times a day for 10 days should be prescribed. This patient has early stage Lyme disease when fever, headache, and myalgias are common, along with the hallmark erythema chronicum migrans. Amoxicillin is not effective against the spirochete that causes Lyme disease. Thirty-day treatment is appropriate for disseminated infection. Serologic and cerebrospinal fluid tests, which would produce false-negative results, are avoided here. Enzyme-linked immunosorbent assay (ELISA) is not used at this point because IgM antibodies detectable by ELISA first appear 2–4 weeks after exposure.

11. The answer is D. Intravenous drug users are at the greatest risk for AIDS, which has become the strongest risk factor for tuberculosis. Homeless individuals, indigent urban populations, and new immigrants from countries where tuberculosis is endemic are also at increased risk. In addition, migrant workers are at risk, perhaps because of poor health care access and crowded living conditions, and prisoners are susceptible because of crowded living conditions. Alcoholics are at risk because of poor nutrition and episodes of pulmonary aspiration. Middle-aged smokers are not among high-risk groups.

12. The answer is D. Tuberculosis cannot be excluded in this situation. The skin test is useful only if it is positive, which is especially true here because control skin tests were not applied at the same time. The lower threshold (5 mm) of induration constitutes a positive purified protein derivative (PPD) in immunologically vulnerable patients, but it is useful only if the test is positive. The 15-mm induration threshold for a positive PPD test is used for immunologically normal patients. False-negative skin tests are common in patients who have AIDS and tuberculosis. If patients have tuberculosis, a chest x-ray would not necessarily be positive, whether or not AIDS is present. Prophylaxis is only for asymptomatic individuals with skin test conversions and negative chest x-rays.

13. The answer is E. Obtain no smears or cultures, and prescribe no treatment for this woman. How long ago her skin test converted is unknown, but probably years ago. The highest risk after conversion is the first year. Isoniazid (INH) prophylaxis is not indicated because, at this age, it could cause her to develop hepatitis. Morning

sputa for acid-fast bacillus and tuberculosis cultures, standard for symptomatic individuals in whom tuberculosis is suspected, are not indicated in asymptomatic patients, especially ones without a cough. The same applies to gastric aspirate for acid-fast bacillus and tuberculosis cultures.

14. The answer is D. Isoniazid (INH) 300 mg each day and rifampin 600 mg each day for 6 months is the appropriate treatment for this patient. Immunocompromised skin test converters are treated with 6 months of the same combination regimen used for immunocompetent individuals who have active tuberculosis. Ethambutol is reserved for use as a third drug in three-drug therapy for patients who have symptomatic, proven, active tuberculosis, especially when resistance to INH is suspected or demonstrated.

15. The answer is C. The patient has typical Rocky Mountain spotted fever (RMSF) based on the incubation period (after exposure to the wilderness and possible tick bites), severe headache, and a macular rash about the wrists and ankles that become purpuric. Meningococcemia is a legitimate concern. However, this condition has a much more rapidly progressive course and moribund prostration by the time (within 48 hours) that the purpuric coalescent rash appears. Lyme disease is not indicated because the lesion does not resemble the classic erythema chronicum migrans and the incubation period is usually about 7 days. Although rubeola occasionally occurs in underimmunized young adults, it is characterized by a morbilliform rash (streaking redness, blanching) and photophobia, which starts on the face. The absence of pruritus rules out urticaria, as does the macular description (urticarial hives are raised and palpable) and evolution to purpura.

16. The answer is A. Wheezing is NOT typical of tuberculosis (the diagnosis in this case), although productive cough, chest pain, and hemoptysis are seen. Fatigue, anorexia, and weight loss are common symptoms of tuberculosis (thus, the earlier, long-held name, "consumption").

BIBLIOGRAPHY

Haddy RI: Less common infectious diseases in primary care. In *Family Medicine* (House Officer Series). Edited by Rudy DR, Kurowski K. Baltimore, Williams & Wilkins, 1997, pp 501–512.

Jacobs RA: Infectious diseases: spirochetal. In *Current Medical Diagnosis and Treatment,* 33rd ed. Edited by Tierney LM, McPhee SJ, Papadakis MA. East Norwalk, CT, Appleton & Lange, 1994.

Endocrinology in Primary Care

Test 31

Diabetes Mellitus

DIRECTIONS (Items 1–18): Each of the numbered items or incomplete statements in this section is followed by answers or by completions of the statement. Select the ONE lettered answer or completion that is BEST in each case.

1. Which of the following is the estimated range of the prevalence (in the United States) of diabetes mellitus, a major public health problem?

(A) 3–5 million
(B) 5–10 million
(C) 10–20 million
(D) 20–30 million
(E) 30–40 million

2. What is the approximate proportion of undiagnosed cases of diabetes?

(A) 10%
(B) 20%
(C) 25%
(D) 33%
(E) 50%

3. The presence of which human leukocyte antigen (HLA) type(s) are thought to pose a risk for type I diabetes?

(A) B17
(B) DR3, DR4
(C) A2, B7
(D) A3, B62
(E) B27

4. In diabetes mellitus, type I and type II disease are best distinguished from each other by the association of type II disease with which of the following?

(A) Insulin resistance
(B) Dyslipidemia
(C) Neuropathy and nephropathy complications
(D) Ready responsiveness to insulin
(E) Peripheral vascular disease

5. A 45-year-old African-American woman has recurrent urinary frequency and burning without systemic symptoms. She denies polyuria and polydipsia. She has never been hospitalized or been in a coma. No costovertebral angle tenderness is present. The patient's weight is 240 lb (109 kg); her height is 5′5″ (1.6 m); and her blood pressure is 170/105 mm Hg. Urinalysis shows white blood cells (WBCs) too numerous to count, glucose present chemically at "2+", and a negative result for ketones. The result of a 2-hour fingerstick blood sugar test is 230 mg/dl. You treat the patient's urinary tract infection (UTI) successfully with trimethoprim/sulfamethoxazole twice daily for 1 week. Follow-up 1 week later confirms fasting hyperglycemia (170 mg/dl) and elevated blood pressure. Total cholesterol was 240 mg/dl; HDL cholesterol was 35 mg/dl. With respect to the patient's condition, which of the following regimens is likely to be the most helpful at this time?

(A) Tolbutamide and hydrochlorothiazide
(B) Insulin and verapamil
(C) Exercise training and weight loss
(D) Acarbose, glipizide, and verapamil
(E) Metformin and propranolol

6. You are starting a 25-year-old man with type I diabetes mellitus on insulin. His weight is 177 lb (80.4 kg), and his height is 6′2″ (1.9 m). Which of the following dietary prescriptions is appropriate?

(A) 1200 calories (carbohydrates 200 g; protein 40 g; fat 200 g)
(B) 1800 calories (carbohydrates 250 g; protein 68 g; fat 68 g)
(C) 2400 calories (carbohydrates 800 g; protein 120 g; fat 100 g)
(D) 3000 calories (carbohydrates 1000 g; protein 150 g; fat 150 g)
(E) Demand schedule of dieting that assumes the patient's appetite is appropriate to his metabolic needs

7. For a 140-lb (63.6-kg) patient with newly diagnosed type I diabetes mellitus, whose insulin requirements have not yet been clearly defined, what is the initial estimate of the daily total insulin requirement?

(A) 15 U
(B) 25 U
(C) 32–64 U
(D) 70–140 U
(E) 140 U

8. Assuming that the selected insulin for the patient in question 7 is a combination of short-acting (R) and intermediate-acting (N) human insulin, what is the most currently accepted method (short of a continuous pumped infusion) of injecting the daily requirement of insulin subcutaneously?

(A) Giving it once: in the *morning* as N
(B) Giving it once: in the *morning* as two-thirds N and one-third R
(C) Giving it twice: in the *morning* as two-thirds of the total N and one-third of the total R, and *before dinner* as one-third of the total N and two-thirds of the total R
(D) Giving it twice: in the *morning* as two-thirds of the total N and two-thirds of the total R, and *before dinner* as one-third of the total N and one-third of the total R
(E) Giving it twice: in the *morning* as two-thirds of the total dose—two-thirds N and one-third R—and *before dinner* as one-third of the total dose—two-thirds N and one-third R

9. A 36-year-old man with a 15-year history of type I diabetes mellitus, who has failed to visit his ophthalmologist during the past 3 years, complains of blurred vision in his left eye. The eye chart test shows that his near visual acuity is 20/50 OS and 20/20 OD. His far visual acuity is 20/40 OS and 20/25 OD. One year ago, his near visual acuity was 20/20 OU, and far was 20/25 OU. A random blood sugar performed today is 130 mg/dl. A hemoglobin A1C drawn last week was 8.5%. Which of the following pathophysiologic mechanisms is the cause of his condition?

(A) Retinal surface proliferative changes
(B) Microaneurysms
(C) Dot hemorrhages
(D) Cotton-wool exudates
(E) Hard exudates

10. In evaluation of the renal status of the man in question 9, you estimate the progress of disease by noting the results of a 24-hour urine test for creatinine and for total and complete protein. Which of the following findings of the 24-hour urine test would be most relevant to an assessment of incipient renal failure?

(A) 10 mg albumin/dl
(B) 295 mg albumin/24 hr
(C) 250 mg protein/dl
(D) 2.0 g protein/24-hr urine output
(E) 3.5 g protein/24-hr urine output

11. You decide to consult a dietician about the man discussed in questions 9 and 10. If he weighs 180 lb (82 kg), how much protein intake should be ordered?

(A) 40 g/day
(B) 60 g/day
(C) 80 g/day
(D) 100 g/day
(E) 120 g/day

12. You are examining a 32-year-old man with type I diabetes mellitus who takes 48 U of insulin per day. He has been experiencing diplopia since awakening this morning. He has a history of difficulty in maintaining control of the disease because of personal circumstances. Examination shows the left eye to be turned inward (esotropic), regardless of the direction in which the patient directs his gaze. Which of the following pathophysiologic processes is directly responsible for this complication?

(A) Neural intracellular accumulation of sorbitol
(B) Microvascular-induced ischemia
(C) Neural intracellular myoinositol depletion
(D) Reduced adenosine triphosphatase (ATPase) activity
(E) Neural glycosylation of proteins

13. For diagnosis of diabetic peripheral polyneuropathy, which of the following is most sensitive?

(A) Presence of an asymmetrical hyperactive knee jerk
(B) Loss of knee jerk
(C) Loss of ankle jerk
(D) Presence of Babinski's reflex
(E) Presence of Hoffmann's reflex

14. Gestational diabetes is physiologically related to which of the following?

(A) Type I diabetes mellitus
(B) Type II diabetes mellitus
(C) Pancreatic diabetes
(D) Endocrine disorders
(E) A genetic syndrome

15. At which point in uncomplicated pregnancies should women be screened for diabetes?

   (A) After the first missed menstrual period
   (B) Between the 6th and 12th weeks
   (C) Between the 12th and 24th weeks
   (D) Between the 24th and 28th weeks
   (E) At the onset of contractions

16. A 35-year-old Caucasian woman who has no history of diabetes is in her 25th week of pregnancy. Her weight is 140 lb (63.6 kg), and her height is 5′5″ (1.6 m) in height. One hour after a test dose of 50 grams of glucose, she manifests a blood glucose of 160 mg/dl. A subsequent oral glucose tolerance test, using a 100-gram test load, results in blood glucose levels of 100 mg/dl, 220 mg/dl, 200 mg/dl, and 160 mg/dl, at 0, 1, 2, and 3 hours, respectively. After a 2-week trial of a 2400-calorie American Diabetes Association (ADA) diet, another 1-hour test, following a 50-gram glucose load, results in a blood glucose level of 170 mg/dl. Which of the following steps should be taken next?

   (A) Start the patient on insulin therapy.
   (B) Institute a third-generation sulfonylurea agent.
   (C) Start the patient on metformin.
   (D) Start the patient on troglitazone.
   (E) Prescribe an 1800-calorie ADA diet.

17. Which of the following complications is seen in type II but not in type I diabetes mellitus?

   (A) Ketoacidosis
   (B) Neuropathy
   (C) Retinopathy
   (D) Hyperosmolar coma
   (E) Renal failure

18. A 55-year-old Mexican-American woman is 240 lb (109 kg) in weight and 5′4″ (1.6 m) in height, with a blood pressure of 170/98 mm Hg. Her history includes no regular physician and no medication. Laboratory studies reveal a blood glucose level of 250 mg/dl; a pH of 7.414; a bicarbonate of 24 mEq/L; and a serum triglyceride of 250 mg/dl. What is her insulin level likely to be?

   (A) Lower than normal
   (B) Higher than normal
   (C) Normal
   (D) Inversely related to her triglyceride level
   (E) Directly related to her high-density lipoprotein (HDL) level

---

DIRECTIONS (Items 19–20): Each of the numbered items or incomplete statements in this section is negatively phrased, as indicated by a capitalized word such as NOT, LEAST, or EXCEPT. Select the ONE lettered answer or completion that is BEST in each case.

---

19. Which of the following is NOT an accepted sign of diabetes?

   (A) Two consecutive, fasting blood glucose determinations of ≥ 140 mg/dl
   (B) A finding of glycosuria in a morning fasting specimen
   (C) A random blood glucose determination of 210 mg/dl, with symptoms
   (D) A blood glucose determination of 600 mg/dl and a bicarbonate (HCO_3^-) determination of 12 mEq/L
   (E) Two values exceeding criteria for normal on a 5-hour glucose tolerance test

20. A 65-year-old Caucasian man who has had type II diabetes mellitus for 20 years has had imperfectly controlled hypertension for the past 10 years. You order a serum creatinine test and a 24-hour urine test for creatinine and for total and complete protein. The patient's weight is 180 lb (81.7 kg), and his height is 6′0″ (1.8 m). From these data, you calculate a creatinine clearance of 50 ml/hr. All of the following statements are relevant to this finding EXCEPT

   (A) Closer blood sugar control is indicated.
   (B) More cases of this condition are caused by type II than by type I diabetes.
   (C) Blood pressure control is important.
   (D) Medication to raise the glomerular filtration rate is indicated.
   (E) Dietary protein control is indicated.

ANSWERS AND EXPLANATIONS

1. The answer is C. An estimated 10–20 million people in the United States have diabetes mellitus. The *Family Medicine* (House Officer) text states that more than 10 million Americans have the disease, and other sources give higher estimates to include many undiagnosed cases.

2. The answer is E. An estimated 50% of the total cases of diabetes mellitus, perhaps as many as 10 million, most of which are mild, are undiagnosed. (The implication is that when diabetes remains undiagnosed, individuals are not experiencing symptoms.)

3. The answer is B. Human leukocyte antigen (HLA) types DR3 and DR4 are thought to represent a risk for type 1 diabetes mellitus. Although type I disease is caused by an autoimmune response to an external assault such as viral infection, the tendency for it to occur is constitutional and likely to be inherited. HLA markers may be strong circumstantial indicators of this tendency. HLA-B17 is associated with psoriasis, more specifically with psoriatic arthritis. HLA types A2 and B7, as well as A3 and B62, are associated with hemochromatosis. HLA-B27 is associated with ankylosing spondylitis.

4. The answer is A. Insulin resistance is characteristic of type II diabetes mellitus. Ready responsiveness to insulin is not a characteristic of type II diabetes. Physicians often resort to insulin in attempts to manage type II diabetes, but insulin is seldom effective in glycemic control in type II disease. The hyperinsulinemia that results from homeostatic responses to hyperglycemia has other detrimental effects such as contributing to hypertension and dyslipidemia. Dyslipidemia, association with neuropathy, nephropathy, and peripheral vascular disease are not restricted to either type I or type II diabetes.

5. The answer is C. Exercise training and weight loss are likely to be the most helpful regimen for this woman, who has a classic case of syndrome X. This syndrome is characterized by type II diabetes, hypertension, and, often, by dyslipidemia. The underlying pathophysiology is thought to involve hyperinsulinemia as a common cause. Weight loss, when successful, helps the greatest number of individuals with type II diabetes, 80% of whom are obese; insulin resistance often remits with weight control. The hypertension also responds to weight loss through reduction of insulin levels, as does dyslipidemia in most cases.

The other answer choices are directed at control of hyperglycemia and blood pressure individually, with separate pharmacologic agents. With respect to the diabetes, hypoglycemic agents, particularly of the sulfonurea family, are most often no more than partially successful if unaccompanied by weight loss. Of the agents directed at diabetes, only metformin attacks the problem closer to the source, resulting in less insulin resistance. Acarbose acts to reduce glucose from the gut, effectively reducing calorie intake. Troglitazone, a drug not listed in the answer choices, reduces insulin resistance even more than metformin. Insulin therapy is not the ideal solution in refractory cases, because insulin levels are already too high. Although metformin, acarbose, and troglitazone are all excellent drugs for treatment of type II diabetes, none should be used until weight loss has been accomplished or the attempt has failed. Often, insulin in doses higher than required in type I diabetes effects a lowering of blood sugar but with the cost of aggravation of hyperinsulinemia. The antihypertensive medications verapamil, hydrochlorothiazide, and propranolol have varying degrees of success against the hypertension. Verapamil, as a calcium channel blocker, and hydrochlorothiazide hold special promise in an African-American. Both African-American and type II diabetes patients tend to have a higher-than-expected proportion of volume-dependent (salt-retentive) hypertension and thus are responsive to diuretics. However, unless blood pressure exceeds 160/100 mm Hg consistently (stage II by JNC-V standards), diuretics should not be prescribed without full attempts at weight loss.

6. The answer is B. A diet of 1800 calories is appropriate for this man, who has type I diabetes mellitus. The numbers are based on a defined formula, which applies equally to individuals with type I and type II diabetes: total calories = (lean) body weight (lb) $\times$ 10. In this case, 10 $\times$ 177 lb (which is, in fact, ideal for this person) = 1770 calories. Carbohydrate calories make up 55% of the total calories (1800), or 990 calories; 990/4 cal/g $\cong$ 248 g. Protein calories make up 15% of total calories (1800), or 270; 270 cal/4 cal/g = 67.5 g. Fat should make up no more than one-third of total calories (1800), or 540 [1800 − (990 + 270)]; 540/8 cal/g = 67.5 g. For men, ideal weight may be estimated as 106 lb for the first 5 ft of height plus 6 pounds for each additional inch. For women, it may be estimated as 100 lb for the initial 5 ft of height and 5 lb for each additional inch. A larger difference is usually found between ideal weight and actual weight in individuals with type II diabetes than in those with type I diabetes, because 80% of persons with type II disease are overweight.

7. The answer is C. The figure of 32–64 U is based on the estimate of 0.5–1.0 U/kg (140/2.2). Thus, 140 U would be dangerously high; more than 70 U would also be too high; 25 U would probably fall well short of controlling the diabetes; and 15 U is inadequate to control type I diabetes in patients of any age or weight.

8. The answer is E. For example, if the starting dosage is 45 U/day (in the range of 0.5–1.0 U/kg/day), 30 U would be given in the morning as 20 U of human N and 10 U human R, and 15 U would be given in the evening as 10 U human N and 5 U human R [see *Family Medicine* (House Officer Series), pp 526–527]. Generally, the evening dose is given generally before dinner, but some practitioners may further divide this dose depending on a patient's individual needs by administering the second R insulin before dinner and the second N insulin at bedtime.

9. The answer is A. Retinal surface proliferative changes are the cause of visual loss in this patient with type I diabetes mellitus. Because the loss is unilateral and the random blood sugar determination is nearly normal, a temporary refractive change brought about by hyperglycemia is ruled out. The elevated glycolated hemoglobin suggests that long-term control has been less than optimal. Thus, the patient probably suffers from retinopathy. Such retinopathy occurs eventually in approximately one-half of all individuals with diabetes ($\geq$ 10 years after the onset of type I disease, and a varying number of years after the onset of type II). The prevalence of this retinal lesion makes diabetes the leading cause of blindness in the United States, and routine annual ophthalmologic examinations are necessary after 5 years of disease or after the development of a proliferative lesion. Other changes, including microaneurysms, dot hemorrhages, cotton-wool exudates, and hard exudates, are commonly seen in diabetes (microaneurysms are virtually pathognomonic of the disease), but these changes are not known to cause blindness.

10. The answer is B. A finding of 295 mg albumin/24 hr would be the most relevant in this case. A rise to 150–300 mg albumin/24 hr (defining microproteinuria) is the earliest clinical sign of diabetic nephropathy that comes after the initial formation of Kimmelstiel-Wilson basement membrane lesions in the glomeruli. Note the distinction between protein and albumin: Microproteinuria is defined in mg/24 hrs of albumin, a component of urinary protein. [The range of 30–300 mg protein/24 hr

given in *Family Medicine* (House Officer Series) is an error.] In any event, this amount of albumin is rather small and may be suggested by consistent appearances of as little as 20 mg/dl of albumin on sample urinalysis. Albuminuria of 200–500 mg/24 hr is a similar but only slightly more liberal figure used in hypertensive renal disease. Total protein of 250 mg/24 hr is within normal limits. Total protein of 2.0 g/24 hr is excessive and signals approaching nephrotic syndrome; a value of 3.5 g/24 hr defines this syndrome (see Tisher, Table 4.1, page 30). However, it is not the typical pathway for diabetic renal disease. The appearance of microproteinuria is significant and is quite typical. It calls for the same measures in type II as in type I diabetes.

11. The answer is B. The amount of protein that should be ordered is 60 g/day (approximately 0.75 g/kg/day). The patient manifests microproteinuria (albuminuria = 295 mg/24 hr). Prevention of end-stage renal disease in both diabetes and hypertension begins with dietary protein restriction. A protein intake of 55 g/day (or 0.67 g/kg/day) would be more effective than 60 g in prevention of end-stage renal disease, but 55 g is difficult to enforce. An amount of 40 g/day is almost deficient. The average American protein intake is roughly 100 g/day (1.25 g/kg/24 hr). A protein intake of 120 g/day is high.

12. The answer is B. Microvascular-induced ischemia accounts for the development of esotropia in this patient with type I diabetes. (Although this complication is more likely to occur in type I than in type II diabetes, it does occur in type II disease.) The vignette illustrates abducens nerve palsy (cranial nerve VI), a mostly self-limited mononeuropathy that occurs in diabetes. Mononeuropathies are thought to be related to microvascular circulatory change, a sequela of long-term diabetic control. Neural intracellular accumulation of sorbitol, neural intracellular myoinositol depletion, reduced adenosine triphosphatase (ATPase) activity, and neural glycosylation of proteins are biochemical changes known to occur acutely and chronically with hyperglycemia. They may contribute to the pathophysiology of microvascular disease, but they generally lead to changes of a more diffuse nature than esotropia (e.g., retinopathy, polyneuropathy).

13. The answer is C. Loss of the ankle jerk is the most sensitive diagnostic indicator (among reflexes) of diabetic peripheral polyneuropathy. Hyperactive deep tendon reflexes such as the knee jerk and Hoffmann's reflex (a counteractive flexion of the ipsilateral index finger and thumb produced by a quick stretch of the flexor tendon of the hands) are indicators of upper motor neuron disease. Babinski's reflex is indicative of upper motor neuron disease.

14. The answer is B. Gestational diabetes, characterized by insulin resistance brought about by the effects of placental lactogen, is most related to type II diabetes mellitus. Approximately 20% of women who develop gestational diabetes eventually contract type II diabetes. Recent meta-analytical information indicates a woman who has gestational diabetes has a 30%–50% chance of developing type II diabetes within 10 years (see Riddle, pp 659–677).

15. The answer is D. The early part of the third trimester of pregnancy is an appropriate time to test women because if insulin resistance is engendered by placental lactogen, it becomes significant as the fetus enters this period of significant growth. In uncomplicated pregnancies, between the 24th and 28th weeks (sixth and seventh months), women should be screened for diabetes with use of a 1-hour glucose tolerance test following a glucose load of 50 grams. A 1-hour reading of more than 140 mg/dl is an indication for a 3-hour glucose tolerance test following a glucose load of 100 grams.

16. The answer is A. Starting this pregnant woman on insulin therapy is the next step in the management of her gestational diabetes, the condition to which the test results point. Because the value exceeded 140 mg/dl in the 1-hour, 50-gram glucose tolerance screen (performed in the patient's 25th week of pregnancy), a 3-hour test with a 100-gram glucose load was performed. Values that exceeded 105 mg/dl, 190 mg/dl, 165 mg/dl, and 145 mg/dl, at 0, 1, 2, and 3 hours, respectively, provided (in the absence of any history of diabetes) the definitive diagnosis of gestational diabetes. Treatment requires insulin therapy to maximize control of blood sugar in the effort to prevent associated complications: stillbirth; macrosomia; and congenital anomalies (four to five times more than among progeny of nondiabetic mothers), especially sacral agenesis and caudal dysplasia (200 times more than among progeny of nondiabetic mothers). Many oral agents are deemed unsafe for the unborn fetus. Furthermore, the sulfonylurea agents metformin and troglitazone are thought to be insufficiently aggressive in terms of controlling blood sugar to the degree now believed necessary to prevent the previously mentioned complications. Dietary considerations are necessary in both pregnancy and diabetes, but they are hardly the mainstay of treatment of gestational diabetes.

17. The answer is D. In hyperosmolar coma, blood glucose levels reach impressive values (e.g., 800 mg/dl), but pH and bicarbonate levels remain within normal limits. The most rapid improvement results from rapid fluid infusion as insulin therapy is initiated

or adjusted upward, as the case requires. Hyperosmolar coma rarely occurs in patients with type I disease because affected patients in such poor control slip readily into ketoacidosis. Conversely, ketoacidosis rarely occurs in type II disease. Neuropathy, retinopathy, and renal failure occur in both type I and type II diabetes, although they occur earlier and at greater rates in type I disease.

18. The answer is B. Her insulin level is likely to be higher than normal. The normal bicarbonate level rules out ketoacidosis. This woman is typical of a person with type II diabetes; she is morbidly obese and asymptomatic but hyperglycemic. That is, in this case, the hyperglycemia is usually not so extreme that it causes noticeable polydipsia and polyuria, and the serum glucose is in the range of 180–300 mg/dl. Unlike type I diabetes, which is characterized by pancreatic beta-cell failure and insufficient insulin, type II diabetes involves insulin resistance, hence hyperinsulinemia. Secondary to elevated insulin levels is dyslipidemia, including a lowered high-density lipoprotein (HDL) level. Hypertriglyceridemia results from out-of-control diabetes, whether type I or type II. However, in this case (type II), the lack of control is caused by insulin resistance and is associated with an elevated insulin level. (In contrast, triglyceride elevation in type I diabetes is the direct result of insulin insufficiency.)

19. The answer is B. A finding of glycosuria in a morning fasting specimen is NOT a criterion for diagnosing diabetes. Urine testing is unreliable for diagnosis and even more unreliable for following diabetes because of variations in the renal threshold for glucose. Valid criteria include two consecutive fasting blood glucose determinations of greater than or equal to 120 mg/dl; a random blood glucose determination of 210 mg/dl, with symptoms; a blood glucose determination of 600 mg/dl and a bicarbonate determination of 12 mEq/dl; and two values exceeding criteria for normal on a 5-hour glucose tolerance test.

20. The answer is D. Medication to raise the glomerular filtration rate is NOT indicated in a case such as this, in which creatinine clearance is significantly less than expected for the patient's gender, age, and size. (Creatinine clearance in a young adult is normally about 100 ml/hr, and it decreases by approximately 1 ml/hr each year after the individual reaches the age of 20 years.) This 65-year-old man has begun to exhibit renal failure. His creatinine clearance of 50 ml/hr indicates the need for aggressive measures to prevent or delay end-stage renal disease. Aggressive measures consist of reduction of the glomerular filtration rate through the use of angiotensin-converting enzyme (ACE) inhibitor agents; dietary protein control; perfectionistic control of blood sugar; and blood pressure control.

BIBLIOGRAPHY

Riddle, MC: Tactics for diabetes, type II. *Endocrinol Metab Clin North Am* 26(3):659–677, 1997.

Roman SH, Harris MI: Management of diabetes mellitus from a public health perspective. *Endocrinol Metab Clin North Am* 26(3):443–474, 1997.

Tisher CC, Wilcox CS: *Nephrology,* 3rd ed. (House Officer series). Baltimore, Williams & Wilkins, 1995.

Tzagournis M, Rudy DR: Diabetes mellitus. In *Family Medicine* (House Officer Series). Edited by Rudy DR, Kurowski K. Baltimore, Williams & Wilkins, 1997, pp 513–542.

Test 32

Thyroid Problems in Primary Care

DIRECTIONS (Items 1–19): Each of the numbered items or incomplete statements in this section is followed by answers or by completions of the statement. Select the ONE lettered answer or completion that is BEST in each case.

1. Which of the following is most relevant to the fact that tetraiodothyronine (T$_4$) exists in the circulation at a concentration 10 times that of tri-iodothyronine (T$_3$)?

  (A) Metabolism is relatively stable because of the longer biological life of T$_4$.
  (B) Metabolism is relatively stable because of the longer biological life of T$_3$.
  (C) T$_4$ is more responsive than T$_3$ to thyrotropin (TSH).
  (D) T$_3$ is more likely than T$_4$ to be the medium of metabolism involved in thyrotoxicosis.
  (E) T$_3$ is formed entirely in the thyroid gland by the addition to di-iodothyronine of one iodine atom.

2. Direct measurement of free tri-iodothyronine (T$_3$) [as opposed to calculation by measuring total T$_3$ and subtracting protein-bound T$_3$] is best applied clinically to which of the following?

  (A) Graves' disease
  (B) Hashimoto's thyroiditis
  (C) T$_3$ toxicosis
  (D) Euthyroid sick syndrome
  (E) Toxic nodular goiter

3. The autoimmune antibody pathophysiology involved in Graves' disease is best described by which of the following?

  (A) Inflammatory immunoglobulin G (IgG)
  (B) Stimulating IgG
  (C) Blocking IgG
  (D) Anaphylactic IgE
  (E) Secretory IgA

4. The autoimmune antibody pathophysiology involved in autoimmune thyroiditis is best described by which of the following?

  (A) Inflammatory immunoglobulin G (IgG)
  (B) Stimulating IgG
  (C) Blocking IgG
  (D) Anaphylactic IgE
  (E) Secretory IgA

5. A 45-year-old Caucasian man complains of gradual weight loss of several weeks' duration. His wife says he now often lowers the home thermostat setting to a previously uncustomary, cool temperature. The man's thyroid gland is enlarged, but not tender, and both lobes are palpably nodular. External eye examination findings are normal, except for sclerae showing above the superior arc of the limbi of the corneas. This man's disease is preceded by which of the following conditions?

  (A) A single "cold" thyroid nodule
  (B) A single "hot" thyroid nodule
  (C) Autoimmune thyroiditis
  (D) A multinodular goiter
  (E) A colloid goiter

6. The widened palpebral angle seen in thyrotoxicosis is best described as which of the following?

  (A) Periorbital infiltration; exophthalmos
  (B) An indication of an underlying anxiety state
  (C) A result of pupillary mydriasis
  (D) A result of an elevated catecholamine state
  (E) Exposure keratopathy

7. A 38-year-old woman manifests a combination of elevated free tetraiodothyronine (T$_4$), free thyroxine index, and suppressed thyroid-stimulating hormone (TSH), along with sinus tachycardia that does not subside with rest or sleep. No palpable thyroid gland is found. Which of the following is the best next step in the management of this patient's condition?

  (A) Order level of stimulatory antithyroid antibodies.
  (B) Order level of inflammatory antithyroid antibodies.
  (C) Start the patient on propylthiouracil (PTU).
  (D) Start the patient on propranolol.
  (E) Check for ingestion of exogenous thyroid hormone.

8. With respect to the patient in question 7, which of the following can confirm the diagnosis?

  (A) A radioiodine uptake test
  (B) A test for thyroid-stimulating hormone (TSH) receptor antibody
  (C) Tri-iodothyronine (T$_3$) studies
  (D) Examination of a thin-needle biopsy
  (E) Measurements of resting pulse and blood pressure

9. A 45-year-old woman complains of increased nervousness and a 25-lb (11.4 kg), involuntary weight loss (despite an increased appetite) in a period of 4 months. Her height is 5′4″ (1.6 m), her weight is 95 lb (43.2 kg), and her apical pulse is 128 beats/min. A random blood sugar level is 95 mg/dl. The skin is thin, moist, and velvety. An asymmetrical proptosis of the eyes, widened palpebral angles, and sclerae visible above the cornea are evident. Which of the following can confirm the most likely diagnosis?

(A) A radioiodine uptake test
(B) A test for thyroid-stimulating (TSH) receptor antibody
(C) Tri-iodothyronine (T_3) studies
(D) Examination of a thin-needle biopsy
(E) Measurement of resting pulse and blood pressure

10. For the patient in question 9, the recommended agent for rapid relief of thyrotoxicosis symptoms is which of the following?

(A) An angiotensin-converting enzyme (ACE) inhibitor
(B) A benzodiazepine
(C) An alpha-adrenergic blocking agent
(D) A nonselective beta-blocking agent
(E) An isotope of radioactive iodine

11. What is the approximate female-male ratio among individuals afflicted with Graves' disease?

(A) 1:10
(B) 1:5
(C) 1:1
(D) 5:1
(E) 10:1

12. What is the most frequently used definitive treatment for Graves' disease in adult patients in the United States?

(A) Methimazole
(B) Propylthiouracil (PTU)
(C) Members of the thioamide family
(D) Radioactive iodine (^{131}I)
(E) Nonselective beta-blockers

13. A 45-year-old woman complains of fatigue. Her husband notes that at home she has been wearing more or heavier clothing this winter than in previous winters. Her face is slightly puffy, and her thyroid gland is palpable, with irregular surfaces on both lobes. What is the first chronological abnormality (and most sensitive indicator) to appear in the condition that fits this picture?

(A) Tetraiodothyronine (T_4) level
(B) Tri-iodothyronine (T_3) level
(C) Thyroid-releasing hormone (TRH) challenge test
(D) Thyroid-stimulating hormone (TSH) level
(E) ^{123}I uptake

14. Which of the following types of hypothyroidism is most common in the United States?

(A) Postablative hypothyroidism
(B) Primary hypothyroidism
(C) Hypothyroidism caused by thyroid aplasia
(D) Hypothyroidism caused by endemic iodine deficiency
(E) Hypothyroidism caused by goitrogenic agents

15. Treatment of hypothyroidism with levothyroxine or thyroxine takes approximately how long to achieve full effect?

(A) 1 week
(B) 1 month
(C) 2 months
(D) 3 months
(E) 4 months

16. What is the most common form of thyroprivic (primary) hypothyroidism?

(A) Acute thyroiditis
(B) Subacute thyroiditis
(C) Chronic thyroiditis (Hashimoto's disease, struma lymphomatosa)
(D) Athyreotic cretinism
(E) Riedel's thyroiditis

17. Which of the following types of thyroid carcinoma is most prevalent (75%), occurs in females three times more than in males, and has a 20-year survival rate of at least 95%?

(A) Medullary
(B) Anaplastic
(C) Follicular
(D) Papillary
(E) Metastatic from other organs

18. Thyroid nodules are found by autopsy or ultrasound in approximately what percentage of the US population?

    (A) Up to 10%
    (B) Up to 20%
    (C) Up to 35%
    (D) Up to 50%
    (E) Up to 70%

19. Among palpable thyroid nodules, what percent prove cancerous?

    (A) 5%–10%
    (B) 10%–20%
    (C) 20%–35%
    (D) 35%–50%
    (E) 50%–70%

DIRECTIONS (Items 20–22): Each of the numbered items or incomplete statements in this section is negatively phrased, as indicated by a capitalized word such as NOT, LEAST, or EXCEPT. Select the ONE lettered answer or completion that is BEST in each case.

20. Thyroid-releasing hormone (TRH) infusion is NOT used as a test for which of the following dysfunctions?

    (A) Primary hypothyroidism
    (B) Secondary hypothalamic and pituitary hypothyroidism
    (C) Primary hyperthyroidism
    (D) Pituitary failure
    (E) Sick euthyroid syndrome

21. A 38-year-old Caucasian woman has contracted a febrile illness, characterized by swelling at the angles of both jaws and painful swelling of the anterior neck. During the first week of illness, she exhibited a resting sinus tachycardia of 110 beats/min. Examination revealed a mass in the anterior neck, as well as symmetrical, tender masses at the angles of the jaw, extending upward and anterior to the ears, anteriorly along the mandible, and upward posterior to the ear. Thyroid tests yielded a tetraiodothyronine (T_4) level of 16 μg/dl (normal range, 4–11 μg/dl) and a free thyroxin level of 0.2 mU/L (normal range, 0.6–4.6 mU/L). All of the following are likely in the course of her illness EXCEPT

    (A) A 2.5%–5% chance of developing hypothyroidism
    (B) A need for ^{131}I therapy
    (C) Occurrence of an associated human leukocyte antigen (HLA) Bw35
    (D) Many symptoms that respond to aspirin
    (E) A sedimentation rate that exceeds 50 mm/hr

22. With respect to palpable thyroid nodules, all of the following are associated risk factors for carcinoma of the thyroid EXCEPT

    (A) Male gender and age > 60 years
    (B) "Fixed" feeling in the palpated nodule(s)
    (C) "Stony hardness" of the nodule(s)
    (D) Presence of lymphadenopathy
    (E) Elevated thyroid-stimulating hormone (TSH)

ANSWERS AND EXPLANATIONS

1. The answer is A. Tetraiodothyronine (T_4) and tri-iodothyronine (T_3) are secreted from the thyroid gland in a 10:1 ratio. Both T_4 and T_3 are produced originally in the thyroid gland by buildup by addition of iodine atoms from mono- and di-iodothyronine. Thyroid-stimulating hormone (TSH) accelerates the conversion process in response to falling levels of both T_4 and T_3 in the circulation. T_3 is the active form, and it has a half-life that is measured in hours, whereas that of T_4 is measured in weeks. T_4 serves as a reservoir for supply of T_3. Conversion from T_4 to T_3 occurs in the peripheral tissues.

2. The answer is C. Tri-iodothyronine (T_3) toxicosis represents the best clinical application of directly measured free T_3. In T_3 toxicosis, an unusual syndrome, tetraiodothyronine (T_4) is normal. Because T_3 is present at only a fraction of the amount of T_4, it must be measured more sensitively, by direct rather than by indirect methods. Thus, by inference, all the other conditions listed can be evaluated adequately by calculated T_3 levels. Hashimoto's thyroiditis, which may be expressed as transient thyrotoxicosis or long-term euthyroid small goiter or hypothyroidism, has a depressed calculated T_3. In euthyroid sick syndrome, calculated T_3 is spuriously low, a nonspecific finding in some chronically ill individuals whose T_4 level and metabolism are normal. Toxic nodular goiter, as the name implies, is a hyperthyroid condition associated with elevated calculated T_3 (and elevated T_4) levels.

3. The answer is B. Stimulating immunoglobulin G (IgG), specifically, thyroid-stimulating immunoglobulin (TSI), epitomizes Graves' disease (autoimmune stimulated primary thyrotoxicosis associated with exophthalmia). Inflammatory IgG is involved in thyroiditis. Blocking IgG is involved in hypothyroidism. Anaphylactic IgE is invoked in immediate skin test reactions and in anaphylactic reactions. Secretory IgA confers gastrointestinal (GI) immunity.

4. The answer is A. Inflammatory immunoglobulin G (IgG) epitomizes the autoimmune antibody pathophysiology involved in autoimmune thyroiditis. Blocking IgG antibodies are involved in autoimmune hypothyroidism.

5. The answer is D. A multinodular goiter (nontoxic) or a multinodular toxic goiter precedes this patient's disease, which is toxic nodular goiter. (Unlike Graves' disease, this disorder is not characterized by exophthalmos, although the eyes may manifest the stare of thyrotoxicosis.) Toxic nodular goiter begins as a grouping of autonomous nodules [often, apparently, under the influence of an elevated level of thyroid-stimulating hormone (TSH) caused by incipient hypothyroidism], which becomes autonomous and hyperfunctional in a certain proportion of cases. This form of thyrotoxicosis is a less severe form of hyperthyroidism, whether measured in terms of clinical symptoms and signs or laboratory values of tetraiodothyronine (T_4), tri-iodothyronine (T_3), or ^{123}I uptake. By definition, a single "cold" thyroid nodule, which does not take up ^{123}I on an ^{123}I uptake test, is metabolically inert. Its chief significance is its malignant potential. A single "hot" nodule, which produces hormone at a rate greater than surrounding tissue, is rare and is usually part of toxic nodular goiter (where the remaining nodularity is unappreciated by the examiner). Autoimmune thyroiditis, while sometimes causing hyperthyroidism, does so only transiently and is usually associated with gland tenderness during the acute phase. Colloid goiter occurs in a euthyroid or hypothyroid state.

6. The answer is D. The elevated catecholamine state present in all forms of thyrotoxicosis (with the possible exception of thyrotoxicosis in the elderly) is the cause of the widened palpebral angle seen in thyrotoxicosis. The widened palpebral angle, usually accompanied by lid lag, is the cause of the hyperthyroid stare (along with true exophthalmos). Another term for this condition is lid retraction. Exophthalmos is caused by periorbital infiltration associated with Graves' disease, an autoimmune type of thyrotoxicosis. Although anxiety may be associated with a stare, it would not be persistent. Elevated catecholamines may result in pupillary mydriasis along with the stare and lid lag in thyrotoxicosis. Mydriasis is an effect, not a cause. Exposure keratopathy occurs as a result of, not because of, severe forms of exophthalmos.

7. The answer is E. Checking for ingestion of exogenous thyroid hormone is the best next step. A patient who has hypermetabolism [elevated pulse, elevated tetraiodothyronine (T_4), and free thyroxine], along with suppressed thyroid-stimulating hormone (TSH), has thyrotoxicosis. However, in endogenous hyperthyroidism, no matter what causes it, an enlarged or at least a palpable thyroid gland would be present. Therefore, the picture points to ingestion of exogenous thyroid hormone in an amount that produces hypermetabolism. Such a condition may result from the patient's misunderstanding about the prescribed hormone dosage, or it may result from surreptitious ingestion of hormone. Ordering a level of stimulatory antithyroid antibodies would be appropriate if Graves' disease were suspected; however, the absence of true proptosis and of a goiter rule strongly against Graves' disease. Ordering a level of inflammatory antithyroid antibodies would be appropriate if thyroiditis were suspected. Propylthiouracil (PTU), an antithyroid medication, would be appropriate if the condition were Graves' disease. (This drug would be titrated against the thyroid function over several weeks and continued for at least 1 year before a reevaluation.) Propranolol, a beta-adrenergic blocker, would be indicated for rapid relief of thyrotoxic symptoms at the same time that antithyroid drugs are started or that radioiodine therapy is prepared or its actions are awaited.

8. The answer is A. The results of a radioactive iodine (^{123}I) uptake test would be nil (flat curve) in a case of exogenous hyperthyroidism caused by either factitious or accidental overdosing with thyroid hormone. If the patient's condition were acute thyroiditis manifesting transient hyperthyroidism (as hormone is released into the blood stream because of inflammation, as opposed to increased thyroid gland endocrine activity), the ^{123}I uptake would be lower than normal. In that case (unlike the case here), the gland would almost certainly be palpable and probably tender. A test for the presence of thyroid-stimulating hormone (TSH) receptor antibody would be performed if Graves' disease were suspected (results of this test would be normal in exogenous thyrotoxicosis). Tri-iodothyronine (T_3) studies would be normal or elevated in exogenous thyroid excess but would not determine the diagnosis because the elevation would also occur in thyrotoxicosis. Thin-needle biopsy, used for examination of suspicious thyroid nodules, would not be used in the absence of a palpable gland. The elevated resting pulse and systolic blood pressure would reflect hypermetabolism but would not distinguish between an endogenous or exogenous source.

9. The answer is B. A test for the thyroid-stimulating hormone (TSH) receptor antibody confirms Graves' disease, the most likely diagnosis of the patient's thyrotoxicosis. Thyroiditis, although an autoimmune condition, is not associated with TSH receptor antibodies. Radioiodine uptake is increased in Graves' disease, but it is also increased in toxic nodular goiter or toxic adenoma. Tri-iodothyronine (T_3) studies are relevant in the rare case of T_3 toxicosis, but not in this instance. Thin-needle biopsy is indicated only when carcinoma of the thyroid is suspected.

10. The answer is D. A nonselective beta-blocking agent such as propranolol or nadolol gives rapid relief of symptoms of thyrotoxicosis. It is given at the same time that more definitive therapy is bringing the patient's hypermetabolism under control. Angiotensin-converting enzyme (ACE) inhibitors are not used in thyrotoxicosis. Benzodiazepines (e.g., diazepam) are sedatives, and may have limited application in the control of thyrotoxicosis symptoms, but they are not nearly as effective as beta-blockers. Alpha-adrenergic blocking agents are not effective in controlling thyrotoxicosis. Radioactive iodine (^{123}I) in low doses is used as a tracer in scanning the thyroid, whereas ^{131}I is used in large doses to ablate the gland in thyrotoxicosis; neither is used for rapid relief of symptoms.

11. The answer is E. Lifetime incidence (sometime prevalence of Graves' disease) is 2.2% for females and 0.2% in males. In general, a greater proportion of most thyroid problems occur in females than in males.

12. The answer is D. Iodine has an affinity for glandular tissue, and the radioactive isotope located in the gland destroys the parenchyma. Its primary disadvantages are an associated high incidence of post-treatment hypothyroidism and contraindications for pregnancy and breast-feeding. Recent findings ensure that this treatment does not cause cancer. Antithyroid drugs of the thioamide family [methimazole and propylthiouracil (PTU)] are effective treatments, but they must be continued for varying periods of time. These agents may cause neutropenia, which is reversible if detected early, but, if not, leads to agranulocytosis. The thioamide family is the inclusive name for the two antithyroid agents previously alluded to. Nonselective beta-blocking agents are not definitive treatments for thyrotoxicosis, except in mild cases (Graves' disease may have a self-limiting course).

13. The answer is D. Elevated thyroid-stimulating hormone (TSH) [in response to falling tetraiodothyronine (T_4) and tri-iodothyronine (T_3)] is the first abnormality to appear (and most sensitive indicator for) hypothyroidism, the condition that fits this picture. Cold intolerance and fatigability are the most typical symptoms. The puffy face is due to myxedema of hypothyroidism, and the nodular goiter is typical of the response of the hypofunctioning thyroid gland to the elevated TSH. In fact, many types of goiters remain indefinitely associated with a euthyroid state as the rising TSH level stimulates the gland to proliferate in barely successful responses in maintaining eumetabolism.

However, TSH level does not in itself reflect metabolism as does T_4, the hormone directly responsible for metabolism. In some cases, patients may never reach hypometabolism despite elevated TSH. The physician must diagnose and treat such patients as if they were hypothyroid to suppress TSH and prevent multinodular goiter. Although both T_3 and T_4 eventually fall below normal in hypothyroidism, resulting in the symptoms and signs of hypothyroidism, a rise in TSH precedes the actual fall in hormone levels. Thyroid-releasing hormone (TRH) stimulates TSH release. The TRH challenge test, when positive, indicates hypothalamic hypothyroidism. There would be no goiter. ^{123}I uptake is suppressed in hypothyroidism at about the same point in disease development that T_3 and T_4 levels begin to fall.

14. The answer is A. Postablative hypothyroidism (hypothyroidism following radioiodine therapy or partial or complete surgical removal of the thyroid) is the most common type of hypothyroidism. Primary hypothyroidism (failure of the gland itself) is the second most common type. Hypothyroidism caused by thyroid aplasia (congenital absence of the gland), endemic iodine deficiency, and goitrogenic substances (e.g., lithium, phenybutazone, para-aminosalicylic acid, ethionamide) occur less frequently.

15. The answer is B. Treatment of hypothyroidism with levothyroxine and thyroxine achieves full effect in approximately 1 month. Conversely, if such a medication is discontinued for any reason, the condition takes approximately 1 month to return to baseline.

16. The answer is C. Chronic thyroiditis (Hashimoto's disease, also called "struma lymphomatosa") is the most common cause of thyroprivic (primary) hypothyroidism. Acute thyroiditis is defined by infection and is rare; it occurs in physically abnormal glands (e.g., nodular goiters, thyroglossal duct remnants, fistulas). Subacute thyroiditis (synonymous with granulomatous thyroiditis) is uncommon, painful, and usually virus-based. Thyroid aplasia causes athyreotic cretinism, a rare, congenital condition that must be diagnosed early to prevent mental retardation. Riedel's or "woody" thyroiditis, which is also rare, is part of a sometimes generalized condition, idiopathic fibrosclerosis, that can include retroperitoneal and mediastinal, as well as uterine cervical, cholangitic, and orbital sclerosis.

17. The answer is D. Papillary carcinoma accounts for a large majority of cases of thyroid cancer, occurs in three times as many females as males, and has a 20-year survival rate of at least 95%. However, only 61% of mortality from this type of carcinoma occurs in females, in whom the disease takes a less malignant course than in males. Papillary carcinoma has a tendency to occur in individuals who have a childhood history of irradiation to the neck. Follicular carcinoma is the second most common thyroid cancer (16%) and carries a 5-year sur-

vival rate of only 44%–86%. Medullary carcinoma accounts for 5% of thyroid cancers; it is associated with pheochromocytoma, hyperparathyroidism, or both, in multiple endocrine neoplasia type IIA (MEN-IIA) or with neuroma, pheochromocytoma, and marfanoid habitus in MEN-IIB. Anaplastic carcinoma, which is very aggressive and carries a poor prognosis, fortunately accounts for only 3% of thyroid cancers.

18. The answer is D. Up to 50% of the US population examined by autopsy or ultrasound have thyroid nodules. However, palpable nodules are present in only 4%–7% of affected individuals.

19. The answer is A. Between 5% and 10% of palpable thyroid nodules prove cancerous.

20. The answer is E. A thyroid-releasing hormone (TRH) infusion test does NOT help in differentiating euthyroid sick syndrome, a nonspecific condition in some chronically ill individuals whose tetraiodothyronine (T_4) levels (and metabolisms) are normal. In practice, the TRH infusion is used most often in testing for secondary hypothalamic or secondary pituitary hypothyroidism. In this procedure, 400 μg of TRH is infused, and the thyroid-stimulating hormone (TSH) level is drawn 30 minutes later. In primary hypothyroidism, the peak value of TSH is elevated from the normal range of 5–30 mU/L, already in a stimulated state; in pituitary secondary hypothyroidism, TSH does not rise normally in response to TRH; and in hypothalamic secondary hypothyroidism, the TSH rise is adequate in response to TRH infusion. TSH tends to be flat after TRH infusion in the case of hyperthyroidism, as a result of the "disuse" suppression of TSH that precedes the diagnostic test. This test is used much less frequently since sensitive TSH has become available. In pituitary failure, hypothyroidism is one of several secondary endocrine failures, and the TRH stimulation test results in failure of TSH rise in response (as in isolated secondary pituitary hypothyroidism).

21. The answer is B. Therapy with ^{131}I, a definitive therapy reserved for treatment of a permanent or indefinite state of thyrotoxicosis, is NOT required in this case. The woman has subacute thyroiditis, generally associated with viral disease (sometimes mumps, as is suggested in this case). Approximately 80% of cases occur in females; 2.5%–5% of cases result in goiter, hypothyroidism, or both; the sedimentation rate is always elevated; and associated HLA-Bw35 occurs in two-thirds of Caucasian and Chinese patients. Many symptoms may be controlled by aspirin alone. Thus, although the woman is hypermetabolic, her condition is due to "spilled" hormone, not thyroid hyperfunction; in fact, to the contrary. Therefore ^{123}I uptake is low or flat. The disease itself is uncommon, compared to Hashimoto's (chronic) thyroiditis.

22. The answer is E. An elevated thyroid-stimulating hormone (TSH) associated with a palpable thyroid nodule is NOT a risk factor for carcinoma of the thyroid. It represents clinical or incipient hypothyroidism. Male gender, together with 60 or more years of age; a "fixed" feeling with respect to the palpated nodule; stony hard-ness of the nodule; and presence of lymphadenopathy are all regarded (in association with a palpable thyroid nodule) as risk factors for thyroid cancer.

BIBLIOGRAPHY

Rudy DR, Tzagournis M: Thyroid problems in primary care. In *Family Medicine* (House Officer Series). Edited by Rudy DR, Kurowski K. Baltimore, Williams & Wilkins, 1997, pp 543–566.

Test 33

Triage of Problems of the Adrenal Gland

DIRECTIONS (Items 1–12): Each of the numbered items or incomplete statements in this section is followed by answers or by completions of the statement. Select the ONE lettered answer or completion that is BEST in each case.

1. To differentiate between primary and secondary adrenal insufficiency, which of the following tests can be used?

    (A) Baseline serum cortisol
    (B) Peak cortisol postcosyntropin
    (C) Eosinophil count
    (D) Baseline adrenocorticotropic hormone (ACTH)
    (E) Serum potassium

2. A 33-year-old woman has been taking dexamethasone 0.75 mg per day as maintenance therapy for primary adrenal failure caused by autoimmune atrophy. She also has Graves' disease. Her new health insurance plan requires her to accept prescription drugs that are less expensive biological equivalents when they are available. What is the usual replacement dosage for prednisone in adrenal insufficiency (i.e., equivalent of 0.75 mg of dexamethasone)?

    (A) 0.75 mg daily in divided doses
    (B) 5 mg daily
    (C) 7.5 mg daily (5 mg in the morning and 2.5 mg in the afternoon)
    (D) 10 mg daily
    (E) 15 mg daily

3. The patient in question 2, who has been receiving prednisone maintenance for the past 6 months, comes to the office urgently after 12 hours of increasingly severe abdominal pain. You diagnose acute appendicitis. Which of the following management plans is the most relevant in the face of the patient's underlying medical condition?

    (A) Preoperative and intraoperative antibiotics throughout the appendectomy
    (B) Insulin coverage on a 6-hour management regimen
    (C) Close observation, copious intravenous (IV) therapy, high dosages of antibiotics, and avoidance of surgery
    (D) Acceleration of IV administration of glucocorticoid, beginning just before surgery and weaning afterward
    (E) Rapid adrenocorticotropic hormone (ACTH) stimulation test

4. A 35-year-old woman, a new patient, asks you to assume responsibility for treatment of her hypertension and type II diabetes mellitus. She has been maintained on triamterene/hydrochlorothiazide for her blood pressure and on glipizide for her diabetes (with less than adequate control). The woman is obese; her obesity is centripetal, with proximal muscle wasting, associated with plethoric facies and purple striae about the trunk. She complains of menstrual irregularity. You order an overnight 8-mg dexamethasone suppression test; the result shows greater than 50% suppression of 24-hour urine 17-hydroxycorticosteroid (i.e., level falls to 50% of baseline). Her disease originates from which of the following sources?

    (A) Adrenal cortex
    (B) Adrenal medulla
    (C) Pituitary
    (D) An ectopic source (e.g., lung metastasis)
    (E) Thyroid

5. Regardless of whether Cushing's syndrome results from pituitary, autonomous adrenal, or ectopic corticotropin causes, which of the following tests is useful for diagnosing it?

    (A) Serum potassium test
    (B) Overnight 1-mg dexamethasone suppression test
    (C) Magnetic resonance imaging (MRI) of the pituitary
    (D) Plasma aldosterone plasma renin activity (PA-PRA) level
    (E) Plasma adrenocorticotropic hormone (ACTH) level

6. What do the drugs ketoconazole, mitotane, metyrapone, and aminoglutethimide have in common?

    (A) They are all antimycotic agents.
    (B) They are all aldosterone inhibitors.
    (C) They are all adrenocorticotropic hormone (ACTH) inhibitors.
    (D) They are all adrenal glucocorticoid inhibitors.
    (E) They all cause neutropenia.

7. What are the two elements that must be present to make the diagnosis of primary aldosteronism?

    (A) Adenoma in the zona glomerulosa of the adrenal cortex and hypertension

    (B) Abdominal bruit and hypertension

    (C) Hypokalemia and elevated renin

    (D) Hypokalemia and hypertension

    (E) Purple striae and dorsal hump

8. What effect does primary aldosteronism have on renin level?

    (A) It is elevated to levels compatible with renovascular hypertension.

    (B) It is elevated to levels found in "high renin" essential hypertension.

    (C) It is lower than normal in primary aldosteronism.

    (D) It is unchanged from premorbid levels in primary aldosteronism.

    (E) It is elevated early in the course and falls to normal as primary aldosteronism persists over time.

9. A 28-year-old man complains of the onset of alarming attacks of shortness of breath and a pounding, racing heart within the past 4 weeks. During an attack, an office nurse measures a blood pressure of 160/105 mm Hg. You have not been able to examine him during an attack. At present, his blood pressure is 128/88 mm Hg. His pulse rate is 76 and regular. Which of the following tests (or combinations) most accurately diagnoses pheochromocytoma?

    (A) 24-hour urine for free catecholamine level

    (B) 24-hour urine for 5-hydroxyindoleacetic acid (5-HIAA) level

    (C) 24-hour urine for metanephrine level

    (D) 24-hour urine for vanillylmandelic acid (VMA) level

    (E) 24-hour urine for free catecholamine and metanephrine

10. You are evaluating the patient in question 9. Test results for pheochromocytoma are negative, except that plasma catecholamine is elevated at 9 nmol/L (0.3–3 nmol/L). Which of the following is the most likely diagnosis?

    (A) Pheochromocytoma

    (B) Carcinoid syndrome

    (C) Thyrotoxicosis

    (D) Panic disorder

    (E) Supraventricular tachycardia

11. A 45-year-old Caucasian man with hypertension has been followed for 2 months since the condition was discovered during an episodic visit for a viral upper respiratory infection. (Readings during a 1-week period were 170/110 mm Hg, 165/115 mm Hg, and 180/108 mm Hg.) No abdominal bruit was present. The physician first prescribed verapamil, increasing the dosage incrementally to 240 mg long-acting twice daily, and then added captopril, increasing the dosage to 25 mg three times daily. At one point, with propranolol up to 40 mg twice daily, the blood pressure actually rose to 190/120 mm Hg. Finally, the physician added hydrochlorothiazide 50 mg per day. Still, the blood pressure was 160/105 mm Hg. Family history reveals that the patient has a brother with neurofibromatosis and a sister who died of medullary carcinoma of the thyroid. What is logically the best next step?

    (A) Prescribe a sympathetic blocking agent such as methyldopa.

    (B) Perform a cold pressor test.

    (C) Add an alpha-/beta-blocking agent such as labetolol.

    (D) Order a 24-hour urine test for metanephrines and free catecholamines.

    (E) Order an intravenous pyelogram (IVP) with special attention to a 2-minute film.

12. A 10-year-old Caucasian boy gained 2.75 inches (7 cm) in the past year and an average of 2 inches (5.1 cm) per year during the 4 years before that. His sexual development fits Tanner stage 3. Plasma 17α-hydroxyprogesterone measurement is high. One hour after adrenocorticotropic hormone (ACTH) infusion, the elevation of 17α-hydroxyprogesterone is tripled. Which of the following is the most likely diagnosis?

    (A) 3β-Hydroxysteroid dehydrogenase deficiency

    (B) 11β-Hydroxylase deficiency

    (C) 17α-Hydroxylase deficiency

    (D) 21-Hydroxylase deficiency

    (E) Sertoli cell tumor

DIRECTIONS (Items 13–17): For each numbered endocrinological diagnosis in these matching questions, select the letter of the identifying characteristic. Each lettered option may be selected once, more than once, or not at all.

(A) Mineralocorticoid deficit
(B) Vanillylmandelic acid (VMA) elevation
(C) Ambivalent genitalia
(D) Potassium wasting
(E) Pituitary origin

13. Pheochromocytoma

14. Congenital adrenal hyperplasia (CAH)

15. Primary aldosteronism

16. Cushing's disease

17. Primary adrenal insufficiency

ANSWERS AND EXPLANATIONS

1. The answer is D. A baseline adrenocorticotropic hormone (ACTH, corticotropin) level may differentiate between primary versus secondary adrenal insufficiency [see *Family Medicine* (House Officer Series), p 568]. Primary adrenal insufficiency results from failure of the adrenal glands despite adequate stimulation by ACTH. Secondary adrenal insufficiency results from lack of stimulation by ACTH from the pituitary. Measurement of peak aldosterone postcosyntropin (> 16 μg/dl, as opposed to < 16 μg/dl) may also differentiate between the primary and secondary conditions. Neither baseline serum cortisol, which is low in the cases of both primary and secondary adrenal insufficiency, nor peak cortisol postcosyntropin, which is less than 20 μg/dl in both primary and secondary adrenal insufficiency, distinguishes between the two conditions. Likewise, the eosinophil count tends to be elevated in both primary or secondary adrenal insufficiency, reflecting a loss of the inflammation-suppressing effects of glucocorticoid, and serum potassium may also be abnormally high in such situations.

2. The answer is C. Although 0.75 mg daily in divided doses is appropriate for dexamethasone, the much more potent glucocorticoid, all the other dosages are fairly typical mild therapeutic maintenance dosages of prednisone. Dexamethasone is approximately 10 times as potent as prednisone.

3. The answer is D. When such a patient, who has been on maintenance glucocorticoid therapy, develops an indication for surgery, whether emergent or elective, surgery must proceed while glucocorticoids are administered at dosages well above maintenance levels (assuming the indication for surgery is unquestioned). Otherwise, under the stress of surgery, the patient will certainly suffer a crisis of adrenal insufficiency ("adrenal crisis"). A dosage of 100 mg hydrocortisone intravenously (IV) 1 hour before anesthesia and repeated every eight hours until the patient's condition is stable, followed by 100 mg orally three times daily, reducing the dosage by 30%–50% every day for the first 3–5 days, is an accepted regimen [see *Family Medicine* (House Officer Series), Chapter 33]. This is approximately three times replacement (maintenance) dosage three times per day, or nine times maintenance. What about the suitability of "equivalent" dosages of other glucocorticoids (e.g., methylprednisolone IV before

surgery and every 8 hours until stable, followed by prednisone 20 mg three times daily, tapering over 10–20 days toward the original maintenance dose)? Hydrocortisone is chosen because it possesses mineralocorticoid activity, obviating concurrent fludrocortisone.

Preoperative and intraoperative antibiotic therapy may or may not be elected by the surgeon, but it is not relevant to the case. Insulin coverage on a 6-hour management program is effected for insulin-dependent diabetics or for type II diabetes perioperatively, but hyperglycemia, although relevant to Cushing's syndrome, is not a part of adrenal insufficiency. The management of appendicitis without surgery (i.e., close observation) is never elected for treatment of appendicitis, except when rupture has already occurred (2 or more days before diagnosis). This applies whether or not patients are in high-risk states, including exigencies such as prior glucocorticoid therapy or poorly controlled diabetes. A rapid ACTH stimulation test is indicated to rule out or diagnose adrenal insufficiency as newly symptomatic. Given the circumstances, the predicted diagnosis of the present case is relative adrenal insufficiency. Thus, the patient is treated accordingly, without effort spent on diagnosis.

4. The answer is C. The patient has Cushing's disease originating in the pituitary. Clinical features are hypertension, type II diabetes mellitus, centripetal obesity, proximal muscle wasting, plethoric facies, and purple striae. Cushing's disease involves excessive production of adrenal glucocorticoid as a result of overproduction of adrenocorticotropic hormone (ACTH) from an autonomous pituitary adenoma. One criterion for diagnosis is suppression of 17-hydroxycorticosteroid to more than 50% of baseline on the overnight 8-mg dexamethasone suppression test. In Cushing's syndrome, regardless of origin, the same symptoms and signs occur. The most common source is exogenous glucocorticoids given as treatment for a chronic inflammatory disease such as rheumatoid arthritis.

5. The answer is B. The overnight 1-mg dexamethasone suppression test is a standard for diagnosis of Cushing's syndrome, whether it results from pituitary, autonomous adrenal, or ectopic corticotropin factors (the latter typically elevated by regressive adenocarcinomas, often metastasized). The morning serum cortisol level after the night dose of dexamethasone should be normal (i.e., < 5 μg/dl). In Cushing's syndrome, the morning cortisol level would be greater than 10 µg/dl. Serum potassium is low in primary aldosteronism and elevated in adrenal insufficiency, but it is usually normal in Cushing's syndrome. Magnetic resonance imaging (MRI) of the pituitary may diagnose Cushing's disease but is normal in other forms of Cushing's syndrome. The plasma aldosterone–plasma renin activity (PA-PRA) ratio is used to diagnose primary aldosteronism in which it is increased compared to normal. Other tests (e.g., 8-mg overnight dexamethasone suppression test) are useful after a positive result is obtained on the screening 1-mg dexamethasone suppression test.

6. The answer is D. Ketoconazole, mitotane, metyrapone, and aminoglutethimide are all adrenal glucocorticoid inhibitors. Clinically, they are all used for temporary suppression of hypercortisolism in preparation for surgical treatment of pituitary adenoma to remove the source of excess adrenocorticotropic hormone (ACTH). Ketoconazole is also an antifungal agent. Mitotane may be used to effect a medical adrenalectomy in certain cases. Metyrapone is useful for controlling autonomous hypercortisolism in Cushing's syndrome. It is also used in diagnostic testing of hypothalamic-pituitary-adrenal axis function. Aminoglutethamide was originally used as an anticonvulsant. Like metyrapone, it is useful for controlling hypercortisolism from autonomous sources.

7. The answer is D. Hypokalemia and hypertension are always present in primary aldosteronism (autonomous production of aldosterone from the adrenal cortex). Adenoma is the cause in 60% of cases, and the remainder are secondary to bilateral adrenal hyperplasia. Purple striae and dorsal hump are stigmata of Cushing's syndrome, manifestations of hypercorticolism.

8. The answer is C. Renin levels are low as a physiologic response to sodium retention and hypervolemia. This is an indirect and homeostatic result of hyperaldosteronism and a direct result of sodium retention, tending to protect blood pressure on the high side (from the teleological evolutionary perspective). Renin levels remain low so long as the disease persists untreated. Essential hypertension features both low and high levels of renin. However, renin levels in "high renin" essential hypertension are still relatively low compared to those in renovascular hypertension, in which levels are clearly two to three times higher.

9. The answer is E. The combination of 24-hour urine metanephrine greater than or equal to 1000 µg and total urinary catecholamines greater than 150 µg/24 hours is 95% sensitive for pheochromocytoma, especially if determined within 24 hours after an attack. For the major-

ity of patients who are norepinephrine producing, who hence have sustained rather than paroxysmal hypertension, a random determination suffices. A metabolite of propranolol spuriously elevates metanephrines, and drugs such as methyldopa, levodopa, or labetalol spuriously increase catecholamines. Thus, elevation of both substances increases the specificity as well as the sensitivity. Elevation of only one requires further evaluation.

Urinary 5-hydroxyindoleacetic acid (5-HIAA) levels are elevated in carcinoid syndrome, which, like pheochromocytoma, is characterized by paroxysms or attacks of anxiety and flushing. Flushing is perhaps a greater part of the clinical picture with carcinoid syndrome than it is with pheochromocytoma. Other symptoms include bronchoconstriction; gastrointestinal (GI) hypermotility, including diarrhea; and cardiac manifestations such as valvular thickening. Vanillylmandelic acid (VMA) level is less sensitive and specific than either catecholamine or metanephrine levels. VMA has been used in the past and is still used in many centers for diagnosis of pheochromocytoma. However, VMA levels alone are more subject to false-positive results than are catecholamine or metanephrine levels, based on a variety of interfering substances such as sympathomimetic or monoamine oxidase–inhibiting drugs.

10. The answer is D. Pheochromocytoma is highly unlikely, because 24-hour urine catecholamine and metanephrine are within normal limits (see the explanation for question 9). Although the plasma catecholamines are elevated, they are in an intermediate zone that overlaps with levels that may occur in anxiety or panic states. Thyrotoxicosis causes tachycardia and often the subjective sensation of pounding heart. However, the tachycardia does not subside with rest, as it has in this case. Other symptoms and signs that would likely emerge in thyrotoxicosis (purposely not mentioned in the clinical scenario) are heat tolerance weight loss despite increased appetite, thyrotoxic stare, probable goiter, and possible exophthalmos. Although carcinoid syndrome and supraventricular tachycardia are part of the differential diagnosis, they are far less likely (in the range of 99% less) than panic attack, the necessary ingredient for panic disorder. Only if an in-depth interview fails to support the diagnosis of panic attack should the possibilities of carcinoid and supraventricular tachycardia be pursued.

11. The answer is D. Ordering a 24-hour urine test for metanephrine and free catecholamines is the best next step, because the patient has two of four indications for pheochromocytoma screening: uncontrollable hypertension and first-degree relatives with possible multiple endocrine neoplasia II (MEN-II). Other indications are paroxysms of hypertension during surgery, labor, or radiologic procedures; and radiologic evidence of a suprarenal mass. Urinary metanephrine of greater than or equal to 1000 μg/24 hours is 75% sensitive; this result together with a finding of urinary free catecholamines of 150 μg/24 hours or more is 95% sensitive. Prescription of additional antihypertensive agents would be futile, especially because a trial of beta-blockade resulted in greater hypertension, a sign of pheochromocytoma. Provocative tests should be avoided because they could precipitate an attack.

12. The answer is D. 21-Hydroxylase deficiency, the most common type of congenital adrenal hyperplasia (CAH), is the most likely diagnosis of this patient's condition. Deficiency of this enzyme prevents the normal rate of conversion of 17α-hydroxyprogesterone to 11-deoxycortisol, a precursor of cortisol in the adrenal cortex. Thus, the relative lack of glucocorticoid leads to increased release of adrenocorticotropic hormone (ACTH) and more stimulation of the faulty reaction that leads to buildup of 17α-hydroxyprogesterone. During the metabolism of 17α-hydroxyprogesterone, androgenic products are released. Treatment consists of exogenous glucocorticoid to suppress the ACTH. Among the other answer choices, 3β-hydroxysteroid dehydrogenase deficiency, 11β-hydroxylase deficiency, and 17α-hydroxylase deficiency are other enzymatic errors involved in CAH. 3β-Hydroxysteroid dehydrogenase deficiency results in elevation of plasma levels of hydroxypregnenolone and dehydroepiandrosterone (DHEA), both of which are elevated further in the ACTH stimulation test. 11β-Hydroxylase deficiency gives rise to elevations of 11-deoxycortisol, the cortisol precursor, one step closer than 17α-hydroxyprogesterone. 17α-Hydroxylase deficiency results in a decrease in α-hydroxysteroids. In this condition, the response to the ACTH stimulation test is poor.

13. The answer is B. Urinary vanillylmandelic acid (VMA) is elevated in pheochromocytoma. Nevertheless, metanephrine and free catecholamines, especially when both are tested together, are the best tests for pheochromocytoma (see explanation for question 11). Diagnostically, urinary VMA testing alone is not nearly as reliable because of its poor sensitivity and specificity.

14. The answer is C. Ambivalent genitalia develop in female fetuses that are exposed in utero to a significant degree of (their own) congenital adrenal hyperplasia (CAH),

an androgenizing disease. The classic form of CAH is diagnosed far more frequently in females than in males.

15. The answer is D. Potassium wasting is associated with primary aldosteronism. Oversecretion of aldosterone results in sodium retention and potassium excretion. Water retention, caused by sodium retention, produces the prototypical, volume-dependent, low renin state (by homeostatic negative feedback, reduced beta-adrenergic stimulation). Patients should be screened when hypokalemia and hypertension coexist, unless a primary cause for potassium loss (e.g., diarrhea, diuresis) is evident.

16. The answer is E. Cushing's disease is of pituitary origin. Although Cushing's disease, like all forms of Cushing's syndrome, is characterized by production of excessive glucocorticoid, Cushing's disease is caused by excessive secretion of adrenocorticotropic hormone (ACTH) from the pituitary.

17. The answer is A. Mineralocorticoid deficiency characterizes primary adrenal insufficiency, a disease with a number of causes: autoimmune atrophy; bilateral adrenal hemorrhage; fungal, tuberculous, or HIV infection; or metastases from cancer of the lung or breast. The latter diseases affect all zones of the adrenal cortex, including the glomerulosa; aldosterone is lacking. Treatment of primary adrenal insufficiency includes repletion of mineralocorticoid (aldosterone), typically in the form of fludrocortisone, in addition to prednisone or dexamethasone. Most adrenal insufficiency (as distinguished from primary adrenal deficiency) is secondary to suppression of the hypothalamic-pituitary-adrenal axis by long-term therapy with glucocorticoid. (Such patients require an increase in maintenance therapy at times of increased need such as the stresses of surgery and disease.) Aldosterone is not usually lacking in secondary adrenal disease. An infrequent cause of secondary disease is pituitary failure, as in Sheehan's syndrome (necrosis of the pituitary as a result of hypotension, usually occurring in intrapartum states).

BIBLIOGRAPHY

Sundaram V, Falko JM: Triage of problems of the adrenal gland. In *Family Medicine* (House Officer Series). Edited by Rudy DR, Kurowski K. Baltimore, Williams & Wilkins, 1997, pp 567–576.

Test 34

Problems of Growth and Development

DIRECTIONS (Items 1–13): Each of the numbered items or incomplete statements in this section is followed by answers or by completions of the statement. Select the ONE lettered answer or completion that is BEST in each case.

1. With respect to human growth, which of the following is correct?

   (A) Children, after infancy, grow approximately 2 inches (5 cm) per year.
   (B) The genetics of the individual is the determinant of growth.
   (C) Growth occurs continuously at a consistent rate throughout childhood.
   (D) The ratio of the upper body segment to lower body segment in the child remains the same despite growth.
   (E) Short stature is defined as one standard deviation (SD) below the mean height for the individual's age and sex.

2. A 5-year-old girl was more than three standard deviations (SDs) below the mean height for her age. Her baseline chemistry profile, karyotype, urine analysis, and sedimentation rate were all normal, and her physical examination showed she was normal except for her small size. The girl had no other complaints and felt well. A growth hormone stimulation test revealed her growth hormone deficiency. Since then you have been treating her with growth hormone injections six times a week. One year after the start of treatment, you find that her growth remains poor. Besides checking for compliance and rechecking the patient's bone age, what is the most appropriate next step?

   (A) Stop growth hormone treatment.
   (B) Check serum cortisol level.
   (C) Order a dexamethasone suppression test.
   (D) Repeat the test for karyotype.
   (E) Order thyroid function studies.

3. You are examining a 14-year-old boy whose parents are concerned that his puberty may be delayed. He has no complaints, and his medical and neonatal histories are unremarkable. On examination, you find he has an enlarged penis, but not of adult size, and pubic hair of full thickness, but not extended onto the thighs. His testes measure approximately 3.5 centimeters bilaterally. The scrotal skin is dark. What is your most appropriate next step?

   (A) Draw follicle-stimulating hormone (FSH) levels.
   (B) Order x-rays for bone age.
   (C) Order a testosterone level.
   (D) Apprise the parents of their son's normal development.
   (E) Institute an empiric trial of testosterone therapy.

4. Almost all girls in the United States start puberty during which age range?

   (A) 7–12 years
   (B) 8–13 years
   (C) 9–14 years
   (D) 10–15 years
   (E) 11–16 years

5. Breast bud development begins to occur in girls during which Tanner stage?

   (A) Stage I
   (B) Stage II
   (C) Stage III
   (D) Stage IV
   (E) Stage V

6. You have examined an obese, 16-year-old girl, who is 2 standard deviations (SDs) below the mean height for her age, has never had a period, and is at Tanner stage I in sexual development. She has no complaints. Results of a thyroid-stimulating test and of a urine pregnancy test are normal and negative, respectively. The girl's bone age is appropriate in a child of her short stature who has not yet begun to grow. Her dehydroepiandrosterone sulfate (DHEAS) level is appropriate for her age. Her follicle-stimulating hormone (FSH) and luteinizing hormone (LH) levels are elevated. Which of the following accounts for her condition?

(A) Prader-Willi syndrome
(B) Prolactinoma
(C) Primary gonadal failure
(D) Constitutional delay
(E) Dramatic recent weight loss (≥ 20% of body weight)

7. A 17-year-old male adolescent is at Tanner stage I. He has no plans for fatherhood in the near future. Which of the following do you recommend?

(A) Patient reassurance only
(B) Oral or intramuscular testosterone
(C) Follicle-stimulating hormone (FSH)
(D) Luteinizing hormone (LH)
(E) Human chorionic gonadotropin (hCG)

8. A 19-month-old girl has unilateral (right) breast bud development. The child has been well, is taking no medications, and is of average height and weight for her age. Her vaginal mucosa appears as expected at her age. Which of the following should you do?

(A) Reassure the parents, and ask them to inform you if other secondary sex characteristics develop.
(B) Order an ultrasound of the right breast.
(C) Order bilateral mammograms.
(D) Request a surgical consultation for excision of the lesion.
(E) Check levels of estradiol, follicle-stimulating hormone (FSH), and luteinizing hormone (LH).

9. Precocious puberty in girls is defined as secondary sexual development before which age?

(A) 13 years
(B) 12 years
(C) 10 years
(D) 8 years
(E) 6 years

10. A 14-year-old girl exhibits virilization, including clitoral enlargement and facial hair. She has no other complaints and has not been ill. Results of motor and sensory examination, including deep tendon reflexes, are normal. No abdominal masses are appreciated. Visual fields are intact to gross confrontation. Which of the following should be part of the initial workup?

(A) Serum testosterone level
(B) Serum progesterone level
(C) Karyotype
(D) Total serum estrogen level
(E) Magnetic resonance imaging (MRI) of the pituitary gland

11. An 8-year-old boy, who has no history of ambiguous genitalia at birth nor use of exogenous estrogen, exhibits bilateral breast bud development. Otherwise, he has been well and is taking no medications. Examination shows that the testes are approximately 1 cm bilaterally and that the penis is small. Breast tissue is palpable bilaterally, and the areolae are increased. No abdominal masses are appreciated. The boy is in the 40th percentile for height and weight. The most appropriate next step is which of the following?

(A) Assure the parents the condition is benign (and probably transient) gynecomastia.
(B) Start the boy on monthly treatment with testosterone enanthate 50 mg intramuscularly (IM).
(C) Begin a search for an estrogen-secreting tumor.
(D) Obtain a surgical consultation for excisional biopsy of breast masses.
(E) Check the boy's thyroid-stimulating hormone (TSH) level to rule out hypothyroidism.

12. Human chorionic gonadotropin (hCG) can be produced by which of the following central nervous system (CNS) tumors?

(A) Astrocytomas
(B) Meningiomas
(C) Craniopharyngiomas
(D) Neurogliomas
(E) Dysgerminomas

13. Regarding treatment of a boy with central precocious puberty, which of the following should be used?

(A) A gonadotropin-releasing hormone (GnRH) agonist
(B) Human chorionic gonadotropin (hCG)
(C) Cyproterone acetate
(D) Medroxyprogesterone acetate
(E) Spironolactone

DIRECTIONS (Items 14–15): Each of the numbered items or incomplete statements in this section is negatively phrased, as indicated by a capitalized word such as NOT, LEAST, or EXCEPT. Select the ONE lettered answer or completion that is BEST in each case.

14. Which of the following disorders is NOT associated with short stature in childhood?

(A) Turner's syndrome
(B) Hypothyroidism
(C) Klinefelter's syndrome
(D) Poorly controlled diabetes mellitus
(E) Renal tubular acidosis

15. Which of the following is NOT a possible etiology for primary ovarian failure?

(A) Polycystic ovary (PCO) syndrome
(B) Radiation to the ovaries of > 3000 rads
(C) Autoimmune gonadal failure
(D) Alkylating agent chemotherapy
(E) Turner's syndrome

ANSWERS AND EXPLANATIONS

1. The answer is A. After infancy (by definition, the age of 1 year), children grow about 2 inches (5 cm) per year. Growth is determined by both genetic and environmental factors. It occurs in spurts, rather than at a consistent rate. With normal growth through infancy and childhood, the ratio of the upper body segment to the lower body segment decreases. Short stature is two or more standard deviations (SDs) below the mean height for the individual's age and sex.

2. The answer is E. Ordering thyroid function studies is the most appropriate next step. Growth hormone sometimes induces hypothyroidism, a likely cause of this patient's continued poor growth despite therapy. (Even patients who are responding to treatment and growing normally should have their thyroid function tested yearly.) The girl's growth hormone treatment should continue, because her growth rate remains an issue. A serum cortisol level should be ordered only if signs or symptoms of adrenal insufficiency or excess are present. The same is true of the dexamethasone suppression test. If the karyotype had not already been tested and found to be normal, it would have been used to rule out Turner's syndrome (XO karyotype) and other chromosome abnormalities. In this case, bone age, a measure of where in the process of long bone growth and epiphyseal closure the patient lies, might provide assurance that lack of growth is not caused by premature or earlier-than-average closure of epiphyses (usually associated with pubescence). Routine chemistries and sedimentation rate are screening tests for the variety of metabolic and inflammatory conditions that may cause growth delay.

3. The answer is D. Parents should be reassured that their son has normal pubertal development for his age. Examination reveals that the boy is in Tanner stage IV of pubertal development. Tanner stages for boys are as follows:

Stage I: no pubic hair; preadolescent genitalia (testes 1–2 cm)

Stage II (9–12.5 years): scanty, slightly pigmented pubic hair; testes > 2 cm; scrotum enlarged

Stage III (10–13.5 years): small amount of darker, coarser, curling pubic hair; longer penis; larger testes

Stage IV [12–15 years): adult type of pubic hair but less than adult quantity; glans widened; testes approaching adult size (3–4 cm), scrotum pigmented

Stage V (14–16 years): pubic hair spread to medial aspects of the thighs; adult genitalia (size varying with body size)

In suspected delayed or failed puberty, an elevated follicle-stimulating hormone (FSH) level would indicate pituitary failure or primary gonadal failure as the cause of the condition. A low testosterone level would confirm delayed puberty and would be commensurate with a lower-than-expected bone age. Testosterone therapy would be appropriate in the management of most types of gonadal failure. (In girls, all Tanner stages occur an average of 6–12 months earlier than in boys.)

4. The answer is B. In 98% of girls in the United States, puberty begins between the ages of 8 and 13 years. It takes an average of 4.2 years to complete. In boys, puberty begins between the ages of 9 and 14 years.

5. The answer is B. Breast bud development, as well as the appearance of sparse pubic hair on the labia, begins in girls during Tanner stage II. Tanner stages for girls are as follows.

Stage I: No pubic hair; preadolescent breasts (elevation of the papilla only); preadolescent genitalia

Stage II: Sparse, long, straight, slightly pigmented pubic hair on labia; visible or palpable breast buds; increased areolar diameter

Stage III: small amount of darker, coarser, curlier, pubic hair spreading over mons pubis; enlargement of breast and areola with no separation of their contours

Stage IV: Adult-type, coarse, curly, pubic hair covering less area than in adult and none on thighs; breast areola and papilla projecting to form a secondary mound

Stage V: pubic hair forming adult inverted triangle, spreading to medial surface of the thigh; adult-contoured breast with projection of the papilla only; areola more pigmented

6. The answer is C. Primary gonadal failure accounts for this girl's condition—delayed puberty despite completion of adrenarchy—as evidenced by normal DHEAS level. The increased luteinizing hormone (LH) and follicle-stimulating hormone (FSH) levels indicate ovarian failure. The possibility of pregnancy having occurred prior to menarche has been ruled out. Short stature is compatible with most causes of delayed puberty. Hypothyroidism is a possible basis of delayed puberty but has been ruled out by the thyroid-stimulating hormone (TSH) test. Turner's syndrome is one likely cause of primary ovarian failure. Weight loss, prolactinoma, and Prader-Willi syndrome can all cause a delay in puberty, but through insufficient hypothalamic release of LH and FSH (thus low levels are detected). Constitutional growth delay also results in low FSH and LH levels.

7. The answer is B. Oral or intramuscular testosterone is appropriate for this patient with delayed puberty, which is the continued absence of secondary sex characteristics by the age of 14 years for boys and 12 years for girls. Treatment is necessary not only to enable the development of secondary sex characteristics, but to minimize tall stature that can result from failure of the growth plates to close. If sperm production were an issue, the gonadotropins [follicle-stimulating hormone (FSH), luteinizing hormone (LH)] would be used. Human chorionic gonadotropin (hCG), which is elevated in pregnancy and in various causes of ectopic production of this hormone of pregnancy, would not be relevant to the study of this case. Patient reassurance without treatment would be inappropriate.

8. The answer is A. Parents should be told that a breast bud can sometimes be seen at this age. Premature thelarche is most commonly seen in children younger than 2 years and older than 6 years. Breast ultrasound, mammograms, surgical consultation, and the checking of estradiol, follicle-stimulating hormone (FSH), and luteinizing hormone (LH) levels are inappropriate in this case. Treatment is unnecessary unless pubertal development in other tissues is evident, or growth or bone age is affected.

9. The answer is D. Precocious puberty is secondary sexual development in girls younger than age 8, or in boys younger than age 9. It is categorized according to whether it is initiated by and dependent on a premature triggering pulse of luteinizing hormone–releasing hormone (LHRH). The LHRH causes otherwise normal gonads to function prematurely, and the sexual precocity is isosexual (i.e., development takes place along the lines of the original sexual phenotype). In 80% of girls and 50% of boys who undergo precocious puberty, sexual precocity is isosexual. In the rest of affected individuals, the condition results from neurologic triggers (traumatic, infectious, or convulsive disorders) that stimulate premature pulsing of LHRH. When LHRH is not involved,

the precocious puberty is due to one of several causes, such as tumors that secrete hormones such as β-human chorionic gonadotropin (β-hCG) and testoterone elaborated by Leydig cell adenomas of the testes. Causes of incomplete isosexual precocity in girls are estrogen-producing tumors in the adrenals [congenital adrenal hyperplasia (CAH)] and the ovaries. Causes in boys are CAH and chorioepithelioma.

10. The answer is A. Clitoral enlargement and facial hair growth are the results of virilization, and ordering a serum testosterone level should be part of the initial workup. Virilization is likely to be the result of an androgen-secreting tumor, congenital adrenal hyperplasia (CAH), hyperprolactinemia, hypothyroidism, or drugs. The abdominal examination is performed to seek evidence of an adrenal mass, and the neurologic examination is done with special attention to visual fields to find evidence of a space-occupying lesion that might affect the pituitary. Checking testosterone, testosterone-binding globulin, and prolactin levels is suitable. An estrogen or progesterone deficiency does not produce virilization, so checking estrogen or progesterone levels is not appropriate. Magnetic resonance imaging (MRI) is indicated only if laboratory studies find hyperprolactinemia or a suspected gonadotropin-dependent disorder. (The rule is that the hormonal abnormality should be defined before imaging studies are ordered.) Although this girl exhibits virilization, she is a phenotypic female, and she has neither Klinefelter's syndrome nor Turner's syndrome. Therefore, checking the karyotype is inappropriate.

11. The answer is C. In contrast to the gynecomastia that occurs at least transiently in more than 30% of pubescent boys, male breast development earlier than puberty suggests estrogen exposure, either from an estrogen-secreting tumor (adrenal, testicular, or bronchogenic) or from an exogenous source. Although breast enlargement sometimes occurs in obese boys, it does so with no palpable breast bud or areolar development. However, this boy is not obese, and areolar changes are present, so reassuring the parents is inappropriate. Treatment with testosterone is premature, as is surgical consultation for excisional breast biopsy. Ruling out hypothyroidism is inappropriate: While hyperthyroidism is sometimes associated with excess estrogen, hypothyroidism is not.

12. The answer is E. Dysgerminomas are tumors of the central nervous system CNS) that can produce human chorionic gonadotropin (hCG). (Other hCG-producing tumors include choriocarcinomas and epitheliomas.) Craniopharyngiomas and neurogliomas can produce precocious puberty by affecting hypothalamic control, but do not produce hCG.

13. The answer is A. A gonadotropin-releasing hormone (GnRH) agonist would be used in the treatment of central precocious puberty in a male child. Chronic use of leuprolide acetate (a synthetic GnRH analog) desensitizes the pituitary to GnRH, leading to a decrease in luteinizing hormone (LH) and follicle-stimulating hormone (FSH) levels. Human chorionic gonadotropin (hCG) has no role in treatment of precocious puberty. Androgen antagonists (e.g., cyproterone) are more appropriate for peripheral precocious puberty. Neither medroxyprogesterone acetate, a progestational agent, nor spironolactone, an aldosterone antagonist, is relevant in this case.

14. The answer is C. Klinefelter's syndrome is NOT associated with short stature in children. Klinefelter's, unlike Turner's syndrome, is a congenital disorder (classically with an XXY karyotype), in which testosterone levels and growth remain normal until patients are approximately 14 years of age. Clinical features, which include small testicle size, greater growth in lower than in upper extremities, and gynecomastia, do not occur until puberty. Individuals with Turner's syndrome exhibit short stature. In addition, hypothyroidism, uncontrolled diabetes mellitus, and renal tubular acidosis are all potential causes of childhood short stature. Some of the most common causes are familial short stature (comparisons with parents are important), constitutional growth delay, and psychosocial deprivation. Constitutional growth delay is characterized by delay in adrenarche and gonadarche and bone age retarded but commensurate with adrenal and gonadal stages. This sets it apart from hypogonadal hypogonadism and other types.

15. The answer is A. Polycystic ovary (PCO) syndrome is NOT an etiology of ovarian failure, although it is a potential etiology of infertility. Other aspects of polycystic ovary (PCO) syndrome include amenorrhea, androgenization, and insulin resistance (leading to type II diabetes). Weight loss is the single best therapy for PCO syndrome. Radiation to the ovaries, autoimmune gonadal failure, alkylating chemotherapy, and Turner's syndrome may account for ovarian failure. Viral infections (such as mumps or Coxsackie B virus) can also produce acute gonadal failure.

BIBLIOGRAPHY

Schuster DP, Falko JM: Problems of growth and development. In *Family Medicine* (House Officer Series). Edited by Rudy DR, Kurowski K. Baltimore, Williams & Wilkins, 1997, pp 577–590.

SECTION **XIII**

Allergies

Test 35

Atopic and Food Allergies

DIRECTIONS (Items 1–13): Each of the numbered items or incomplete statements in this section is followed by answers or by completions of the statement. Select the ONE lettered answer or completion that is BEST in each case.

1. A 30-year-old woman develops wheezing, throat tightness, and urticaria 2 minutes after being stung by a yellow jacket (vespid wasp). Her pulse is 104 beats/min, her respiratory rate is 30 breaths/min, and her blood pressure is 90/60 mm Hg. She appears in significant distress and complains of lightheadedness, and she asks to sit down, lest she faint. She exhibits diffuse expiratory wheezing. Which of the following best describes the pathophysiology of her condition?

    (A) Circulating antigens reacting with tissue-based antigen, producing inflammatory injury
    (B) Deposition of circulating immune complexes into the tissues where they produced inflammatory injury
    (C) Occurrence of an immunoglobulin G (IgG) response to injected antigen
    (D) Release of mast cell granules in response to membrane-bound IgE cross-linking with specific allergen
    (E) Production of a "late phase" reaction through inflammation

2. Atopic dermatitis frequently appears on the facial cheeks in which of the following age-groups?

    (A) Infants
    (B) Children
    (C) Adolescents
    (D) Adults
    (E) Elderly individuals

3. With respect to atopic dermatitis, which of the following statements is correct?

    (A) It generally becomes symptomatic in adulthood.
    (B) Mild childhood cases generally remit by age 20.
    (C) It is associated with allergies to multiple foods and produces several positive results on skin tests and radioallergosorbent tests (RASTs).
    (D) Pruritus is unusual.
    (E) Adult patients with severe relapsing lesions most often had mild disease in childhood.

4. A 30-year-old woman has a few patches of scaly, pruritic erythema on her upper eyelids and on the back of her hands. She is taking no medications or over-the-counter preparations, has received no recent therapy, and is not pregnant. Which of the following is the appropriate treatment?

    (A) A tapering dose of oral glucocorticoid
    (B) A low-dose topical glucocorticoid
    (C) Trial elimination of all milk products from her diet
    (D) Continuous use of a topical antihistamine
    (E) Application of topical ketoconazole

5. Which of the following is a known allergen that frequently precipitates allergic rhinitis?

    (A) Animal dander
    (B) Perfume
    (C) Air pollution
    (D) Tobacco smoke
    (E) Paint

6. With respect to ragweed and its role in allergic rhinitis, which of the following statements is correct?

    (A) Ragweed is second to mold spores as the most common cause of allergic rhinitis in the United States.
    (B) Sunshine lowers ragweed pollen counts.
    (C) Rain lowers ragweed pollen counts.
    (D) Ragweed pollen counts are highest from April through July.
    (E) Ragweed is usually released during lawn mowing and leaf raking.

7. A 25-year-old man is taking erythromycin 500 mg orally 4 times a day for 10 days for urethritis caused by chlamydia. During treatment, seasonal allergic rhinitis symptoms develop. Which of the medications listed below should be avoided because serum levels are excessively high when given with erythromycin (or other macrolide antibiotics) and sometimes produce cardiac dysrhythmia?

    (A) Pseudoephedrine
    (B) Chlorpheniramine maleate
    (C) Terfenadine
    (D) Loratadine
    (E) Cromolyn sodium nasal inhaler

8. A 30-year-old man with severe allergic rhinitis has significant symptoms despite environmental modifications, oral antihistamines, and intranasal steroids. His reactions on skin tests are strongly positive to ragweed and mold. You start him on immunotherapy, but he does not experience symptomatic improvement. How long should you continue the injections before abandoning them?

(A) 1 month
(B) 6 months
(C) 1 year
(D) 5 years
(E) 10 years

9. Which of the following is one of the beneficial effects of immunotherapy on the immune system?

(A) Increase of mast cell and basophil degranulation
(B) Decrease in allergen-specific immunoglobulin E (IgE) antibody levels
(C) Decrease in allergen-specific IgE-blocking antibody
(D) Stimulation of T-lymphocyte suppression of IgE production
(E) Acceleration of the usual increase in seasonal IgE levels

10. Desensitization (immunotherapy) is most effective with which of the following allergens?

(A) Pollen
(B) Molds
(C) Cat dander
(D) Dog dander
(E) Cockroaches

11. A 6-year-old girl has wheezing dyspnea. Which of the following organisms is most consistently linked with provocation of her condition?

(A) Adenoviruses
(B) Herpes viruses
(C) Arboviruses
(D) Respiratory syncytial virus (RSV)
(E) *Streptococcus pneumoniae*

12. A 17-year-old boy with a 12-year history of asthma has been taking short-acting beta-agonist inhalers and cromolyn inhalers. They provide fair control of his daytime symptoms but poor control of the wheezing and dyspnea that awaken him almost every night. Which of the following inhalers has the longest duration of action and, thus, ability to control his nocturnal symptoms?

(A) Albuterol
(B) Terbutaline
(C) Pirbuterol
(D) Ipratropium
(E) Salmeterol

13. Which of the following is more likely than the others to be a food allergen in a 10-year-old child?

(A) Strawberries
(B) Shellfish
(C) Chocolate
(D) Tomatoes
(E) Corn

DIRECTIONS (Items 14–16): Each of the numbered items or incomplete statements in this section is negatively phrased, as indicated by a capitalized word such as NOT, LEAST, or EXCEPT. Select the ONE lettered answer or completion that is BEST in each case.

14. Regarding the patient in question 1, all EXCEPT which of the following is relevant to immediate alleviation of the emergency?

    (A) Placement in the Trendelenburg position

    (B) Administration of epinephrine 0.1–0.2 ml in 1:10,000 solution intravenously (IV) slowly

    (C) Administration of theophylline 5.6 mg/kg IV over 20 minutes

    (D) Administration of diphenhydramine 25–50 mg intramuscularly (IM)

    (E) Administration of methylprednisolone 40 mg IV over 1 minute

15. An 18-year-old Caucasian man living in Ohio complains of rhinorrhea and sneezing that occur during the months of April, May, and June and taper off in July and August. Which of the following statements with regard to his condition is NOT true?

    (A) Nasal eosinophils are increased during the season.

    (B) Exposure to tree pollen is the cause of the symptoms.

    (C) The peak age for symptoms is between 15 and 25 years.

    (D) Both sexes are equally likely to be affected.

    (E) Symptoms can be controlled in a great number of cases by serial injections.

16. A 32-year-old woman with a history of asthma complains of 2 days of shortness of breath and wheezing. She says that she developed a cold 1 week ago. She has been treating herself with over-the-counter, proprietary epinephrine mist but is taking no other medications. She has no allergies to medications. Her temperature is 98.8°F (37.1°C), her respiratory rate is 30 breaths/min, heart rate is 90 beats/min and regular, and her blood pressure is 140/80 mm Hg. She is fully awake and alert but in moderate distress. No accessory muscle use or cyanosis is evident. Tympanic membranes are gray and intact. Pharynx is moist and shows only trace erythema with no exudate. Diffuse expiratory wheezes are evident in all fields of lungs. Percussion is normal. Cardiac examination reveals no murmur, irregular rhythm, or friction rub. The abdomen is soft with no mass and no tenderness. You can recommend several interventions and treatments. Which of the following should you NOT recommend?

    (A) Peak flow measurement before and after therapy

    (B) An inhaled beta-agonist

    (C) Cromolyn inhaler

    (D) Systemic glucocorticoid

    (E) Oxygen

ANSWERS AND EXPLANATIONS

1. The answer is D. This is a classic immediate hypersensitivity response. This woman must have had prior exposure to the antigen (although she may not recall the first uneventful sting) that led to the production of the immunoglobulin E (IgE) antibodies on the mast cell surface.

The early phase response is characterized by capillary permeability and fluid leakage. Other features of this response are capillary permeability and fluid leakage. In susceptible individuals, early phase reactants are responsible for bronchospasm—hence the wheezing. The throat tightness refers to the laryngeal response to the early phase reaction leading to laryngospasm. The sinus tachycardia is a nonspecific response to any acute stress. It is invoked in allergy skin testing as another example of its applicability.

The late phase response, which occurs 3–8 hours later and can last up to 24 hours, involves local invasion by basophils, eosinophils, monocytes, and lymphocytes. Analogous clinical situations include the rapid onset and recovery (15–30 minutes) of bronchospasm in asthmatic exposure to inhaled allergenic antigens. There are mucosal and conjunctival counterparts to these reactions. The late phase resembles the actual clinical picture in asthma, resulting, for example, in air trapping. Deposition of circulating immune complexes into the tissues produces inflammatory injury on an autoimmune basis, as occurs in acute or chronic glomerulonephritis and lupus erythematosus. Circulating antigens reacting with tissue-based antigen combine to form new complexes different from either the foreign antigen or the tissue-based antigen and produced inflammatory injury similar to that which occurs on an autoimmune basis. IgG is ultimately manufactured normally in response to injected antigen to form true protective immunity. It is involved pathologically in serum sickness, a systemic immune reaction characterized by urticarial rash and even subacute glomerulonephritis. None of the reactions among the incorrect choices results in anaphylaxis.

2. The answer is A. Atopic dermatitis frequently appears on the cheeks, as well as on the abdomen and extensor surfaces of the legs, in infants. Although atopic dermatitis may appear on other parts of the body in individuals of all ages, when the tendency for it is strong, the typical patches of atopic dermatitis seen on the cheeks of susceptible infants are seldom seen on the cheeks in other age-groups.

3. The answer is B. The great majority of cases become asymptomatic in childhood, and almost all cases (90%) of children with mild atopic dermatitis remit fully by age 20. However, severe disease in childhood is associated with persistent chronic disease in adulthood. Most children with atopic dermatitis are allergic to only one or two foods, despite testing positive to multiple foods on skin tests and radioallergosorbent tests (RASTs). Intense pruritus is a hallmark of atopic dermatitis.

4. The answer is B. A low-dose topical glucocorticoid is appropriate for this woman, who has either nummular eczema or contact dermatitis caused by a cosmetic. (The former is more likely because the patient has symptoms on the hands as well as the eyelids.) The case is not severe enough to institute a systemic (oral) glucocorticoid. Milk allergy is rarely expressed as a facial eczematoid eruption, so milk elimination will not help. Topical antihistamines do not control allergic response or give relief to pruritus. Ketoconazole, an antifungal agent, is not used in the treatment of allergies.

5. The answer is A. Animal dander is a known allergen that frequently precipitates allergic rhinitis. Perfume, air pollution, tobacco smoke, and paint may be irritants that produce similar symptoms, but they are not allergens for allergic rhinitis. Many other allergens cause allergic rhinitis such as ragweed and grass pollens, mold spores (*Hormodendrum* and *Alternaria*) and house dust (primarily products of mites).

6. The answer is C. Rain lowers ragweed pollen counts by temporarily wringing the particles from the air and into the ground. Wind also lowers ragweed pollen counts by temporarily moving the air away from the source of the ragweed pollen. In North America, the peak season for release of ragweed pollen (the leading cause of allergic rhinitis) occurs from mid-August to the first drop in temperature to less than or equal to 40°F (4.4°C) [approximately], often in October. Sunshine promotes drying and therefore results in increased pollen counts. Because ragweed is not normally present in domestic yards, it is not normally released in lawn mowing or leaf raking.

Mold spores, the most prevalent being *Alternaria* and *Hormodendrum*, enter the breathable atmosphere over the eastern half of the United States in May and June, peak the first week of July, and remain until the cool weather of fall. They are second only to ragweed as causing the most cases of symptomatic rhinitis.

7. The answer is C. Erythromycin and other macrolide antibiotics, as well as ketoconazole and itraconazole, decrease the clearance of a terfenadine acid metabolite. Terfenadine should be avoided. Elevated terfenadine levels are associated with QT interval prolongations on electrocardiograph (EKG) and can produce torsades de pointes and other cardiac dysrhythmias. Torsades de pointes is a polymorphous ventricular tachycardia with shifting QRS axis which is difficult to treat and may deteriorate to ventricular fibrillation.

8. The answer is C. Patients who do not respond at least partially to 1–2 years of treatment are unlikely to respond to further immunotherapy. Patients who do respond can be treated for up to 4–5 years.

9. The answer is D. A beneficial effect of immunotherapy on the immune system is the stimulation of lymphocyte suppression of immunoglobulin E (IgE) production, leading to a decrease in mast cell and basophil degranulation. Effects of desensitization are not directly on the specific IgE antibody levels but rather indirectly on the lymphocytes that are producing the specific IgE. Increasing IgE would be a detrimental, rather than a therapeutic, effect. Increasing mast cell and basophil degranulation would be a pathologic effect.

10. The answer is A. Of the answer choices, desensitization to pollen is most effective. Such therapy is also much more likely to alleviate allergic rhinitis than asthma. Desensitization is effective against mold spore allergy, but not as effective as against ragweed. Desensitization to animal dander is not only less likely to be successful, but the required vaccine inoculations can cause severe systemic reactions. Desensitization is much less effective against cockroaches and to house dust, a mixture of mite parts and excreta.

11. The answer is D. Respiratory syncytial virus (RSV) has consistently been linked with wheezing dyspnea (asthma). Up to 50% of children with RSV bronchiolitis have recurrent wheezing until 3 years of age. Bacteria are less likely than viruses to provoke asthma. Most children with a history of RSV infection and subsequent asthma have atopic constitutions (genetic tendencies toward allergic rhinitis and/or asthma) and family histories of similar problems. RSV bronchiolitis aggravates the inherited tendency, but it can also cause wheezing in individuals without such tendencies. This may be one reason why the term "reactive airway disease" (sometimes used in place of asthma) has appeared in the medical vocabulary in recent years. Adenoviruses attack people of all ages, including children. Although they are implicated in bronchitis, bronchiolitis, croup, and pneumonia, they are not associated with later onset of asthma. Her-

pes viruses cause localized vesicular infections with long-standing chronic asymptomatic occupation of sites between flare-ups. There are only two types, 1 and 2, which infect predominantly oral and genital mucosa, respectively. They do not cause respiratory infections unless such a development is a part of systemic infection in immunologically defenseless individuals (e.g., patients with cancer, blood dyscrasias, AIDS; patients on anti-cancer chemotherapy). Arboviruses cause various encephalitides, including eastern equine, western equine, St. Louis, and California encephalitides. Their species are also causes of yellow fever, jungle fever, dengue fever, and several other diseases. None of these is a respiratory infection. Although streptococcal pneumonia is likely to cause infection as a complication of reactive airway disease, it is not a particular cause of asthmatic attacks.

12. The answer is E. Salmeterol inhaler (a β_2 agonist) has the longest duration of action (up to 30 hours). It is many times stronger than albuterol, and lasts longer than terbutaline or pirbuterol (all β_2 agonists). It also lasts longer than anticholinergic medications (including ipratropium), which are rather short-acting (4–6 hours).

13. The answer is B. Shellfish is one of the most likely food allergens in children. Nuts, peanuts, and fish are also common food allergens. Contrary to reputation, chocolate, strawberries, and tomatoes rarely cause allergic symptoms. Corn and other foods are much less certainly linked to food allergy. Elimination diets are used to discover empirically what food may be a cause of symptoms. A practical approach involves elimination of all of the suspected allergenic foods for up to 1 week or until symptoms abate. Then, the most desired foods are added back individually with at least 2 days between additions. A food allergen is one that produces symptoms within minutes to 1 hour from the time of ingestion.

14. The answer is E. Glucocorticoids are an integral part of management of any severe allergic reaction, but they do not begin to work soon enough to have an immediate effect during life-threatening emergencies such as anaphylaxis or acute asthma. Placement in the Trendelenburg position may preserve consciousness when the brain is otherwise not being perfused due to hypotension. Epinephrine, usually given subcutaneously, is indicated in all allergic emergencies. However, when hypotension exists as part of the clinical picture, as in the clinical scenario, epinephrine may better be given intravenously (IV) both for quicker onset and because of more assured absorption. In shock states, absorption of medications given subcutaneously may be indefinitely delayed from the peripheral source of injection. Aminophylline is indicated for the bronchospasm in the present case. Diphenhydramine, as an H_1 histamine blocking agent, takes effect quickly and is indicated for all truly allergic emergencies in the first wave of medications (those given in rapid succession, if not simultaneously). It is also indicated in acute and subacute nonemergencies.

15. The answer is B. This patient's allergic rhinitis with seasonal onset is NOT caused by tree pollen. In the United States, the tree pollenating season begins roughly in March and continues through April. The months in which this patient is affected represent the season of grass allergy in US temperate regions. In North America, allergic symptoms to mold spores begin in June, peak in early July, and subside gradually throughout the autumn months. The peak age range for symptoms is 15–25 years, and both sexes are equally affected. Desensitization by serial injections of upwardly graduated concentrations and volumes of solutions of the offending antigen leads to alleviation of symptoms in a vast majority of cases of allergic rhinitis (but not of allergic asthma).

16. The answer is C. A cromolyn inhaler should NOT be recommended for this patient. Cromolyn is effective in preventing asthma, particularly in children, but it does not relieve acute asthmatic attacks. Moreover, it is irritating and may aggravate acute symptoms. Peak flow measurement before and after therapy is the quickest way of assessing success of therapeutic measures. For acute asthma, inhaled beta-agonists are standard treatment, as are glucocorticoids and oxygen. Oxygen therapy is standard care in any dyspneic patient. In addition, systemic glucocorticoids, while requiring longer to take effect (4–6 hours) than beta-agonists, are an important part of acute asthma management. Use of accessory muscles (e.g., intercostals, pectorals) and presence of cyanosis would be indicators of increased severity of obstructive disease and of dyspnea.

BIBLIOGRAPHY

Schwer WA: Atopic, food, and contact allergies. In *Family Medicine* (House Officer Series). Edited by Rudy DR, Kurowski K. Baltimore, Williams & Wilkins, 1997, pp 591–604.

SECTION XIV

Preventive Care, Health, and Efficiency

Test 36

Preventive Care, the Patient, and the Doctor

DIRECTIONS: (Items 1–8): Each of the numbered items or incomplete statements in this section is followed by answers or by completions of the statement. Select the ONE lettered answer or completion that is BEST in each case.

1. Which of the following constitutes primary prevention?

   (A) Papanicolaou (Pap) smear in asymptomatic women to detect abnormalities that could lead to carcinoma of the cervix.
   (B) Percutaneous coronary angioplasty in individuals who have symptoms with exercise but no myocardial damage to prevent coronary disease
   (C) Removal of adenomatous polyps during screening colonoscopy to prevent progression of a precancerous process
   (D) Routine blood pressure surveillance to prevent coronary artery disease
   (E) Smoking cessation after myocardial infarction to prevent progression of coronary disease

2. Which of the following statements expresses sensitivity?

   (A) Papanicolaou (Pap) smears diagnose 60% of cervical cancers in one determination.
   (B) A fasting blood sugar in which the normal cut-off point is set downward yields more false-positive results.
   (C) Stool occult blood tests produce negative results in 95% of normal individuals who have no polyp or cancer of the colon.
   (D) Positive mammographic readings (suspicious for cancer) are based on carcinoma of the breast in 23% of cases.
   (E) Negative results on test "X" for disease "A," which is prevalent at 2/1000, indicate a 99.9% chance that the disease is not present.

3. Which of the following is an example of specificity?

   (A) Papanicolaou (Pap) smears diagnose 60% of cervical cancers in one determination.
   (B) Transferrin saturation greater than or equal to 62% diagnoses 95% of hemochromatosis.
   (C) Papanicolaou (Pap) smears are negative in 98.9% of women who have no cervical cancer.
   (D) Positive mammographic readings (suspicious for cancer) are based on carcinoma of the breast in 23% of cases.
   (E) Negative results on test "X" for disease "A," which is prevalent at 2/1000, indicate a 99.9% chance that the disease is not present.

4. Which of the following is an example of prevalence (US population)?

   (A) The annual number of new cases of colorectal cancer is 131,000.
   (B) The number of individuals with diabetes mellitus is 11–15 million.
   (C) Testicular cancer strikes 4 of 100,000 men per year.
   (D) The annual number of cases of herpes simplex genitalis is 200,000–500,000.
   (E) The annual number of deaths from smoking-related causes is 420,000.

5. Which of the following is an example of incidence?

   (A) Essential hypertension is present in 15% of the population of the United States and 25% of the population of Japan.
   (B) Either hypothyroidism or hyperthyroidism is present in 1%–4% of the US population.
   (C) New cases of carcinoma of the cervix in the United States number 16,000 per year (8/100,000 population and 4/100,000 women).
   (D) Ischemic heart disease causes 490,000 deaths per year in the United States (245/100,000 population).
   (E) Depression is found in 5%–13% of patients in a primary care practice.

6. You are inventing a new disposable thermometer (of chemically impregnated hemp) whose color changes at sites along the strip reflect a temperature spectrum of 97°F–104°F (36.1°C–40°C). You test it against incubators with known, constant temperature settings within a certain spectrum. Use of your thermometer in an incubator whose confirmed setting and temperature is 99°F (37.2°C) produces five consecutive readings of 100.9°F, 100.9°F, 101.0°F, 101.0°F, and 101.1°F. Which of the following is true of your thermometer?

   (A) Its precision is unacceptable.
   (B) The reproducibility of its results is unacceptable.
   (C) Its accuracy is unacceptable.
   (D) Its accuracy is acceptable.
   (E) The test is inapplicable in the clinically significant range of temperatures.

7. In community "A," with 10,000 men, the incidence of prostate cancer is 15 cases per year. In community "B," with 15,000 men (same age distribution as in community "A"), the incidence of prostate cancer is 45 cases per year. The odds ratio (OR) of carcinoma of the prostate in community "B" compared to community "A" is approximately which of the following?

  (A) 0.5
  (B) 1.0
  (C) 1.5
  (D) 2.0
  (E) 2.5

8. A research question has been raised regarding whether dietary fiber offers protection against cancer of the colon. Which of the following studies would most reliably answer this question?

  (A) One that calculates the rate of colon cancer in Africa, where a high-fiber diet is consumed, and in the United States, where a relatively low-fiber diet is consumed
  (B) One that compares the calculated values of the fiber content of the diet in a large group of patients with colon cancer with that of a carefully matched control group that does not have cancer
  (C) One that seeks a correlation between the fiber content in the diet of people from a certain country and the incidence of colon cancer in that same country
  (D) One that puts a large number of individuals who are at risk for colon cancer on either high- or low-fiber diets and evaluates the appearance of colon cancer in both groups over a long period of time
  (E) One that observes two populations, one that normally consumes a high-fiber diet (i.e., Seventh Day Adventists) and another that normally consumes a low-fiber diet, for a sufficiently long period to determine the incidence of cancer

QUESTIONS 9–12.

Disease "X" has a prevalence of 10/1000. The sensitivity of test "T" for disease "X" is 95% for denoting serum "Y" levels when they exceed the normal range. The specificity is 90%.

9. In a population of 100,000, approximately how many individuals have disease "X"?

  (A) 1
  (B) 10
  (C) 100
  (D) 1000
  (E) 10,000

10. If the entire population of 100,000 were tested with test "T," how many individuals would test positive for the disease?

  (A) 5
  (B) 95
  (C) 950
  (D) 9900
  (E) 10,850

11. In the population of 100,000, how many would test negative?

  (A) 95
  (B) 89,150
  (C) 89,915
  (D) 90,000
  (E) 99,900

12. The positive predictive value (PPV) is

  (A) 5.3%
  (B) 8.8%
  (C) 10.6%
  (D) 90.2%
  (E) 95.7%

DIRECTIONS (Item 13): Each of the numbered items or incomplete statements in this section is negatively phrased, as indicated by a capitalized word such as NOT, LEAST, or EXCEPT. Select the ONE lettered answer or completion that is BEST in each case.

13. Which of the following is NOT a prerequisite for screening?

  (A) The test is reasonably inexpensive.
  (B) The disease is a significant threat to life or quality of life.
  (C) The disease has a long asymptomatic phase.
  (D) The test is completely sensitive and completely specific.
  (E) The test is readily tolerated.

ANSWERS AND EXPLANATIONS

1. The answer is D. The other answer choices are examples of secondary or tertiary prevention. Positive Papanicolaou (Pap) smears discover disease already in progress but still asymptomatic; hence, they are part of the process of secondary prevention. Percutaneous coronary angioplasty that interrupts a symptomatic coronary disease already in progress is tertiary prevention. Removal of adenomatous polyps (i.e., by definition, the condition is asymptomatic) during screening colonoscopy prevents progression of a precancerous process, and is, therefore, secondary prevention. Smoking cessation to prevent conditions that do not yet exist is primary prevention, but after myocardial infarction has already occurred, smoking cessation is another example of tertiary prevention (to prevent a symptomatic recurrence).

2. The answer is A. The ability of Papanicolaou (Pap) smears to diagnose 60% of cervical cancers in one determination is an example of sensitivity (i.e., measure of ability to diagnose the presence of disease). Setting the fasting blood sugar normal cutoff point downward results in more false-positive results or a decrease in specificity (i.e., measure of ability to be truly negative in the absence of disease). Negative results of stool occult blood tests in 95% of normal individuals who have no polyp or cancer of the colon are an expression of specificity. The 23% chance that a positive mammographic reading (suspicious for cancer) is based on carcinoma of the breast is an example of positive predictive value (PPV) [i.e., chance that a positive test actually indicates presence of disease]. The 99.9% chance that disease "A," which is prevalent at 2/1000, is absent if test "X" is negative is an example of negative predictive value (NPV) [i.e., chance that a negative test indicates absence of disease].

3. The answer is C. Negative Papanicolaou (Pap) smears in 98.9% of women who have no cervical cancer is an expression of specificity (i.e., measure of ability to be truly negative in the absence of disease). The ability of Pap smears to diagnose 60% of cervical cancers in one determination and the ability of transferrin saturation of greater than or equal to 62% to diagnose 95% of hemochromatosis are expressions of sensitivity (i.e., measure of ability to diagnose the presence of disease). The 23% chance that a positive mammographic reading (suspicious for cancer) is based on carcinoma of the breast is an example of positive predictive value (PPV)

[i.e., chance that a positive test actually indicates presence of disease]. The 99.9% chance that disease "A", which is prevalent at 2/1000, is absent if the results of test "X" are negative is an example of negative predictive value (NPV) [i.e., chance that a negative test indicates absence of disease].

4. The answer is B. The presence of diabetes mellitus in 11–15 million people is an example of prevalence (i.e., number of cases that exist in a population at a given point in time). (Prevalence is usually, but not always, expressed as a numerator and denominator to form a rate.) The 131,000 new cases of colorectal cancer each year, the testicular cancer that strikes 4 of every 100,000 men each year, and the 200,000–500,000 cases of herpes simplex genitalis that occur each year are examples of incidence. [Incidence is the number of new occurrences of a disease, per unit of time (usually 1 year), per known population of a country or per unit of population]. The number of smoking-related deaths per year is an example of cause-specific mortality; it is also a rate of occurrences per unit of time, similar in that regard to incidence. Looking at incidence and prevalence together, it is apparent that a disease of high incidence, but of slow progression, subsidence, or remission, has a larger prevalence than a disease of the same incidence that either abates quickly or kills quickly.

5. The answer is C. The 16,000 new cases of carcinoma of the cervix per year is an example of incidence expressed three different ways. The percentages of the US and Japanese populations that have essential hypertension, the percentage of the US population that has hypothyroidism or hyperthyroidism, and the percentage of depressed patients in a primary care practice are all examples of prevalence. The 490,000 deaths per year from ischemic heart disease is an example of cause-specific mortality data.

6. The answer is C. The accuracy of the thermometer is, of course, unacceptable. This explanation offers an easy review of the difference between "accuracy" on the one hand, and "precision" and "reproducibility" on the other. Accuracy is an assessment of how close an instrument (or test result) comes to the known "truth" or "gold standard." In the scenario, the test results are regularly approximately two degrees Fahrenheit from the temperature of the known heat source, so the degree of accuracy is unacceptable. "Precision" and "reproducibility" are synonymous: They represent the degree of variability among repeated measurements, irrespective of how far the results may be from the true value. The five temperature readings varied only 0.2°F, an acceptable level of precision or reproducibility. If this thermometer's accuracy were as good as its precision, the new invention would be acceptable in clinical practice. The difference between accuracy and precision is important in preventive medicine.

7. The answer is D. The problem is one of comparing the odds of contracting cancer of the prostate in males in community "B" (the community with the higher incidence rate) with that in community "A". It is solved by setting up a 2 × 2 table:

	Community B	Community A
Disease	45 (cell a)	15 (cell b)
No disease	14055 (cell c)	9085 (cell d)

Cross-multiplying yields the following:

$$\text{Odds ratio (OR)} = ad/bc, \text{ or}$$
$$(45 \times 9085)/(15 \times 14055) = 1.939$$

When the compared incidences are quite low (and only then), as in this case, dividing the incidence of the test population (B) by that of the standard population (A) yields virtually the same result:

$$\text{Incidence in community "B"} = 45/15{,}000 = 0.0030$$

$$\text{Incidence in community "A"} = 15/10{,}000 = 0.0015$$

$$\text{Incidence in community "B"} \div \text{incidence in community "A"} = 0.0030/0.0015 = 2$$

This calculation happens also to define relative risk (RR) [i.e., the ratio of risk in the test population compared to the expected risk (in the standard population)]. Thus, in this instance, OR closely approximates RR.

8. The answer is D. This is an example of a prospective interventional study. Thus, true incidences can be calculated in both the interventional group and the control group and compared for statistical differences (if there are differences) by such tests as the two-sample Student's T test. In an appropriately designed interventional study, the subjects are assigned to the treatment and control groups in two ways: by a random process or matching for such characteristics as sex, age, and socioeconomic status. If the study sample population is sufficiently large, either method can generally be assumed to be similar for the population characteristics. Random assignment has one advantage: control for confounding factors not considered by the investigator (e.g., number of children, occupation, smoking habits).

Regarding the other answer choices: Choice A—calculating the rate of colon cancer in Africa and comparing it to that in the United States is an example of an ecological study. An ecological study, which cannot yield an incidence in either comparison population, is not intended to be applicable for definitive answers to a research question. Because this type of study is relatively inexpensive, however, it may form the basis for more definitive investigations such as the interventional study.

Choice B—comparing the calculated values of the fiber content of the diet in a large group of patients with colon cancer with that of a carefully matched control group that does not have cancer is an example of a case control study, a retrospective investigation. Best suited to study of a relatively rare disease, it is inexpensive compared to either of the prospective types of investigations. A case-control study could be used in a medical center or ward that specializes in rare diseases (e.g., amyotrophic lateral sclerosis). In a case control study, the rate of presence of the suspected risk factor is calculated and compared in the diseased group and a control group that is matched for every conceivable trait except for the risk factor being investigated. The odds of contracting colon cancer can be compared between the two groups, but an incidence cannot be calculated.

Choice C—Seeking a correlation between the fiber content in the diet of people from a country with the incidence of colon cancer in the same country is an example of a cross-sectional or prevalence study. In a cross-sectional investigation, populations are simply studied for the prevalence of the disease in question and for suspected risk factors (and other factors that might conceivably turn out to be risks).

Choice E—Observing one population that normally consumes a high-fiber diet (i.e., Seventh Day Adventists) and another that normally consumes a low-fiber diet (E) for a sufficiently long period to determine the incidence of cancer is a prospective study, which is similar to the interventional study with one critical difference. This prospective study is a passive process. Thus, although it compares incidences, it does not define or control for other differences between the two populations besides diet that could account for variation in incidences (e.g., smoking). Smoking would be a confounding factor.

9. The answer is D. Approximately 1000 people in a population of 100,000 have the disease whose prevalence is 10/1000, or 1%.

10. The answer is E. If all the population of 100,000 were tested, 10,850 individuals would test positive for the disease. Among the 1000 individuals who have the disease, a test that is 95% sensitive would be positive in

950 people. Among the 99,000 individuals who do not have the disease, a test that is 90% specific (which would show true negative results in 90%) would show false-positive results in 10%, or 9900. 950 + 9900 = 10,850.

11. The answer is B. In the population of 100,000, those who would test negative number 89,150. This is arrived at by the following process: Of those who have the disease, 1000, 5% would be falsely negative, or 50. Of those who do not have the disease, 99,000, the test with 90% specificity would show true negative results in 90% of cases, or 89,100. 50 + 89,100 = 89,150.

12. The answer is B. The positive predictive value (PPV) [i.e., chance that a positive test actually indicates presence of disease] is 8.8%. The number of true positives, divided by the sum of true positives and false positives, and multiplied by 100, equals the PPV. Thus, 950/(950 + 9900) = 0.08755. This figure, multiplied by 100, and rounded to one decimal place, yields a PPV of 8.8%.

13. The answer is D. Complete sensitivity and complete specificity (together) do NOT constitute a prerequisite for the use of a screening test. No such tests exist other than surgical exploration or similarly invasive procedures in which the expense and the risks are unacceptable in asymptomatic patients. Prerequisites for screening include an acceptable level of expense; disease that poses a significant threat to life, quality of life, or the public welfare; a disease that manifests a long asymptomatic phase (during which the disease is amenable to discovery by the applicable technology); ready tolerability of the test, so that asymptomatic individuals permit themselves to be screened.

BIBLIOGRAPHY

Bloch DJ, Aukerman GF: Preventive care, the patient, and the doctor. In *Family Medicine* (House Officer Series). Edited by Rudy DR, Kurowski K. Baltimore, Williams & Wilkins, 1997, pp 605–616.

Test 37

Preoperative Clearance and Preparation

DIRECTIONS (Items 1–19): Each of the numbered items or incomplete statements in this section is followed by answers or by completions of the statement. Select the ONE lettered answer or completion that is BEST in each case.

1. In preparation for elective surgery, routine preoperative tests [hemoglobin, electrolytes, blood urea nitrogen (BUN), creatinine, urinalysis, serum albumin, chest x-ray] are considered unnecessary for healthy individuals who are

   (A) < 21 years
   (B) < 30 years
   (C) < 40 years
   (D) < 50 years
   (E) < 60 years

2. You have referred a 55-year-old Caucasian man for elective cholecystectomy. He is otherwise healthy and takes no medication. His weight is 185 lb (68 kg); his height, 5′9″ (1.8 m); and his blood pressure, 138/88 mm Hg. Routine preoperative blood urea nitrogen (BUN) and serum creatinine are considered necessary for this individual because

   (A) his age is ≥ 21 years
   (B) his BMI is ≥ 24
   (C) his age is ≥ 40 years
   (D) his age is ≥ 50 years
   (E) his BP is ≥ 130/80

3. Routine electrolyte determination and chest x-ray before major surgery (e.g., entrance to the peritoneal or pleural cavities, dissection of the neck or limbs, or amputation) are justified in otherwise healthy individuals whose age is

   (A) ≥ 30 years
   (B) ≥ 40 years
   (C) ≥ 50 years
   (D) ≥ 60 years
   (E) ≥ 70 years

4. Urinalysis and a serum albumin test should be performed preoperatively (before major surgery) in healthy individuals whose age is

   (A) ≥ 25 years
   (B) ≥ 35 years
   (C) ≥ 45 years
   (D) ≥ 55 years
   (E) ≥ 65 years

5. A routine preoperative electrocardiogram (EKG) should be required before major surgery in healthy individuals who are

   (A) patients of any age
   (B) adults of any age
   (C) men older than 35 years or women older than 50 years
   (D) men older than 40 years or women older than 45 years
   (E) men older than 45 years or women older than 50 years

6. A 63-year-old woman is scheduled for an operation in 1 week to relieve a partial bowel obstruction caused by a carcinoma in the descending colon. For approximately 6 weeks she has experienced alternating periods of constipation (cessation of normal daily movements) for 2–3 days, followed by diarrhea for 1–2 days, during which time her appetite has waned. Her weight is 120 lb (54.5 kg) and her height is 5′6″ (1.67 m). With respect to her nutritional needs before surgery, what are the minimum dietary amounts of calories and protein she should be able to ingest daily to make an oral liquid supplement (e.g., Ensure) or other delivery of nutrition unnecessary?

   (A) 35 kcal/kg, of which 20% is protein
   (B) 30 kcal/kg, of which 30% is protein
   (C) 40 kcal/kg, with 80 grams of protein
   (D) Amounts judged by the patient to be adequate
   (E) Amounts that need to be calculated only if the patient's serum albumin and transferrin are outside of normal limits

7. The woman in question 6, who canceled her semi-elective surgery for personal reasons, returned 3 weeks later with a totally obstructed large bowel. She has been anorectic and in colicky pain for the past 7 days. The surgeon says she requires a temporary colostomy. Her weight is now 110 lb (50 kg). Skin turgor is normal, but mucosae are "sticky" although not dry. Laboratory findings include: serum albumin, 2.9 g/dl (3.5–5.5 g/dl); serum transferrin, 150 mg/dl (250–430 mg/dl); and total lymphocyte count, 1200/mm³ (1500–3000/mm³). Surgery is scheduled for the next morning. Under these circumstances, which is the most appropriate nutritional program for this patient?

(A) Oral liquid–nutriment supplementation, 200 ml by mouth 4 times per day today and for 10 days after surgery

(B) Total parenteral nutrition (TPN), starting now and for 7 days after surgery

(C) A low-residue diet, starting 2 days after surgery

(D) Nasogastric tube feedings, 2100 calories per day for the first 7 postoperative days

(E) Clear liquid diet, for a total of 3 liters prior to surgery

8. Patients are considered to be severely malnourished when their serum albumin level is

(A) $\leq$ 4.0 g/dl
(B) $\leq$ 3.5 g/dl
(C) < 3.0 g/dl
(D) < 2.0 g/dl
(E) < 1.5 g/dl

9. Patients are considered to be severely malnourished when their serum transferrin level is

(A) $\leq$ 300 mg/dl
(B) < 220 mg/dl
(C) < 170 mg/dl
(D) < 100 mg/dl
(E) < 75 mg/dl

10. Patients are considered to be severely malnourished when their level of serum prealbumin is

(A) < 20 mg/dl
(B) < 17 mg/dl
(C) < 12 mg/dl
(D) < 7 mg/dl
(E) < 5 mg/dl

11. Severe malnutrition is indicated by a total lymphocyte count of

(A) < 500 cells/mm³
(B) < 1000 cells/mm³
(C) < 1500 cells/mm³
(D) < 2000 cells/mm³
(E) < 2500 cells/mm³

12. Detsky's modified risk index for surgery evaluates such patient conditions as history of coronary artery disease, congestive heart failure (including pulmonary edema), valvular disease, and dysrhythmias, as well as age and general medical status [see Table 37.4 in *Family Medicine* (House Officer Series)]. Points may be accumulated up to a maximum of 120. Above which of the following scores do the majority of complications occur?

(A) 10
(B) 16
(C) 32
(D) 64
(E) 96

13. A 52-year-old white man suffers crushing chest pain for 4 hours before coming to the hospital emergency department. Findings include elevated ST segments and Q waves 10 mm deep in leads V_5 and V_6. The man is admitted to the hospital, where his course remains uncomplicated, and 10 days later he is discharged for convalescence at home. During his hospitalization, he and his surgeon cancel an elective inguinal herniorrhaphy that had been scheduled prior to his emergency visit. What is the minimum time that this patient should wait before having the elective surgery?

(A) 6 weeks
(B) 3 months
(C) 9 months
(D) 12 months
(E) 18 months

14. A 56-year-old man, who has a 75% stenosis of his left common carotid artery at a point just below the bifurcation, requires a carotid endarterectomy. He has been treated for hypertension, which is partially controlled by sustained-release verapamil. The endarterectomy can be performed if this man's stable diastolic blood pressure is no higher than

(A) 90 mm Hg
(B) 95 mm Hg
(C) 100 mm Hg
(D) 110 mm Hg
(E) 120 mm Hg

15. A 45-year-old woman, who is new to you, complains of light-headedness that occurs when she arises from sitting. She has a history of a "heart murmur" that is not further delineated. You hear a crescendo/decrescendo murmur, loudest at the left second interspace. Her blood pressure is 110/88 mm Hg. You order an echocardiogram. The day after the echocardiogram appointment, the patient complains that she has begun to experience shortness of breath when she is lying down. You find moist rales (i.e., "crackles") at both bases. You admit her to the hospital and treat her with furosemide 40 mg daily. After 2 days, she is no longer symptomatic. The echocardiogram shows aortic stenosis of a congenital nature. How long should valve replacement surgery be delayed?

- (A) 1 day
- (B) 1 week
- (C) 2 weeks
- (D) 3 weeks
- (E) 3 months

16. What is a safe cutoff point for pulmonary function to clear for most operations?

- (A) Forced vital capacity (FVC) > 50% of predicted (normal for age and height)
- (B) Maximal voluntary ventilation (MVV) > 50% of predicted
- (C) Forced expiratory volume in 1 second (FEV_1) > 2 liters
- (D) Diffusion capacity of lung for carbon monoxide (DLCO) > 40% of predicted
- (E) All of the above

17. Which of the following combinations of pulmonary function tests is a safe cutoff point to clear for pulmonary resection (e.g., to determine whether a right lower lobectomy would be safe and would spare the patient chronic maintenance on a ventilator)?

- (A) Forced expiratory volume in 1 second (FEV_1) > 1 liter, forced vital capacity (FVC) > 50% of predicted (normal for age and height), and maximal voluntary ventilation (MVV) > 50% of predicted
- (B) MVV > 50% of predicted and diffusion capacity of lung for carbon monoxide (DLCO) > 40% of predicted
- (C) FEV_1 > 2 liters, MVV > 50% of predicted, and DLCO > 60% of predicted
- (D) DLCO > 40% of predicted and FVC > 60% of predicted

18. Preoperative antibiotic prophylaxis against bacterial endocarditis is recommended for patients who have which of the following?

- (A) A history of coronary bypass surgery
- (B) A history of Kawasaki's disease
- (C) Hypertrophic cardiomyopathy
- (D) A cardiac pacemaker
- (E) An implanted defibrillator

19. Which of the following areas carries the highest risk of being the portal of entry for bacterial endocarditis?

- (A) Genitourinary tract
- (B) Gastrointestinal (GI) tract
- (C) Oral cavity
- (D) Skin above the waist
- (E) Skin below the waist

DIRECTIONS (Item 20): The incomplete statement in this section is negatively phrased, as indicated by the capitalized word EXCEPT. Select the ONE lettered answer or completion that is BEST.

20. The general rule is that hypertensive patients scheduled for surgery should be maintained on their antihypertensive medications through the period of surgery. This is true with all of the following categories of medication EXCEPT

- (A) beta-adrenergic blocking agents
- (B) alpha-adrenergic blocking agents
- (C) calcium channel blocking agents
- (D) antidysrhythmic agents
- (E) diuretic agents

DIRECTIONS (Items 21–23): For each numbered anticoagulant, select the letter of the correct perioperative time period in which it should be withheld.

(A) From 4 weeks before surgery to 2 weeks after surgery

(B) From 3–5 days before surgery to 3–5 days after surgery for atrial fibrillation, deep venous thrombosis (DVT), and cerebrovascular disease

(C) From 1 week before surgery to 1 week after surgery

(D) From 2 weeks before surgery to 48 hours after surgery

(E) From 1 week before surgery to 48 hours after surgery

21. Aspirin

22. Ticlopidine

23. Warfarin

ANSWERS AND EXPLANATIONS

1. The answer is C. Forty years is the age under which, for elective surgery, routine preoperative tests are now considered unnecessary in healthy individuals.

2. The answer is D. Routine preoperative blood urea nitrogen (BUN) and serum creatinine tests are indicated for healthy individuals whose age is 50 years or more. For younger patients, these preoperative tests are indicated if the patient has been taking diuretics, digoxin, or glucocorticoids; is known to have renal disease, diabetes mellitus, or alcohol dependency; or has major organ system disease [see Table 37.1 in *Family Medicine* (House Officer Series)]. Because this patient is over 50 years old, he should have preoperative tests for BUN and creatinine.

3. The answer is D. Routine electrolyte measurements and chest x-rays are justified before major surgery in otherwise healthy individuals who are 60 years of age or older. They are also indicated for patients who have been taking diuretics, digoxin, or glucocorticoids; who are known to have renal disease, diabetes mellitus, alcohol dependency, or major organ system disease; who have a history of pulmonary disease, cardiac disease, or malignancy; or who are at high risk for tuberculosis [see Table 37.1 in *Family Medicine* (House Officer Series)]. The 55-year-old man in question 2 needs neither routine preoperative electrolyte testing nor chest x-ray.

4. The answer is E. At 65 years and older, even healthy individuals require preoperative urinalyses and serum albumin tests [see Table 37.1 in *Family Medicine* (House Officer Series)]. The 55-year-old man in question 2 does not need such routine preoperative tests.

5. The answer is C. A routine preoperative electrocardiogram (EKG) is required before major surgery for healthy men older than 35 years or healthy women older than 50 years. A preoperative EKG is also indicated for patients who have cardiac or pulmonary disease (or significant risk factor for such disease), peripheral atherosclerosis, electrolyte disturbance, as well as for those who take medication(s) that may have cardiologic ramifications (e.g., tricyclic antidepressants, phenothiazines, anthracycline chemotherapeutic agents). An EKG is warranted for patients who are about to undergo high-risk surgery (e.g., thoracic, abdominal, or major emergency surgery) [see Table 37.2 in *Family Medicine* (House Officer Series)]. In addition, a preoperative EKG is advisable for alcoholics or suspected alcoholics.

Based on his age of 55 years, the patient in question 2, an otherwise healthy man, requires a routine preoperative EKG.

6. The answer is A. If the woman cannot ingest a minimum of 35 kcal/kg, of which 20% is protein, she should receive oral or other preoperative supplementation. Many patients who orally consume nutrients of adequate quantity but insufficient quality can be fed oral supplements that correct for inadequate protein and other nutrients. It may be unsafe to rely on the patient's impression of her intake. If levels of serum albumin or transferrin are abnormal, the patient may be moderately or severely malnourished [see Table 37.3 in *Family Medicine* (House Officer Series)]. In such a situation, total parenteral nutrition (TPN) may be indicated.

7. The answer is B. Total parenteral nutrition (TPN) should be administered now and for 7 postoperative days (or for as long as necessary for delivery of adequate calories, protein, and fluid). This patient, who is moderately malnourished (10%–20% weight loss, albumin < 3.0 g/dl, transferrin < 170 mg/dl, lymphocyte count < 1500 cells/mm^3), will not be able to take nutrients orally for at least 7 days after her surgery. Because of the projected enteral malfunction during the early postoperative period, oral liquid–nutriment supplement, low-residue diet, tube feedings, and clear liquids are ruled out. A clear liquid diet would not even provide maintenance calories and no protein whatever, to say nothing of the required calories and protein repletion.

8. The answer is D. A serum albumin level of less than 2.0 g/dl indicates severe malnourishment. A level of 2.0–3.0 g/dl is a sign of moderate malnourishment, and a level of less than 3.5 g/dl but more than 3.0 g/dl indicates mild malnourishment. (However, special circumstances may exist to account for the measurement as an isolated finding.)

9. The answer is D. Severe malnourishment is indicated by a serum transferrin level of less than 100 mg/dl. Moderate malnourishment is indicated by a serum transferrin level of 100 mg/dl to less than 170 mg/dl, and mild malnourishment by a serum transferrin level of 170 mg/dl to less than 220 mg/dl.

10. The answer is D. Severe malnourishment is indicated by a serum prealbumin level of less than 7 mg/dl.

Moderate malnourishment is indicated by a serum prealbumin level of 7 mg/dl to less than 12 mg/dl, and mild malnourishment by a serum prealbumin level of 12 mg/dl to less than 17 mg/dl.

11. The answer is B. A total lymphocyte count of less than 1000 cells/mm^3 indicates severe malnutrition [if no special circumstances (e.g., a blood dyscrasia) are responsible for an isolated finding]. A count of 1000 cells/mm^3 to less than 1500 cells/mm^3 indicates moderate malnutrition, and a count of 1500 cells/mm^3 to less than 2000 cells/mm^3 indicates mild malnutrition.

12. The answer is B. A score of 16 points (out of a possible 120) on Detsky's modified risk index evaluation appears to be an important threshold above which signals significant risk for surgery [see Table 37.4 in *Family Medicine* (House Officer Series)]. Although the criteria that establish this index seem arbitrary, certain principles can be extracted. Among some 19 categories and subcategories, cardiac valvular disease and class IV angina [symptoms from any activity (Canadian Cardiovascular Society)] each confer 20 points. The following conditions are also accorded 10 points each: myocardial infarction (MI) within 6 months; class III angina (symptoms from walking 1–2 blocks or climbing stairs); pulmonary edema within 1 week; or emergency surgery.

13. The answer is B. Three months is the minimum time after myocardial infarction (MI) that one should wait for elective surgery. This rule applies to any diagnosed MI regardless of its location. During the first 3 months, the risk of perioperative recurrent MI or death is 8%–30%; after 6 months, the risk falls to 3.5%–5%.

14. The answer is D. A stable diastolic blood pressure no higher than 110 mm Hg is required for surgery in patients who have a history of hypertension. This criterion applies to major surgery, especially of a vascular nature, but not to procedures requiring only local anesthesia or a brief period of general anesthesia. (Of course, urgent need for emergency surgery may take precedence over this and other criteria.)

15. The answer is B. One week is presently the accepted delay for elective surgery after stabilization of congestive heart failure. This permits observation and confirmation of the compensated state and allows sufficient time so that hurried and aggressive therapy is less likely to result in hypokalemia or hypovolemia. (Absence of orthostatic hypotension is the clinical checkpoint for hypovolemia.)

16. The answer is E. All of the answer choices are safe cutoff points for pulmonary function to clear for most operations. Forced expiratory volume in 1 second (FEV$_1$) greater than 2 liters is the most appropriate screen. The other measures are supplemental and used particularly to define high risk for pulmonary complications in major surgery. Indicators of high risk include forced vital capacity (FVC) that is less than or equal to 50% of predicted for age and height; maximal voluntary ventilation (MVV) that is less than or equal to 50% of predicted, and diffusing capacity of the lung for carbon monoxide (DLCO) that is less than or equal to 40% of predicted.

17. The answer is C. A combination of forced expiratory volume in 1 second (FEV$_1$) greater than 2 liters, maximal voluntary ventilation (MVV) greater than 50% of predicted for age and height, and diffusing capacity of the lung for carbon monoxide (DLCO) greater than 60% of predicted constitutes a safe cutoff point for pulmonary function studies to clear for pulmonary resection. Even if FEV$_1$ is greater than 2 liters and MVV is greater than 50% of predicted, a DLCO that is less than or equal to 60% of predicted indicates the patient's status is high-risk. If FEV$_1$ is greater than 2 liters, but MVV is less than or equal to 50% of predicted, and DLCO is less than or equal to 60%, the patient is at high risk for resection.

18. The answer is C. Surprisingly, patients with hypertrophic cardiomyopathy warrant preoperative antibiotic prophylaxis against bacterial endocarditis, possibly on the basis of relative stagnation of blood due to the obstructive component. Other patients who merit such preoperative prophylaxis include those who have prosthetic cardiac valves, rheumatic and other valvular dysfunction, a history of bacterial endocarditis, and a history of significant congenital cardiac malformations even if they have been repaired. A past history of coronary bypass or Kawasaki's disease and presence of cardiac pacemaker or implanted defibrillator do not indicate a need for prophylactic antibiotics.

19. The answer is C. The oral cavity carries the greatest risk of being the portal of entry for bacterial endocarditis. The genitourinary tract carries the next highest risk, and the gastrointestinal (GI) tract carries significantly less risk than either of these two. Skin incisions are not considered to put patients at risk for bacterial endocarditis.

20. The answer is E. Diuretic agents are the exception to the general rule that hypertensive patients should be maintained on antihypertensive medications throughout the period of surgery. Diuretic medications are discontinued mainly because of the catastrophic sequelae of hypokalemia. Beta- and alpha-adrenergic blocking agents, calcium channel blocking agents, and antidysrhythmic agents may be continued up to and through the period of surgery.

21. The answer is E. Aspirin is withheld from 1 week before surgery until 48 hours after surgery. This interval is considered adequate to reduce the chances of intraoperative and postoperative bleeding due to the effects of aspirin on platelet aggregation.

22. The answer is D. Ticlopidine is withheld from 2 weeks before surgery until 48 hours after surgery. The effects of this agent on platelet aggregation are longer lasting than those of aspirin.

23. The answer is B. Warfarin is withheld from 3–5 days before surgery to 3–5 days after surgery in patients with atrial fibrillation, deep venous thrombosis (DVT), and cerebrovascular disease. In patients at high risk for thromboembolism (e.g., those with certain prosthetic valves or recent pulmonary embolism as reasons for warfarin therapy), anticoagulation is continued until the day of surgery and discontinued for 12–24 hours. Anticoagulation with intravenous heparin therapy is then resumed until the transition back to warfarin has occurred.

BIBLIOGRAPHY

Vanderhoff BT: Preoperative clearance and preparation. In *Family Medicine* (House Officer Series). Edited by Rudy DR, Kurowski K. Baltimore, Williams & Wilkins, 1997, pp 617–636.

Test 38

Obesity and Dyslipidemia

DIRECTIONS (Items 1–13): Each of the numbered items or incomplete statements in this section is followed by answers or by completions of the statement. Select the ONE lettered answer or completion that is BEST in each case.

1. A 22-year-old woman, whose height is 5′5″ (1.65 m) and weight is 143 pounds (65 kg), inquires about approaches to weight loss. You calculate her ideal weight to be 125 pounds (57 kg). Which is the most appropriate next step?

- (A) Reassure the patient that her present weight poses no risk to her health.
- (B) Order the patient onto a diet of 1300 calories, consisting of 175 g carbohydrate, 50 g fat, and 50 g protein.
- (C) Place the patient on a very low-calorie diet (VLCD).
- (D) Prescribe phentermine.
- (E) Obtain more information to enable you to formulate a plan.

2. A 45-year-old woman who has never before confronted her weight problem, consulted a physician about it, or been informed of the health risks posed by it, is discussing weight loss with you. Her weight is 180 lb (82 kg), and her height is 5′5″ (1.65 m). Her body mass index is 30, or 38% above ideal weight. Which of the following is the best next treatment step?

- (A) Refer the patient to a noncommercial self-help group (e.g., Overeaters Anonymous).
- (B) Reassure the patient that her health is not at risk.
- (C) Prescribe phentermine.
- (D) Place the patient on a very low-calorie diet (VLCD).
- (E) Refer the patient to a commercial weight loss program (e.g., Weight Watchers).

3. A 50-year-old white man, whose weight has not changed in 10 years, now weighs 240 lb (109 kg) and stands 5′10″ (1.8 m) tall. Which of the following statements is most true?

- (A) He consumes more calories than a nonobese individual.
- (B) The chance that he has a binge eating disorder is 30%.
- (C) His rate of energy expenditure is the same as that of a nonobese individual.
- (D) His level of physical activity is the same as that of a nonobese individual.
- (E) The likelihood that he has psychological problems is higher than that of a nonobese individual, even when he is not dieting.

4. A 38-year-old male African-American mail carrier, who is a nonsmoker, has blood pressures consistently in the range of 145/90 to 150/95 mm Hg. His weight is 184 lb (83.6 kg), and his height is 5′11″ (1.8 m). His total cholesterol is 240 mg/dl and his high-density lipoprotein (HDL) cholesterol is 28 mg/dl, despite a diet that includes less than 200 mg of cholesterol and less than 30% fat (of which less than 7% is saturated fat). The man has a history of substance abuse (1 year during his early twenties). Both his mother and sister are obese and have non–insulin-dependent diabetes. To rectify this man's dyslipidemia, which of the following steps is most appropriate?

- (A) Recommend no new interventions now, and require another lipid panel in 6–12 months.
- (B) Decrease the patient's dietary cholesterol to less than 100 mg/day and fat to 20% or less of all calories.
- (C) Encourage the patient to drink a small amount of alcohol each day to raise his HDL cholesterol.
- (D) Start the patient on a bile acid sequestrant medication.
- (E) Start the patient on niacin or on a 3-hydroxy-3-methylglutaryl coenzyme A (HMG-CoA) reductase inhibitor ("statin").

5. A very low-calorie diet (VLCD) contains how many kilocalories per day?

- (A) 800
- (B) 1000
- (C) 1200
- (D) 1500
- (E) 2000

6. A 51-year-old man has significant dyslipidemia despite adhering to a low-fat, low-cholesterol diet. You prescribe gemfibrozil and request another lipid profile in 2 months. In which of the following lipids do you expect to see the greatest decrease?

- (A) Total cholesterol
- (B) Triglycerides
- (C) High-density lipoprotein (HDL) cholesterol
- (D) Low-density lipoprotein (LDL) cholesterol
- (E) Chylomicrons

7. A 32-year-old man last had his total cholesterol checked 2 years ago, and then it was 180 mg/dl. He is in good health, is taking no medications, and is at the same weight and activity level as before. He has no history of smoking and no family history of stroke, coronary artery disease, or dyslipidemia. His blood pressure is 130/80 mm Hg, and his pulse is 72 beats/min and regular. Cardiac examination reveals S_1, S_2, and no extra sounds. No bruits are present. Radial and dorsalis pedis pulses are normal bilaterally. According to the National Cholesterol Education Panel and American College of Physicians, which of the following screenings should be recommended for this man?

(A) No screening at this time; total cholesterol in 3 years
(B) Total cholesterol
(C) Total cholesterol and high-density lipoprotein (HDL) cholesterol
(D) Fasting lipid panel, including levels of total and HDL cholesterols as well as triglycerides
(E) Lipoprotein electrophoresis (LPE)

8. Which is the principal advantage of using bile acid sequestrants such as cholestyramine or colestipol?

(A) They are the most potent cholesterol-lowering agents on the market.
(B) They can be taken with medications such as warfarin and digoxin without causing drug interactions.
(C) They produce little bloating or constipation.
(D) They require no mixing with water or juice.
(E) They are not absorbed systemically.

9. You are treating a 55-year-old man with a history of angina and a previous coronary angiogram that showed a 60% stenosis of the left anterior descending artery. He has been on a step II low-cholesterol diet for 3 months. A current lipid profile shows that his total cholesterol is 295 mg/dl, his high-density lipoprotein (HDL) cholesterol is 30 mg/dl, and his triglycerides are 220 mg/dl, despite full compliance with his diet (corroborated by his wife). You have ruled out secondary causes of dyslipidemia. This patient is taking only nitroglycerin (as needed) and 325 mg aspirin each day. Which of the following is the most appropriate next step?

(A) Continue the patient on his cholesterol-lowering diet, and recheck lipid levels in 3 months.
(B) Prescribe colestipol.
(C) Prescribe niacin.
(D) Prescribe gemfibrozil.
(E) Prescribe an HMG-CoA reductase inhibitor.

10. An HMG-CoA reductase inhibitor and gemfibrozil should not be taken together because the combination produces which of the following effect(s)?

(A) Increased risk of hepatotoxicity
(B) Paradoxical rise in serum cholesterol
(C) Increased risks of myopathy and rhabdomyolysis
(D) Paradoxical increase in cardiovascular mortality
(E) Increased risk of nonmyoglobin-related renal failure

11. Which of the following is compatible with the Step 1 American Heart Association (AHA) diet?

(A) 30% of calories as fat, of which at least one-third should be unsaturated
(B) 30 grams of fat, of which one-third should be saturated
(C) Less than 30% of calories as fat, of which less than one-third should be saturated
(D) 20% of calories as fat, of which one-tenth should be saturated
(E) 20% of calories as fat, of which less than one-half should be saturated

12. Which of the following possible beneficial effects of estrogen replacement therapy (ERT) most reduces mortality in postmenopausal women (statistically)?

(A) Reduction in incidence of coronary artery disease
(B) Reduction in incidence of hip fracture
(C) Reduction in severity of atrophic vaginitis
(D) Reduction in incidence of breast carcinoma
(E) Prevention of vasomotor effects of estrogen deficiency

13. A 27-year-old Caucasian man weighs 275 lb (125 kg) and stands 5'7" (1.7 m) tall. His total cholesterol is 250 mg/dl, with high-density lipoprotein (HDL) cholesterol of 35 mg/dl and serum triglycerides of 200 mg/dl despite taking lovastatin 40 mg daily. He suffers from traumatic arthritis of both knees and has a family history of coronary heart disease [acute myocardial infarction (MI) in father at 48 years and in paternal uncle at 55 years]. The man professes a keen desire to lose weight, feeling he is unattractive and ineffective in his work in criminology. In the several diet programs he has tried, including Overeaters Anonymous, Take Off Pounds Sensibly, and Weight Watchers, he lost approximately 20 pounds each time, only to regain them after 6 months. In addition, he has tried counseling that uses cognitive and then behavioral therapy. Which of the following is the most logical next step?

(A) Prescribe simvastatin.
(B) Prescribe benzphetamine.
(C) Prescribe cholestyramine.
(D) Obtain consult for gastric bypass.
(E) Prescribe gemfibrozil.

DIRECTIONS (Item 14): The incomplete statement in this section is negatively phrased, as indicated by the capitalized word EXCEPT. Select the ONE lettered answer or completion that is BEST.

14. Obese individuals are subject to an increased incidence of all of the following conditions EXCEPT

- (A) Breast cancer
- (B) Endometrial carcinoma
- (C) Chronic obstructive pulmonary disease
- (D) Osteoarthritis of the knees
- (E) Gallstones

ANSWERS AND EXPLANATIONS

1. The answer is A. Reassure this woman that her present weight poses no health risk and that she is not even mildly obese. A person must be at least 20% overweight to be considered mildly obese, and she is only 14% heavier than her ideal body weight, which is calculated at 100 pounds plus 5 pounds for each inch over 60 inches (guidelines for females). This patient's ideal weight is $100 + 5 \times 5 = 125$ pounds. At 143 pounds she is only 18 pounds, or 14% over ideal body weight, and not an appropriate candidate for an aggressive weight loss program. Her weight of 143 pounds corresponds to a body mass index of 24, which is in the acceptable range. (Body mass index is calculated by dividing the weight in kilograms by the square of the height in meters.) By body mass criteria, moderate obesity is defined as 30–40 and high obesity as 40 or more.

A diet of 1300 calories, consisting of 175 g carbohydrate, 50 g fat, 50 g protein, is a well-designed, modest, weight reduction diet: 1300 calories meets a guideline for the maintenance needs of a 125-pound woman; 175 grams of carbohydrate approximates 55% of total calories, and 50 grams of fat provides less than 30% of total calories. This diet meets the American Heart Association (AHA) recommendations and satisfies the requirements for managing diabetes. A very low-calorie diet (VLCD), which consists of 800 calories, is normally reserved for severe cases such as morbid obesity (100% above ideal weight). Phentermine or any other appetite suppressant is reserved for more severe cases such as those in which weight is 40% or more above the ideal. The information given in the vignette is sufficient to select a treatment choice.

2. The answer is E. You should refer this moderately obese patient to a commercial weight loss program, a good option for an individual who appears to need social support. (You, a trained nurse, or a dietitian can assess the nutritional component and make modifications.) Patients typically lose 11–22 pounds in commercial programs. The downside is that attrition is high, and eventual regain of lost weight is common. In addition, these programs are often expensive. Participants in noncommercial self-help programs do not achieve as much weight loss as in commercial programs. A weight loss program, rather than reassurance, is appropriate for a moderately obese patient. Very low-calorie diets (VLCDs) and pharmacotherapy such as phentermine should not be tried before more conservative measures have failed.

3. The answer is B. This man has a 30% chance of having a binge eating disorder. He is in the static phase of obesity: neither gaining nor losing weight. In general, physical activity and energy expenditure are lower-than-normal in obese individuals, and caloric consumption is actually lower as well. Thus, they metabolize at a lower rate and find it more difficult to remain in calorie balance while eating at rates similar to peers of their age and sex. Obese patients have no greater number of diagnosed psychological problems than do the rest of the population.

4. The answer is E. Drug therapy with niacin or an HMG-CoA reductase inhibitor (a "statin" such as atorvastatin) is the best step for correction of dyslipidemia in this 38-year-old male nonsmoker with mild hypertension, a poor total cholesterol:high-density lipoprotein (HDL) cholesterol ratio (240:28, > 8.5:1), and a family history of diabetes. A man should have a ratio of ≤ 4.5:1. This patient exhibits dyslipidemia at a young age and the possible inheritance of syndrome X (hyperinsulinemia and insulin resistance). Waiting for another lipid panel in 6–12 months is inadvisable because the patient's status is not likely to change without therapy. Among the numerous risk factors are none that can be approached reasonably by changes in life style: The patient is near his ideal weight; he is eating a recommended diet; and he gets sufficient exercise in his job as a mail carrier. Although people who drink alcoholic beverages moderately tend to have more favorable lipid profiles than do nondrinkers, daily alcohol to raise HDL cholesterol is not only unconventional and potentially dangerous, it is precluded in this patient because of his history of previous substance abuse. The patient's HDL level is very low; therefore, niacin or one of the "statins" is a better choice than a bile acid sequestrant (the latter is relatively ineffective at raising the HDL cholesterol level).

5. The answer is A. The caloric limit in a very low-calorie diet (VLCD), which is instituted in cases of severe obesity, is 800 kilocalories per day. Patients remain on this diet for 12–16 weeks. This diet is reserved for patients who are at least 30% overweight in whom more conservative measures have failed. Side effects include hair loss, chilly sensation, and thinning of the skin.

6. The answer is B. This patient's triglycerides are likely to show the greatest decrease. Gemfibrozil (a member of the fibric acid group) reduces triglyceride levels dramatically and also raises high-density lipoprotein (HDL) cholesterol 10%–30% but reduces total cholesterol only mildly. Effects on low-density lipoprotein (LDL) cholesterol are unpredictable. The ideal candidate for gemfibrozil therapy is an individual who has only modestly elevated total cholesterol but low HDL cholesterol (despite adherence to dietary measures) and marked hypertriglyceridemia.

7. The answer is A. Screening is unnecessary at this time, and total cholesterol can be checked again in 3 years. Having ruled out a history of risk factors for coronary heart disease and a family history of hyperlipidemia, you can screen this patient once every 5 years as long as cholesterol levels remain in the desirable range. (Nevertheless, suggesting a reduction of fat and cholesterol intake may benefit any American, even one with desirable cholesterol levels.) A lipoprotein electrophoresis (LPE) allows the complete differentiation of lipids found in the lipid profile [total cholesterol, high-density lipoprotein (HDL) and low-density lipoprotein (LDL) cholesterol, and triglycerides]. In addition, LPE permits differentiation of intermediate-density lipoprotein (IDL) and very low-density lipoprotein (VLDL) [the band in which triglycerides reside]. IDL, which is a mergence on electrophoresis between LDL and VLDL, is an uncommon type of dyslipoproteinemia that poses a significant vascular risk.

8. The answer is E. The principal advantage of bile acid sequestrants is that they are not absorbed systemically. These medications may interfere with absorption of some other medications, especially if taken concurrently. They should not be taken with agents such as warfarin and digoxin, with which they interact. Bile acid sequestrants frequently produce bloating, abdominal cramping, and constipation. (Gradual increases from a small starting dose may diminish these effects.) These medications are tolerated better when mixed with water or juice. The HMG-CoA reductase inhibitors ("statins"), not the bile acid sequestrants, are the most potent cholesterol-lowering agents on the market.

9. The answer is E. An HMG-CoA reductase inhibitor ("statin") such as fluvastatin, pravastatin, lovastatin, simvastatin, or atorvastatin should be prescribed for this patient; the high-density lipoprotein (HDL)-raising effect of such an agent is warranted in the presence of the low levels of HDL, high total cholesterol:HDL cholesterol ratio, and documented coronary artery disease. The low-cholesterol diet is not aggressive enough in the face of the patient's known heart disease and highly unfavorable lipid profile. Colestipol, niacin, and gemfibrozil, although useful in various types of dyslipidemia, are not as effective as "statins" in raising HDL cholesterol.

10. The answer is C. An increased risk of myopathy and even rhabdomyolysis exists when a "statin" is taken with gemfibrozil. (This increased risk also exists when a "statin" is taken with cyclosporine, erythromycin, or niacin.) The combination of a "statin" and gemfibrozil does not particularly increase the risk of hepatotoxicity, elevated serum cholesterol, or cardiovascular mortality. A risk of renal failure with the "statins" is myoglobinuria-related.

11. The answer is C. The Step 1 American Heart Association (AHA) diet consists of less than 300 mg cholesterol and less than 30% total calories of fat, of which less than one-third (10% of total calories) should be saturated fat; 50%–60% of calories in carbohydrate; and 10%–20% of calories in protein [see Table 38.3 in *Family Medicine* (House Officer Series)].

12. The answer is A. Coronary artery disease (CAD) is the ranking cause of death among postmenopausal women (> 10,000/100,000 per year). Reduction of the risk of CAD is the direct result of improvement in the lipid profile effected by ERT. It is estimated that estrogen replacement therapy (ERT) reduces the incidence and mortality due to coronary artery disease by one-half. Hip fracture, with a one-third lifetime incidence for women who live to the age of 80, has a 20% first-year mortality in postmenopausal women (> 900 deaths/100,000 per year). Atrophic vaginitis does not carry a measurable mortality. The incidence of endometrial carcinoma increases slightly with ERT, although hormone replacement therapy (HRT) [estrogen replacement with cycled progesterone] actually results in a reduced incidence. However, the expected deaths decrease only from 188/100,000 to 37/100,000 per year. Deaths from breast carcinoma are estimated at 1406/100,000 per year. The prevailing opinion is that both ERT and HRT lead to a significant increase in mortality to 2250/100,000 per year. The decrease in mortality from hip fractures due to osteoporosis and coronary artery disease more than offset this increase.

13. The answer is D. Gastric bypass surgery should be arranged. This patient has severe dyslipidemia, much of which may be assumed to be secondary to his severe, morbid obesity, defined as 100% or 100 pounds overweight. The ideal body weight for this patient is 148 pounds [see explanation for question 1 and use 106 pounds, instead of 100, and 6 pounds, instead of 5, for each inch of height over 5 feet ("rule" for males)]. The morbid obesity is the more critical problem. Weight loss efforts, consisting of two self-help programs, as well as a commercial program have failed. Without judging the behavioral versus genetic and humoral causes of this patient's morbid obesity, it may be that invasive measures are warranted, if the patient is motivated. Besides gastric bypass, the other invasive intervention is vertically banded gastroplasty.

The severe dyslipidemia is indicated by the man's total cholesterol:high-density lipoprotein (HDL) cholesterol ratio of 7:1, and in a young man, the expected ratio is no more than 4.5:1. The best pharmacologic agent for this aberration is one of the HMG-CoA reductase inhibitors ("statins") such as simvastatin, which research has recently endorsed as a proven protector against coronary artery events. He is already taking lovastatin, however, and he is not likely to benefit further from a member of the same class of drugs until the obesity is corrected. The same applies to gemfibrozil. Gemfibrozil is particularly effective against hypertriglyceridemia, but his condition is particularly sensitive to weight loss. The patient's triglycerides have already proved to be relatively impervious to the lovastatin.

14. The answer is C. Obesity is not associated with an increased incidence of chronic obstructive pulmonary disease, although it is associated with an increased incidence of sleep apnea and restrictive lung disease. Obesity is a risk for breast cancer because of the increased storage of estrogens in adipose tissue. For the same reason, obesity is also a risk for endometrial carcinoma. This risk may be related to the higher storage levels of estrogen; circulating estrogen stimulates both breast and uterine tissues. Obesity is also a risk for osteoarthritis of the knees and hips, because the joints of overweight people bear heavier loads. In addition, it is a risk for gallstones, especially cholesterol stones, most likely because of the statistically higher cholesterol levels among the obese.

BIBLIOGRAPHY

Smith PO, Noble SL, Johnson WG: Obesity and dyslipidemias. In *Family Medicine* (House Officer Series). Edited by Rudy DR, Kurowski K. Baltimore, Williams & Wilkins, 1997, pp 637–648.

Test 39

Smoking Cessation

DIRECTIONS (Items 1–9): Each of the numbered items or incomplete statements in this section is followed by answers or by completions of the statement. Select the ONE lettered answer or completion that is BEST in each case.

---

1. A 25-year-old woman in her first trimester of pregnancy smokes one pack of cigarettes per day. You advise her that if she continues to smoke, her baby will be at increased risk for which of the following conditions?

  (A) Preterm birth
  (B) Macrosomia
  (C) Transient tachypnea of the newborn (TTN)
  (D) Congenital birth defect(s)
  (E) Congenital hypothyroidism

2. Which of the following statements regarding physician efforts to encourage smoking cessation is correct?

  (A) It may be assumed that smokers have already been told of the adverse effects by their previous physicians.
  (B) Smoking in the physician's office should be permitted only in partitioned, ventilated smoking areas.
  (C) Counseling smokers should involve full, detailed discussion of smoking cessation.
  (D) Smoking should be listed on the problem list of any smoker and on the chart of any child who lives with smokers.
  (E) Conducting surveys concerning smoking habits of new patients is no more effective than simply telling patients to quit.

3. After smoking cessation, patient risk is reduced most quickly for which of the following cancers?

  (A) Bladder cancer
  (B) Lung cancer
  (C) Breast cancer
  (D) Malignant melanoma
  (E) Prostate carcinoma

4. A 25-year-old woman who comes to the office for a routine gynecologic examination is taking birth control pills and has no plans to have children in the near future. She has no complaints. She has been smoking one-and-one-half packs of cigarettes per day since age 19; has not considered quitting; and has never set a stop date. Which of the following is your most appropriate next step?

  (A) Avoid the topic of smoking cessation, because the patient may not be receptive to it.
  (B) Discuss adverse health effects briefly; give the patient smoking cessation literature; and mention your availability to pursue the subject further.
  (C) Firmly ask the patient to pick a stop date and follow through with quitting.
  (D) Prescribe sustained-release bupropion.
  (E) Recommend a nicotine patch.

5. The following five patients are all actively committed to quitting smoking. Which one is likeliest to benefit from a nicotine patch?

  (A) Patient A, a smoker who always has his first cigarette of the day at his noon lunch hour
  (B) Patient B, a smoker of approximately one-half pack of cigarettes at clubs or parties one or two times per week (but none on other occasions)
  (C) Patient C, a smoker of three packs of cigarettes per day at home beginning before breakfast and at work
  (D) Patient D, a smoker who quit but relapsed after exposure to a situation that made her want to smoke
  (E) Patient E, a smoker primarily at particular times of need for solace or reward or as part of certain social rituals

6. A 50-year-old man, who has been smoking one-and-one-half to two packs of cigarettes per day for 20 years, wants to stop smoking. A contraindication to the use of a nicotine patch in this patient is that he

(A) Sometimes noted pruritus at the patch sites when he tried patches 5 years ago

(B) Noted some erythema at the patch sites when he tried patches 5 years ago

(C) Is already under smoking cessation treatment with oral, sustained-release bupropion

(D) Has a history of hypertension and poorly controlled diabetes mellitus

(E) Suffered a myocardial infarction (MI) 2 weeks ago

7. A woman stops smoking and starts using nicotine patches. She applies a new patch each day. How long must she wait before applying a patch to a skin site that had previously held a patch?

(A) 1 day

(B) 2 days

(C) 3 days

(D) 1 week

(E) 2 weeks

8. With regard to the appropriate use of nicotine gum, which of the following is true?

(A) Use of the gum enables patients to taper smoking gradually.

(B) The urge to smoke should prompt patients to place the gum next to the buccal mucosa and chew it for about 30 minutes.

(C) The maximal use of the gum is 50 pieces per day.

(D) The gum is more effective if used with coffee.

(E) The gum is used as a cigarette substitute that helps patients to smoke less per day.

9. In children whose parents (or other permanent occupants of the home) smoke, the incidence of which of the following childhood diseases is increased?

(A) Otitis media

(B) Croup

(C) Sudden infant death syndrome (SIDS)

(D) Leukemia

(E) Lymphoma

DIRECTIONS (Item 10): The numbered item in this section is negatively phrased, as indicated by the capitalized word NOT. Select the one lettered answer that is BEST.

10. Which of the following is NOT a symptom of nicotine withdrawal?

(A) Sleepiness

(B) Irritability

(C) Hunger

(D) Anxiety

(E) Difficulty concentrating

ANSWERS AND EXPLANATIONS

1. The answer is A. The infant will be at increased risk for preterm birth. Smoking during pregnancy is associated with newborns that are premature or smaller than normal in size but not with specific birth defects or hypothyroidism. There is no known association between maternal smoking and transient tachypnea of the newborn (TTN).

2. The answer is D. Smoking should be included on the problem list of any smoker and on the chart of any child who lives with one or more smokers to keep smoking in the forefront as a possible cause of problems such as worsening asthma, recurrent otitis media in a child, or coronary artery disease. Recording patient's smoking habits by survey and sharing results with patients is more effective than other types of explanation. Survey results quantify the problem, and sharing this information demonstrates how important the physician views the impact of smoking on patient health. Telling smokers to quit is also important—some smokers say that their physicians never told them to quit. The physician need not wait for an opportunity for a lengthy, complete discussion; some smokers will respond to brief interventions. A smoke-free office is preferable to one in which smoking is permitted, even in special areas. Scare tactics often backfire, either through incitement to rebellion or through generation of a defeatist attitude in patients who already are proven to be weak willed.

3. The answer is A. The risk of bladder cancer is reduced by 50% within 3 years after the patient stops smoking. The risk of lung carcinoma is also reduced by smoking cessation, but the 50% reduction takes about 10 years. Breast cancer, malignant melanoma, and prostate carcinoma have not been linked to cigarette smoking.

4. The answer is B. Briefly discuss adverse health effects, provide smoking cessation literature, and mention your availability to pursue the subject further when she is interested. She is unlikely to be sufficiently motivated at this time to stop. An oral agent, nicotine patch, or nicotine gum is unlikely to be successful when the patient has not made a personal commitment. Nevertheless, a smoker should be advised and reminded periodically of the health risks of smoking and should be reminded of the opportunities for help.

5. The answer is C. Patient C, the smoker of three packs of cigarettes per day, who smokes both at home, beginning early, and at work, is the likeliest of these patients to benefit from a nicotine patch. Pharmacologic therapy with nicotine is most appropriate for patients who are physically addicted to nicotine (including smokers of more than one pack per day, early morning smokers, and smokers who experience physical withdrawal symptoms when they stop). Patients who relapse after situational exposure are better candidates for behavioral therapy than for the patch. Patients who begin smoking relatively late in the day or who smoke only on certain types of occasions are not pharmacologically addicted. (Patient E is psychologically, not pharmacologically, addicted.)

6. The answer is E. A recent myocardial infarction (MI) is a contraindication to the use of a nicotine patch due to the vasoconstrictive action of nicotine. [The length of the critical period after an MI is not well established; however, 3 months is a good estimate.] Recent MI, recent cardiac dysrhythmia, and true hypersensitivity reaction to the patch (rather than local erythema or pruritus) are the only real contraindications to the use of the patch. Current treatment with bupropion, history of hypertension, and presence of diabetes mellitus are not contraindications.

7. The answer is D. To avoid contact irritation, a delay of 1 week is recommended before application of a nicotine patch to an area of skin that had already held a patch.

8. The answer is B. When nicotine gum is used correctly, the urge to smoke prompts a patient to place the gum next to the buccal mucosa and chew for about 30 minutes. Patients must stop (not taper) their smoking when they begin using nicotine gum (or nicotine patches), and they must not use the gum as a cigarette substitute. The free alkaloid form of nicotine polacrilex in nicotine gum is best absorbed through the oral mucosa. If acidic coffee or juice is taken less than 15 minutes before chewing, it hinders, rather than boosts, absorption. Patients should not chew more than 30 pieces of regular-strength (2 mg) polacrilex per day, and not more than 20 pieces of the higher strength (4 mg).

9. The answer is A. Otitis media increases in incidence in children who live with smokers. Ear and upper respiratory infections decrease if the smoking stops. Although second-hand smoke in the household is not known to cause childhood asthma, it can be a respiratory irritant that can precipitate asthma. No causal relationship has been established between parents' cigarette smoking and sudden infant death syndrome (SIDS) or childhood malignancies, including leukemia or lymphoma.

10. The answer is A. Sleepiness is NOT a symptom of nicotine withdrawal; insomnia may be a problem. Irritability, hunger, anxiety, and inability to concentrate are symptoms of nicotine withdrawal.

BIBLIOGRAPHY

Bope ET: Smoking cessation. In: *Family Medicine* (House Officer Series). Edited by Rudy DR, Kurowski K. Baltimore, Williams & Wilkins, 1997, pp 649–656.

Test 40

Exercise and Health

DIRECTIONS (Items 1–10): Each of the numbered or incomplete statements in this section is followed by answers or by completions of the statement. Select the ONE lettered answer or completion that is BEST in each case.

1. A 50-year-old man, who feels well, visits his physician for his annual physical examination. He has no symptoms of angina and no history of heart disease. He is taking no medications. He is 6′0″ (1.8 m) and weighs 154 lb (70 kg). Although he considers himself to be physically active at work, he follows no exercise regimen. According to the Centers for Disease Control and Prevention (CDC), how much time each week should he spend in moderate-intensity physical activity?

(A) 15 minutes 3 days per week
(B) 15 minutes 5–7 days per week
(C) 30 minutes 3 days per week
(D) 30 minutes 5–7 days per week

2. To be engaged in moderate physical activity, what minimal pulse rate does the man in question 1 need to achieve?

(A) 70 beats/min
(B) 119 beats/min
(C) 130 beats/min
(D) 150 beats/min
(E) 170 beats/min

3. Approximately how many metabolic equivalents (METs) are typically consumed during moderate physical activity (e.g., brisk walking)?

(A) 1–2
(B) 2–3
(C) 3–6
(D) 6–10
(E) 10–15

4. A 150-lb (68.2-kg) woman expends 100 calories walking 1 mile. In the 30 minutes she takes to walk this distance, she maintains a pulse rate of 100 beats/min. How many calories does she burn if she cycles fast for 1 hour, maintaining a pulse rate of 150 beats/min?

(A) 100
(B) 200
(C) 300
(D) 500
(E) 600

5. A 30-year-old physically inactive woman who has not been exercising is now going to begin a daily activity program of racquetball and conditioning exercises. After how much regular exercise can she expect to see a decrease in her resting pulse rate?

(A) As soon as she begins exercising
(B) 2–3 weeks
(C) 4–6 weeks
(D) 8–10 weeks
(E) At no time, because this type of exercise does not produce a change in the resting pulse rate

6. The woman in question 5 asks you how long she needs to follow her exercise program before she begins to notice improved exercise endurance (i.e., ability to engage in exercise for longer periods or at greater intensity). Which of the following do you tell her?

(A) As soon as she begins exercising
(B) After 2–3 weeks
(C) After 4–6 weeks
(D) After 8–10 weeks
(E) At no time, because this type of exercise does not produce improvements in exercise endurance

7. A 55-year-old man has a 20% stenosis of the right coronary artery and a 30% stenosis of the left anterior descending artery. He is asymptomatic and wants to start an exercise program. Which of the following statements concerning exercise and risk factors for coronary artery disease expresses the correct perspective?

(A) Hypertension, a risk factor for coronary artery disease, is more prevalent than sedentary lifestyle, another risk factor, in the United States.
(B) Hypercholesterolemia, a risk factor for coronary artery disease, is more prevalent than sedentary lifestyle, another risk factor, in the United States.
(C) This man's total and high-density lipoprotein (HDL) cholesterol are expected to decrease with exercise.
(D) The risk of developing coronary artery disease is five times greater in physically inactive individuals.
(E) The incidence of cardiac arrest is lower in individuals who exercise.

8. A 53-year-old female attorney who has never engaged in a formal exercise program consults you about starting an exercise regimen. She frequently walks to the courthouse near her office and to adjacent buildings as well as about four blocks to the grocery store every day. She does not smoke. She has no history of coronary artery disease and experiences no chest discomfort, syncope, or dyspnea with her daily activities. She is taking a diuretic for hypertension and is following a low-cholesterol diet for hypercholesterolemia.

She is 5'7" (1.7 m) tall and weighs 130 lb (59 kg). Her blood pressure is 130/80 mm Hg, her pulse rate is 68 beats/min and regular, and her respiratory rate is 16 breaths/min. You do not appreciate any murmurs. Which of the following is an example of an exercise program she could start without your recommending an exercise stress test?

(A) No exercise program
(B) Carpet cleaning using a vacuum cleaner
(C) Lawn mowing with a hand mower
(D) Conditioning exercises and general calisthenics

9. Which of the following statements best applies to the cool-down component of an exercise program?

(A) It allows a net clearing of lactic acid from the muscles.
(B) It has four characteristics (frequency, intensity, type, and time), as described by the mnemonic FITT.
(C) It is necessary only in vigorous-intensity programs.
(D) It represents the aerobic phase of a workout.
(E) It increases peripheral blood pooling in muscles.

10. At what time post-myocardial infarction (MI) is it appropriate to begin exercise testing?

(A) 72 hours post-MI (during "step down" care)
(B) 1–2 weeks post-MI
(C) 2–4 weeks post-MI
(D) 3–6 weeks post-MI
(E) 13 weeks post-MI

DIRECTIONS (Item 11): The question in this section is negatively phrased, as indicated by the capitalized word NOT. Select the ONE lettered answer that is BEST.

---

11. Which of the following statements is NOT a reason to decrease the level of exercise activity of a patient in a moderate-intensity exercise program?

(A) Inability to carry on a conversation comfortably while exercising
(B) Increase in pulse rate to up to 70% of predicted maximum value
(C) Persistent headache
(D) Fatigue for more than 1 hour after termination of exercise
(E) Joint pain

ANSWERS AND EXPLANATIONS

1. The answer is E. Moderate activity for at least 30 minutes, preferably 7 days a week, is recommended. Examples of moderate activity include brisk walking [3–4 miles per hour (mph)], cycling (≤ 10 mph), swimming with moderate effort (i.e., more than slow treading of water and less than a steady crawl), table tennis, canoeing (2–4 mph), general home cleaning, and lawn mowing with a power mower.

2. The answer is B. Moderate activity (e.g., brisk walking) produces about 70% of the predicted maximum pulse rate, which may be defined as 220 minus age. Thus, $220 - 50 = 170 \times 0.70 = 119$ beats/min.

3. The answer is C. In moderate physical activity, 3–6 metabolic equivalents (METs) are consumed. A MET is a measure of energy. One MET—the amount of oxygen consumed per unit time —equals 3.5 ml/kg/min. Generally, an individual burns about 1 kcal/hr/MET. Light physical activity involves less than 3 METs, and vigorous activity more than 6 METs.

4. The answer is C. The correct answer may be calculated using the following formula:

$$C_X = C_W \times P_X/P_W \times T_X/T_W, \text{ where}$$

C_W = Energy consumed in locomotion of 1 mile at any pace (calories)
P_X = Pulse rate during new exercise (beats/min)
P_W = Pulse rate during 1-mile walk (beats/min)
T_X = Time spent at new exercise (min)
T_W = Time spent walking 1 mile (min)

$$= 100 \times 150/100 \times 60/30$$
$$= 100 \times 1.5 \times 2$$
$$= 300 \text{ calories}$$

5. The answer is C. After beginning a moderate exercise program, a decrease in resting pulse rate takes 4–6 weeks, when other cardiorespiratory improvements such as a higher threshold for exertional dyspnea occur. Beneficial effects such as weight control and stress reduction may be noticed immediately. Improvements in muscle strength take 2–3 weeks.

6. The answer is C. Like cardiorespiratory improvement, increased exercise endurance takes about 4–6 weeks. Endurance has several physiologic components, the most noticeable being a cardiorespiratory effect, which is manifested by more elapsed time before feeling "winded." This is accompanied by a gradual reduction in pulse rate, which reaches the exercise baseline in about the same time. No clear etiologic explanation of endurance appears in the literature, but the cause probably involves strengthening of cardiac muscle fibers with exercise, as occurs in skeletal muscle (intensity of endurance). The suppleness as well as strength of skeletal muscles also increases, so that the tendency for sprains is diminished.

7. The answer is E. Individuals who exercise are less likely to experience cardiac arrest. Sedentary lifestyle, a risk factor for coronary artery disease, is more prevalent than hypertension, smoking, or hypercholesterolemia. The relative risk (RR) of coronary heart disease for sedentary lifestyle is 2.0, and it is 2.5 for smoking, 3.1 for hypertension, and 2.4 for hypercholesterolemia. Total cholesterol tends to decrease with exercise, but high-density lipoprotein (HDL) increases.

8. The answer is D. General calisthenics is an example of moderate-intensity exercise. Examples of such exercise include those given in answer 1, as well as golfing using a pull-cart; fishing while standing and casting; and home repair, including painting. If the woman had symptoms of ischemic chest pain, dyspnea, or dizziness on exertion, she would need further evaluation (possibly including a stress test) even before starting a moderate-intensity program. When she cannot comfortably carry on conversation during the exercise or if she notices dizziness, shortness of breath, persistent headache, or joint pain during exercise, a decrease in exercise activity level is indicated. Fatigue that lasts more than 1 hour after exercise termination is also an indication for a reduction in intensity level [see *Family Medicine* (House Officer Series), p 663].

Note that this woman is not sedentary, even though she is not following a formal exercise program. Because she has the risk factors of age, hypertension, and dyslipidemia, she should undergo stress testing before engaging in vigorous exercise (e.g., conditioning using stair ergometer or ski machine, singles racquet sports, moving furniture, lawn mowing using a hand mower).

9. The answer is A. The cool-down period is the voluntary deceleration of the exercise activity over several seconds to 1 minute. During this time, a net clearing of lactic acid from the muscles occurs as a result of resumption of normal venous return. Lactic acid contributes to muscle soreness during the early phase of conditioning, and the cool-down period decreases peripheral blood pooling in muscles. The return to normal venous circulation also minimizes lightheadedness and nausea as circulation returns to the head and splanchic bed. Characteristics such as frequency, intensity, type, and time (FITT) refer to the defining characteristics of an exercise program. The aerobic phase applies to the activity phase of the workout, not the cool-down period.

10. The answer is C. At 2–4 weeks post-MI, regular attendance at a rehabilitation center should begin. At this time, electrocardiography (EKG)-monitored stress testing is not performed with exertion of maximum stress. A protocol allows for EKG-monitored stress testing for 9 minutes of incremental work on a treadmill or stationary bicycle. The target heart rate is 60%–80% of maximum predicted (220 minus age in years) rather than 90%.

Regarding the other answer choices: The most dangerous period has passed after 72 hours, when patients with uncomplicated conditions have left the coronary care unit. However, it is far too early for cardiac stress testing because of the danger of precipitating threatening dysrhythmias. To a lesser extent, this also applies to the 1–2 week period, with the additional danger of possible rupture of necrotic myocardium before significant fibroblast infiltration has occurred. At 3–6 weeks, the previously described exercise program is safe, assuming no preexisting complications. However, this unnecessary delay limits psychological and, to some extent, conditioning-related benefits.

Note: This subject is not covered in the reference material.

11. The answer is B. The desired pulse rate for a patient during a moderate-intensity exercise program is 70% of predicted maximum pulse rate. Attainment of this pulse rate is not a reason to reduce the intensity of the program. A decrease in exercise activity level is indicated when an individual cannot comfortably carry on conversation during the exercise or if dizziness, shortness of breath, persistent headache, or joint pain occur as a result. Fatigue that lasts more than 1 hour after exercise termination is also a reason for decreasing the intensity level [see *Family Medicine* (House Officer Series), p 663].

BIBLIOGRAPHY

Coleman MT: Exercise and Health. In *Family Medicine* (House Officer Series). Edited by Rudy DR, Kurowski K. Baltimore, Williams & Wilkins, 1997, pp 657–668.

Test 41

Preventive Care and Triage of the Infant and Newborn

DIRECTIONS (Items 1–9): Each of the numbered or incomplete statements in this section is followed by answers or by completions of the statement. Select the ONE lettered answer or completion that is BEST in each case.

1. With respect to circumcision of neonates, which of the following statements is correct?

   (A) The procedure results in an increased incidence of urinary tract infections (UTIs) in male infants.
   (B) The procedure results in an increased incidence of phimosis.
   (C) The procedure gives rise to a decrease in the lifetime incidence of penile cancer.
   (D) Control of postoperative bleeding after circumcision usually requires penile artery ligation.
   (E) Infants with hypospadias should undergo circumcision to decrease their chances of developing a UTI.

2. Which of the following infant sleeping positions is believed to increase the risk for sudden infant death syndrome (SIDS)?

   (A) Prone
   (B) Supine
   (C) On the left side
   (D) On the right side
   (E) With head in partial flexion

3. Shortly after an infant's birth, an obstetric nurse puts drops of 1% silver nitrate into the infant's eyes. This is a prophylactic measure against which type of neonatal conjunctivitis?

   (A) Chlamydia conjunctivitis
   (B) Gonococcal conjunctivitis
   (C) Staphylococcal conjunctivitis
   (D) Pneumococcal conjunctivitis
   (E) Herpes simplex conjunctivitis

4. You are counseling an expectant couple about the pros and cons of breastfeeding. Which of the following are recognized benefits of breastfeeding?

   (A) Reduction in neonatal jaundice
   (B) Relative increase in weight gain (compared with formula-fed infants)
   (C) Increase in immunoglobulin G (IgG) antibodies
   (D) Faster return of mother's uterus to normal size
   (E) Absence of need for fluoride supplementation in term infants

5. You see a 1-month-old male infant who was born at 39 weeks' gestation and required no resuscitation. He is his parents' first child. For the last week he has had several episodes of protracted screaming and crying, and he has had no fever. The infant, who has been growing well, now weighs 11 lb (5 kg). He produces two formed stools each day. On examination, he is afebrile with normal tympanic membranes and pharynx. The lungs are clear. Heart sounds are normal, and the abdomen is nontender and has no masses.

   The child's mother has been giving him Enfamil formula. Another mother has suggested that he might have a milk allergy, and the parents are seeking your advice on formula choice. What do you recommend?

   (A) Continuing using Enfamil
   (B) Switching to Isomil
   (C) Switching to Nursoy
   (D) Switching to Nutramigen
   (E) Switching to Alimentum

6. How much food (formula or breast milk) does a newborn (i.e., 24 hours in age) need, assuming the infant feeds about seven times a day?

   (A) 1/4 to 1/2 ounce
   (B) 1/2 to 1 ounce
   (C) 2 ounces
   (D) 4 ounces
   (E) 6 ounces

7. You are examining a 4-month-old African-American girl whose parents both have sickle cell trait. Her neonatal history is unremarkable, her growth has been normal, and she has not been ill. Which of the following statements regarding her situation is correct?

    (A) If she has sickle cell disease, she would have had sickle cell crises (which would not occur with sickle cell trait).

    (B) If she has sickle cell disease, she is at particular risk for gram-negative sepsis from *Escherichia coli*.

    (C) If she has sickle cell disease, her spleen would not be affected at this age.

    (D) To determine whether an infant has sickle cell disease or sickle cell trait, the baby should undergo hemoglobin electrophoresis at age 2 months.

    (E) If an infant has sickle cell disease, penicillin prophylaxis should begin by age 2 months.

8. You are deciding whether it is appropriate to give a diphtheria-tetanus-pertussis (DTP) vaccination to a 4-month-old infant on a well-child visit. Assuming that the child has otherwise been healthy and is taking no medications, which of the following represents a true contraindication to administration of the vaccine at this time?

    (A) Presence of otitis media but absence of fever

    (B) Father with a history of an allergic reaction to pertussis vaccine

    (C) Temperature of 102.5°F (39.2°C) and a right-sided pneumonia

    (D) Development of a fever [temperature to 102°F (39°C)] after receiving DTP at 2 months

    (E) Administration of oral polio vaccine at the same visit

9. Which of the following is more characteristic of pathologic jaundice rather than physiologic jaundice of infants?

    (A) Total bilirubin level peaking at 11 mg/dl

    (B) Appearance of jaundice on the first day of life

    (C) Direct bilirubin level < 1.0 mg/dl

    (D) Serum bilirubin levels rising by about 1 mg/dl/day until the peak is reached

    (E) Possible necessity for exchange transfusion if total bilirubin levels are severely elevated (> 20–25 mg/dl) or do not decrease with phototherapy

---

DIRECTIONS (Item 10): The incomplete statement in this section is negatively phrased, as indicated by the capitalized word EXCEPT. Select the ONE lettered answer that is BEST.

10. Newborns are frequently screened for all the following metabolic disorders EXCEPT

    (A) phenylketonuria

    (B) hypothyroidism

    (C) galactosemia

    (D) hemochromatosis

    (E) biotinidase deficiency

ANSWERS AND EXPLANATIONS

1. The answer is C. Circumcision results in a decreasing lifetime incidence of penile cancer. Circumcision in infancy leads to a decrease, not an increase, in childhood urinary tract infections (UTIs) and phimosis. Postoperative bleeding after the procedure is usually controlled with local pressure at the bleeding site. Circumcision should not be performed on any child with an anatomical abnormality of the penis. With hypospadias, the urologist usually uses the foreskin tissue to reconstruct the urethral orifice.

2. The answer is A. The prone position has been associated with occurrence of sudden infant death syndrome (SIDS). Side or supine sleeping positions are recommended.

3. The answer is B. The Centers for Disease Control and Prevention (CDC) recommends application of silver nitrate, erythromycin, or tetracycline drops *or* erythromycin or tetracycline ointment at birth for prevention of neonatal gonorrhea. Conjunctivitis from chlamydia must be treated with oral erythromycin, and that due to herpes simplex should be treated with acyclovir.

4. The answer is D. The uterus returns to normal size more rapidly in mothers who breastfeed because the sucking reflex results in oxytocin release. Although some breast-fed infants develop jaundice, neonatal jaundice from breastfeeding is thought to be benign and is not believed to produce kernicterus. Breast-fed infants also have decreased weights relative to formula-fed babies during the initial months, but this does not affect their final stature or weight. Breast milk supplies secretory immunoglobulin A (IgA), not IgG, and macrophages. Although breast-fed term infants do not need iron supplementation, they do require fluoride.

5. The answer is A. Enfamil, a cow's milk–based infant formula, should be continued. The described syndrome is colic, which is not related to milk allergy. Soy formulas such as Nursoy and Isomil are not indicated in cow's-milk allergy. Protein hydrolysate formulas such as Nutramigen or Alimentum are useful in true cow's-milk allergy but not with colic.

6. The answer is B. An expected volume for initial feeding is 1/2 to 1 ounces every 2 1/2 to 4 hours. By the age of 3 days, feeding volumes are up to about 2 ounces.

7. The answer is E. Penicillin prophylaxis should start by age 2 months in infants with sickle cell disease. Affected children are usually asymptomatic for the first 3 or 4 months because of persistent fetal hemoglobin. They are functionally asplenic by age 2 and at greatest risk for sepsis from encapsulated organisms, especially pneumococci. Symptoms of sickle cell disease rarely occur before the age of 4 months.

8. The answer is C. A temperature of 102.5°F (39.2°C) and pneumonia constitute a contraindication to diphtheria-tetanus-pertussis (DTP) vaccine. Moderate-to-severe active bacterial illness associated with fever represents a contraindication. Known personal (not familial) hypersensitivity to the vaccine and a history of encephalopathy after pertussis vaccination (not a history of fever after vaccination) are other contraindications even to acellular pertussis vaccination. In contradistinction to past thinking, administration of a another vaccine in addition to DTP (or any other vaccine) at the same visit is not a contraindication. There is no competition for vaccine antigens for the attention of the immune system.

9. The answer is B. With pathologic jaundice, the jaundice may appear on the first day, bilirubin levels may rise by more than 5 mg/dl/day, and the peak may exceed 12 mg/dl and last for more than 10 days. With physiologic jaundice, jaundice never occurs on the first day. Physiologic jaundice resolves in 10 days and does not require treatment such as phototherapy, because bilirubin levels peak at 12 mg/dl or less. The condition should be recognized and distinguished from pathologic jaundice precisely to avoid unnecessarily expensive follow-up.

10. The answer is D. Neonatal screening does NOT check for hemochromatosis, which is a common genetic cause of liver disease in adults. The disease must be present for 4–6 decades of life before excess storage of iron leads to symptoms and irreversible organ damage. All of the conditions listed are considered inborn errors of metabolism. All states require screening of newborns for phenylketonuria and hypothyroidism, and most states require checking for galactosemia and biotinidase deficiency.

BIBLIOGRAPHY

Gegas BG: Preventive care and triage of the infant and newborn. In *Family Medicine* (House Officer Series). Edited by Rudy DR, Kurowski K. Baltimore: Williams & Wilkins, 1997, pp 669–688.

Test 42

Preventive Care of the Preschool Child (1–5 Years)

DIRECTIONS (Items 1–10): Each of the numbered or incomplete statements in this section is followed by answers or by completions of the statement. Select the ONE lettered answer or completion that is BEST in each case.

1. Which of the following age ranges is associated with the highest death rate from drowning?

   (A) 0–1 year
   (B) 1–3 years
   (C) 3–6 years
   (D) 6–12 years
   (E) 12–18 years

2. Which of the following accounts for the largest number of injury-related deaths in children?

   (A) Motor vehicle accidents
   (B) Falls
   (C) Burns
   (D) Violence (e.g., gunshots, knife wounds, strangulation)
   (E) Drowning

3. Which of the following conditions may cause both microcephaly and macrocephaly?

   (A) Perinatal asphyxia
   (B) Infections with agents that cause TORCHS (TOxoplasmosis, Rubella, Cytomegalovirus, Herpes simplex, Syphilis) syndrome
   (C) Trisomy 18
   (D) Cornelia de Lange's syndrome
   (E) Maternal phenylketonuria

4. Normal serum lead levels in children are no higher than which of the following values?

   (A) 10 μg/dl
   (B) 20 μg/dl
   (C) 30–40 μg/dl
   (D) 60–80 μg/dl
   (E) 100 μg/dl

5. A 2 1/2-year-old boy has poor speech development, and you are concerned that he may have lead toxicity. He has had no vomiting, abdominal pain, or constipation. Which of the following tests or signs is the most sensitive indicator of lead toxicity?

   (A) Complete blood count (CBC) that shows a hypochromic anemia with basophilic stippling
   (B) Flat plate of abdomen that reveals specks of lead in the intestine
   (C) Blood lead levels that are mildly elevated
   (D) Burton's lines on physical examination
   (E) Long bone x-rays that show disturbed lines of osteogenesis in the metaphyses

6. In which of the following children would a lead screening test be most appropriate?

   (A) A 2-year-old boy who demonstrates a great deal of hand-to-mouth activity but has no symptoms
   (B) An 8-month-old boy who is asymptomatic but lives in an apartment complex built in 1971
   (C) A 4-month-old girl who has had several episodes of loose stools
   (D) A 3-year-old girl who lives next to a sewage plant
   (E) A 6-month-old boy who is asymptomatic and has no known environmental exposures to lead

7. You are concerned about iron deficiency in an asymptomatic 1-year-old girl who was born 4 weeks premature and was taking formula supplemented with cow's milk for the first 6 months. If she does have iron deficiency, which of the following laboratory results would indicate the problem at the earliest stage?

(A) Increase in total iron-binding capacity
(B) Decrease in serum ferritin
(C) Increase in red blood cell distribution width (RDW)
(D) Development of thrombocytosis
(E) Decrease in hemoglobin

8. Besides prematurity, which of the following scenarios predisposes children to iron deficiency?

(A) Breastfeeding in an infant
(B) Feeding with Enfamil formula in a 4-month-old term infant
(C) Feeding with Isomil formula in a 3-month-old postdates infant
(D) An allergy to cow's milk protein in a 10-month-old infant
(E) 6 months of eating vitamin C–rich solid foods in an infant

9. There is currently an epidemic of measles in the community in which you are practicing. In this situation, at what age should you start giving measles vaccine to unimmunized children?

(A) 2 months
(B) 6 months
(C) 12 months
(D) 15 months
(E) 18 months

10. A healthy 4-year-old boy, who has had no prior immunizations, lives in the same house with his 16-year-old brother, who is HIV-positive. Which of the following principles is most applicable to immunization of the younger boy?

(A) Measles-mumps-rubella (MMR) vaccine and oral polio vaccine (OPV) should not be given together because of competition for antibody-producing sites.
(B) No live vaccine should be given to this child.
(C) No immunizations should be given to the child until his 16-year-old brother moves out of the house.
(D) Bacille-Calmette Guérin (BCG) vaccine should be given to the child because of his brother's susceptibility to tuberculosis (TB).

DIRECTIONS (Item 11): The question in this section is negatively phrased, as indicated by the capitalized word NOT. Select the ONE lettered answer that is BEST.

---

11. You are evaluating a 1-year-old child who is short (less than fifth percentile on growth curves) even after correcting for midparental height. Which of the following is NOT one of the many potential causes of short stature?

(A) Parental deprivation
(B) Intrauterine growth retardation
(C) HIV infection
(D) Klinefelter's syndrome
(E) Familial short stature

ANSWERS AND EXPLANATIONS

1. The answer is B. Children who are 1–3 years old have the highest death rate from drowning, probably because they are old enough to move about but too young to comprehend danger. In-ground pools are a far greater risk than above-ground pools. Pool fences reduce the drowning and near-drowning rates by 50%.

2. The answer is A. Motor vehicle accidents (with children as vehicle occupants or pedestrians) account for about 47% of injury deaths in children.

3. The answer is B. Although all of the choices listed may cause microcephaly, only agents that cause TORCHS (TOxoplasmosis, Rubella, Cytomegalovirus, Herpes simplex, Syphilis) syndrome can result in macrocephaly as well.

4. The answer is A. Ongoing studies have resulted in steady reduction of lead level cutoff points over the past 30 years, and tolerable lead levels are now defined as less than 10 μg/dl. Even lead exposures to levels ranging from 10–15 μg/dl, if prolonged, can produce behavioral and cognitive effects.

5. The answer is C. In cases of mild lead toxicity, only the blood lead level is abnormal (range, 10–20 μg/dl). Symptoms of anorexia, vomiting, constipation, and abdominal pain, as well as Burton's lines (i.e., blue-black lines visible at the dental insertion margins) and x-ray abnormalities usually require levels of at least 30–40 μg/dl. Such levels result in hypochromic anemia with basophilic stippling. This anemia is differentiated from iron-deficiency anemia by manifestation of a normal transferrin saturation (serum/total iron-binding capacity).

6. The answer is A. Although this boy has no symptoms of lead toxicity, he displays a great deal of hand-to-mouth activity. The serum lead levels of children of any age should be checked if they have symptoms of lead poisoning or demonstrate much hand-to-mouth activity. Routine screening starts at age 1 year with checks at 6 months only for high-risk children. Residence in houses built before 1960, which contain lead-based paint, and nearby industry that includes lead smelting and battery manufacturing puts children at high risk. In neighborhoods where lead toxicity is rare, some physicians use a written questionnaire instead of automatic level checks to assess risk factors.

7. The answer is B. The first event that occurs in iron deficiency is a depletion of iron stores in the liver and marrow, with an associated decrease in serum ferritin. A complete blood count (CBC) is the usual screening tool for iron deficiency in children, but attention-related and behavior-related problems may occur in those who have iron deficiency even without anemia. In this particular child, who would be considered high-risk, a CBC is obtained at 6 months. As the hemoglobin begins to become affected, the total iron-binding capacity rises even as the serum falls (thus transferrin saturation declines). In addition, the red blood cell distribution width (RDW) then increases. Microcytosis would be an earlier sign than decreased hemoglobin, but it would occur after a drop in serum ferritin.

8. The answer is D. The reaction to the cow's mild protein causes inflammation in the intestine and resultant chronic, low-grade gastrointestinal (GI) blood loss that predisposes to iron deficiency. Although the iron in breast milk is not high in concentration, it is well absorbed because the lactoferrin in the milk enhances absorption. Vitamin C also increases intestinal iron absorption. Normal term and postdates infants, who are not at increased risk for anemia, are receiving "standard" formulas, which are iron fortified.

9. The answer is B. The measles vaccine should be given at the age of 6 months in this situation. Normally, the first dose is administered as part of the measles-mumps-rubella (MMR) vaccine at the age of 15 months, because seroconversion is less likely at an earlier age. In the face of an epidemic, however, it can be given to children as young as 6 months. To ensure seroconversion, children should still receive MMR at 15 months.

10. The answer is B. No live vaccine preparations should be given to the child, because his HIV-positive brother living under the same roof is presumed to be immunodeficient. Because the older brother is HIV-positive, he may be more susceptible to tuberculosis (TB). Bacille-Calmette Guérin (BCG), a live attenuated mycobacterial vaccine, should not be given to the younger boy when they are living in the same house. Except for these considerations, any primary series may be initiated in children of any age, simultaneously with other primary series. Live preparations may be given with killed [e.g., diphtheria-tetanus-pertussis (DTP)] or with other live preparations [measles-mumps-rubella (MMR) vaccine]. After many years of observation, no diminution of antigenic activity or antibody response of any involved vaccines is apparent with the administration of more than one vaccine at the same visit.

11. The answer is D. Klinefelter's syndrome is associated with tall stature, with disproportional increases in long bones. All the other diseases result in growth retardation. Parental deprivation leads to starvation, sometimes through anorexia; intrauterine growth retardation, by definition, is characterized by starting life in a

growth-retarded state; HIV infection exerts a nonspecific effect of failure to thrive; and familial short stature, which exerts its effects at birth, could account for short stature in a 1-year-old child.

BIBLIOGRAPHY

Kurowski K: Preventive Care of the Preschool Child (1–5 Years). In *Family Medicine* (House Officer Series). Edited by Rudy DR, Kurowski K. Baltimore, Williams & Wilkins, 1997, pp 689–702.

Test 43

Preventive Care of the Child Through the Latent Years (5–12)

DIRECTIONS (Items 1–6): Each of the numbered or incomplete statements in this section is followed by answers or by completions of the statement. Select the ONE lettered answer or completion that is BEST in each case.

1. After motor vehicle accidents, what is the second most common cause of death in children of all ages?

    (A) Homicide
    (B) Fires and burns
    (C) Drowning
    (D) Firearms
    (E) Poisoning

2. A 5-year-old boy falls off his bicycle, striking his head. His mother has brought him to you 1 1/2 hours after the fall. She says he was "woozy" for half an hour but then vomited and seemed to feel better. What proportion of fatalities associated with bicycle accidents are due to this type of injury?

    (A) 13%–18%
    (B) 23%–48%
    (C) 32%–55%
    (D) 58%-85%
    (E) 90%-95%

3. What proportion of head injuries in bicycle accidents can be prevented by use of helmets?

    (A) 20%
    (B) 30%
    (C) 40%
    (D) 50%
    (E) 80%

4. In adults, 95% of hypertension is primary (i.e., essential hypertension), and 5% of hypertension results from secondary causes. In children, what percentage of hypertension is secondary?

    (A) 5%
    (B) 10%
    (C) 18%
    (D) 28%
    (E) 42%

5. During the age of 5–10 years, children maintain a steady growth rate of about

    (A) 0.5–1.0 inches per year
    (B) 1.0–2.0 inches per year
    (C) 2.0–2.5 inches per year
    (D) 2.5–3.5 inches per year
    (E) 3.0–4.0 inches per year

6. Scoliosis is associated with a male:female ratio of

    (A) 1:4
    (B) 1:2
    (C) 1:1
    (D) 2:1
    (E) 4:1

DIRECTIONS (Items 7–11): For each of the numbered immunizations, select the letter that corresponds to the recommended age/status of immunization. Each lettered option may be selected once, more than once, or not at all.

    (A) Over 2 years of age, in high-risk groups (especially those in an institutional or endemic setting)
    (B) Older children to prevent complications of primary disease in adults
    (C) For all children who are not already immunized; requires a total of three injections (congenital passage)
    (D) 11–13 years for children who did not receive a booster at an earlier age (4–6 years)
    (E) 4–6 years [first booster (after primary series)]

7. Diphtheria-tetanus-acellular pertussis (DTaP) vaccine

8. Measles-mumps-rubella (MMR) vaccine

9. Hepatitis B vaccine

10. Varicella vaccine

11. Hepatitis A vaccine

ANSWERS AND EXPLANATIONS

1. The answer is B. Fires and burns are second to motor vehicle accidents as the leading cause of death in children. Most incidents occur in residential situations. Therefore, matches and lighters should be stored out of reach of children.

2. The answer is D. The estimated range of proportion of fatalities associated with bicycle accidents that are due to head injury is 58%–85%. Head injury is, by far, the predominant cause of mortality in bicycle accidents. In this clinical scenario, the boy has suffered a mild cerebral concussion, as evidenced by the period of nausea and vomiting.

3. The answer is C. The proportion of head injuries in bicycle accidents that can be prevented by helmet use is 40%. Therefore, it is important that parents be counseled strongly about requiring helmet use for their children who ride bicycles. Parents should also be told to caution children about avoiding riding in areas where automobile traffic is present; 95% of bicycle fatalities in children are the result of auto–bicycle collisions.

4. The answer is D. In children, 28% of hypertension is secondary, which says more about the rarity of essential hypertension in young individuals than it does about the relative frequency of secondary hypertension.

5. The answer is C. The general rate of growth in children at this age is 2–2.5 inches per year. Generally, at the age of 5, the growth rate is 2.5 inches per year, and it decreases to about 2 inches per year by the age of 10, prior to the growth spurt that occurs during puberty.

6. The answer is E. The male:female ratio for prevalence of scoliosis is 4:1. The age of onset is between 8 and 10 years, and the most severe degrees of curvature occur before the age of 16 years (i.e., before closure of the epiphyses). The American Academy of Pediatrics (AAP) recommends screening for scoliosis in children of both sexes, using physician observation of forward bending at ages 1, 12, 14, and 16 years. A positive test, with the child bending forward 90°, consists of asymmetry in the height of the ribs. Correction through bracing is indicated for curvatures of 20° to 40°, and surgery is recommended for curvatures greater than 40°.

7. The answer is E. For diphtheria-tetanus-acellular pertussis (DTaP) vaccine, the first booster should occur at 4–6 years of age, the primary series having been given in the first 6 months of life.

8. The answer is D. A measles-mumps-rubella (MMR) booster is given at 11–13 years only if one was not given at 4–6 years. The primary injection should be given at 12–15 months [see *Family Medicine* (House Officer Series), Appendix I].

9. The answer is C. Hepatitis B vaccine is indicated for all children who are not already immunized. Immunization requires two injections 1 month apart and a third injection 6 months after the second one. Hepatitis B in children is most often transmitted congenitally through the placenta.

10. The answer is B. Varicella vaccine should be considered for older children to prevent complications of primary disease such as encephalitis and varicella pneumonia in adults.

11. The answer is A. The newly available hepatitis A vaccine is recommended in children over 2 years of age who are in high-risk groups, defined especially as those living in crowded conditions such as institutions or in endemic areas.

BIBLIOGRAPHY

Welker MJ: Preventive Care of the Child Through the Latent Years (5–12). In *Family Medicine* (House Officer Series). Edited by Rudy DR, Kurowski K. Baltimore, Williams & Wilkins, 1997, pp 703–712.

Test 44

Preventive Care of the Adolescent (12–20 Years)

DIRECTIONS (Items 1–9): Each of the numbered or incomplete statements in this section is followed by answers or by completions of the statement. Select the ONE lettered answer or completion that is BEST in each case.

1. The reported percentage of adolescent boys in the United States who attempt suicide is

   (A) 1%–2%
   (B) 4%–6%
   (C) 10%–15%
   (D) 15%–20%
   (E) 20%–25%

2. Which of the following statements regarding teenage pregnancy in the United States is correct?

   (A) Most teenage mothers who leave high school for delivery and child care return to graduate.
   (B) Infants of teenage mothers are at increased risk for child abuse.
   (C) Nearly 75% of teenage pregnancies are ended by spontaneous or elective abortion.
   (D) About 15% of teenage girls are pregnant before leaving high school.
   (E) About 5% of teenage pregnancies occur within 1 month of first having sexual intercourse.

3. You are seeing a 16-year-old boy for a physical examination for school, and you decide to use some of the interaction time to discourage him from starting smoking. You want to tell him what chance he has of becoming a regular smoker if he smokes just two cigarettes completely. The correct percentage is

   (A) 25%
   (B) 50%
   (C) 60%
   (D) 70%
   (E) 85%

4. You are deciding about preventive screening measures for a young woman whose age at menarche was 13 years. Her menstrual cycles are every 30 days with 4 days of moderate flow, and her last menstrual period (LMP) was 2 weeks ago. She denies any sexual activity, any vaginal discharge, or any pelvic area pain. After what age should she have her first Papanicolaou (Pap) smear?

   (A) 13 years
   (B) 15 years
   (C) 18 years
   (D) 22 years
   (E) 25 years

5. Which of the following is characteristic of normal late adolescent development?

   (A) Beginning of separation from parents
   (B) Increasing concern with intimate relationships and careers
   (C) Participation in greater risk-taking behaviors
   (D) Increased involvement with peer groups
   (E) Increased involvement in substance abuse, sexual activity, and delinquency

6. The mother of a 13-year-old boy who believes that her son is not drinking enough milk asks you about calcium intake requirements. What are the current daily recommendations concerning calcium intake for adolescents?

   (A) 300–500 mg/day
   (B) 600–1000 mg/day
   (C) 1200–1500 mg/day
   (D) 1500–2000 mg/day
   (E) 2000–2500 mg/day

7. A 15-year-old girl is considering starting a weight-lifting program at school. Her last menstrual period (LMP) was 1 week ago. What Tanner stage of pubertal maturation should she have reached before she begins such a program?

   (A) Tanner stage I
   (B) Tanner stage II
   (C) Tanner stage III
   (D) Tanner stage IV
   (E) Tanner stage V

8. A 16-year-old girl comes to the office for a physical examination for school. She is presently menstruating. You check her immunization history and find that she completed her primary series and boosters for both diphtheria-tetanus-pertussis (DTP) vaccine and oral polio vaccine (OPV) during childhood. Five years ago, she received a tetanus-diphtheria (Td) booster in an emergency department after helping her parents clean out a flooded basement. At age 16 months, she received one dose of measles-mumps-rubella (MMR) vaccine. By age 6 she had completed the series of hepatitis B vaccinations. She was diagnosed with chickenpox by a physician at age 4. She never had the *Haemophilus influenzae* type b (Hib) vaccine. Which of the following preventive measures is most strongly indicated?

(A) Varicella antibody titer
(B) Hepatitis B vaccine booster dose
(C) Hib vaccine
(D) Td booster
(E) MMR booster

9. The patient referred to in question 8 asks you about what vitamin supplements she should take. She drinks four glasses of milk each day and is not a vegetarian. She eats salads at least four times per week. Assuming she has no intestinal disorders or malabsorption, what supplements do you recommend?

(A) Vitamin A
(B) Vitamin E
(C) Folic acid
(D) Vitamin B_{12}
(E) Vitamin C

DIRECTIONS (Item 10): The question in this section is negatively phrased as indicated by the capitalized word LEAST. Select the ONE lettered answer that is BEST.

10. Which of the following is the LEAST common cause of death in adolescents?

(A) HIV and AIDS
(B) Gunshot wounds
(C) Drowning
(D) Motor vehicle accidents
(E) Suicide

ANSWERS AND EXPLANATIONS

1. The answer is C. The attempted suicide rate among male adolescents is 10%–15%, and an even higher percentage report seriously considering suicide. Although girls attempt suicide at a rate four times that of boys, successful suicides in girls occur at only one-fourth the rate in boys. In both sexes, risk factors include substance abuse, chronic illness (males), depression, psychosis, gender identity issues, and previous attempts. Family concerns such as disruption, divorce, parental separation, parental death, substance abuse in the family, and family history of attempted or successful suicide also play a role.

2. The answer is B. Infants of teenage mothers are at increased risk for child abuse. Only about 40% of teenagers who leave high school secondary to pregnancy return to graduate. Only 50% of teenage pregnancies end in spontaneous or elective abortions. About 20% of teenage pregnancies occur within the first month of intercourse.

3. The answer is E. Of the teenagers who smoke two cigarettes completely, 85% become regular smokers. Surveys show that most adolescents are sorry they began smoking.

4. The answer is C. Papanicolaou (Pap) smears should begin after age 18. New research shows an even stronger link between cervical dysplasia and the acquisition of human papilloma virus. Conversely, Pap smears may be recommended less frequently for low risk women.

5. The answer is B. In their late teens, adolescents normally become more concerned about intimate relationships and careers. The beginning of parental separation and more involvement with peers, cited in choices A and D, are characteristic of earlier phases of development. The behaviors identified in choices C and E (e.g., risk-taking actions, substance abuse, sexual activity, delinquency) are abnormal patterns.

6. The answer is C. The new recommended level for calcium intake in adolescents of 1200–1500 mg/day is close to the 1500 mg/day amount that is recommended for adults to help prevent osteoporosis.

7. The answer is E. In Tanner stage V, adolescents have full adult secondary sex characteristics.

8. The answer is E. A measles-mumps-rubella (MMR) booster is indicated, because it is likely that her immunities to rubella as well as to measles and mumps have partially faded since she received the MMR vaccine about 14 years ago. She is now starting her reproductive years and the vaccine is avoided during pregnancy (live viral vaccine), so the time to boost her immunity is now, to avoid the adverse effects of the congenital rubella syndrome. Varicella immunity can be assumed because of the girl's previous history of the disease, which usually confers lifelong immunity. *Haemophilus influenzae* type b (Hib) vaccine is indicated in children only up to age 6. She is not due for another tetanus-diphtheria (Td) booster for 5 years.

9. The answer is C. Adequate pre- and periconception folic acid levels may diminish neural tube defects in the fetus if the girl becomes pregnant. There are no recommendations for exogenous vitamin supplements for the other listed vitamins in adolescents.

10. The answer is A. The primary causes of death in adolescents (in order of frequency) are accidents, homicide, and suicide. Although a large number of adolescents become infected with HIV, they do not die during the teenage years.

BIBLIOGRAPHY

Sternback M, Lipsky MS: Preventive Care of the Adolescent (12–20 Years). In *Family Medicine* (House Officer Series). Edited by Rudy DR, Kurowski K. Baltimore, Williams & Wilkins, 1997, pp 713–720.

Test 45

Preventive Care of the Young Adult (20–40 Years)

DIRECTIONS (Items 1–6): Each of the numbered or incomplete statements in this section is followed by answers or by completions of the statement. Select the ONE lettered answer or completion that is BEST in each case.

1. Which of the following categories among the following accounts for the largest proportion of deaths in individuals younger than 45 years of age?

   (A) Cardiovascular disease
   (B) Accidental injury
   (C) Pneumonia
   (D) Suicide
   (E) HIV infection

2. What is the second most common cause of death in individuals in the 25- to 44-year age group?

   (A) Cardiovascular disease
   (B) Accidental injury
   (C) Pneumonia
   (D) Suicide
   (E) HIV infection

3. What percent of motorists in the United States wear seat belts when driving an automobile?

   (A) 10%
   (B) 25%
   (C) 33%
   (D) 50%
   (E) 67%

4. Cancers are the third leading cause of death in the 25- to 44-year age group. The leading cause of cancer death among individuals in this group is

   (A) lung cancer
   (B) breast cancer
   (C) prostate cancer
   (D) leukemia
   (E) cervical cancer

5. Approximately what drop in the average mean blood pressure of the American population would result in a 25% reduction in the incidence of coronary artery disease and a 50% decline in incidence of stroke?

   (A) 4 mm Hg
   (B) 7 mm Hg
   (C) 15 mm Hg
   (D) 20 mm Hg
   (E) 25 mm Hg

6. How frequently does the Guide to Clinical Preventive Services (US Preventive Services Task Force) [see Table 45.1 in *Family Medicine* (House Officer Series)] recommend that total cholesterol (TC) be screened in the 20- to 40-year age group (assuming normal baseline result)?

   (A) Every year
   (B) Every 2 years
   (C) Every 3 years
   (D) Every 5 years
   (E) Every 10 years

7. You are counseling a 40-year-old white man, a successful real estate salesman, 1 week after you performed a comprehensive history and physical examination. You discovered that he has been married for 7 years (second time) and that he has four children in all [two boys (ages 14 and 16 years) by the first marriage; two girls (ages 4 and 6 years) by the second marriage]. He reported that he has smoked one pack-per-day for 20 years and said that he drinks 1–3 glasses of wine daily (plus more socially). You learned that he has received two drinking-while-intoxicated (DWI) citations.

The man's past medical history includes an appendectomy at age 12 and maxillofacial traumatic surgery during his first marriage following an auto accident in which he was cited and found to have an illegally high blood alcohol level. In addition, he received treatment for sexually transmitted disease (STD) twice: once for gonorrhea (between marriages) and once for chlamydia (after the second marriage).

The man's father, who smoked 1 1/2 packs per day for 45 years, died at 65 years of age of coronary artery disease. His mother [5′5″ (1.7 m) and 130 lb (59.1 kg)] has type II diabetes mellitus.

A review of systems was unremarkable. The man, whose height is 5′9″ (1.8 m) and weight is 180 lb (81.7 kg), had a blood pressure of 145/88 mm Hg and regular and a respiration rate of 16 breaths/min. The physical examination, including rectal examination for prostate size and shape, was entirely within normal limits. As part of the examination, you ordered a comprehensive series of laboratory tests. Laboratory findings were: complete blood count (CBC) within normal limits; total cholesterol (TC), 240 mg/dl; high-density lipoprotein (HDL) cholesterol, 38 mg/dl; low-density lipoprotein (LDL) cholesterol, 140 mg/dl; blood urea nitrogen (BUN), 18 mg/dl, creatinine, 1.2 mg/dl; and serum triglycerides, 200 mg/dl.

What is the order of importance of risk factors (i.e., most urgent and timely to the least pressing) that deserve your attention, assuming patients can commit effort for change in only one area at a time period of 6 months?

- (A) Smoking, alcohol intake, dietary fats, lack of use of seat belts, calorie restriction
- (B) Alcohol intake, lack of use of seat belts, smoking, dietary fat
- (C) Dietary fat, smoking, alcohol intake, calorie restriction
- (D) Calorie restriction, alcohol intake, dietary fats, smoking
- (E) Calorie restriction, smoking, alcohol intake, dietary fats, lack of use of seat belts

---

DIRECTIONS (Item 8): The incomplete statement in this section is negatively phrased, as indicated by the capitalized word NOT. Select the ONE lettered answer or completion that is BEST.

8. Suicide occurs in a complex variety of settings. Which of the following statements regarding suicide, the fifth leading cause of death in the 25- to 44-year age group, is NOT true?

- (A) Victims have often been in contact with medical services in the period just prior to suicide.
- (B) Firearms are a significantly prevalent method in men, adolescents, and young adults.
- (C) Previous suicidal "gestures" (previous half-hearted attempts) place patients in a normal risk category.
- (D) HIV infection and AIDS confer significant risk status.
- (E) Drug addiction is a leading risk factor.

DIRECTIONS (Items 9–13): For each numbered immunization, select the letter of the correct condition under which it should be offered. Each letter option may be selected once, more than once, or not at all.

- (A) Individuals with chronic medical conditions
- (B) Individuals born after 1956 who lack evidence of immunity
- (C) Health care workers and recipients of blood products
- (D) All adults every 10 years
- (E) Before travel to a foreign country

9. Tetanus-diphtheria (Td) vaccine

10. Measles-mumps-rubella (MMR) vaccine

11. Hepatitis B vaccine

12. Pneumococcal vaccine

13. Influenza vaccine

ANSWERS AND EXPLANATIONS

1. The answer is B. The category of accidental injury is the most common cause of death in individuals under the age of 45 years. One-half of these fatal accidents involve motor vehicles. In young adults, impulsiveness remains an issue. Vascular disease, the "great killer," does not affect most individuals until they are in their 50s.

2. The answer is E. HIV infection is the second most common cause of death in individuals in the 25- to 44-year age group, and AIDS is the leading cause of death of men in this age group. The immediate basis for this is intravenous (IV) drug use, which no doubt also contributes to the accidental death rate. After the age of 40 years, the prevalence of drug abuse markedly decreases.

3. The answer is E. It is unfortunate that more American motorists do not wear seat belts when driving, because they are 60% effective in preventing fatalities from automobile accidents. Perfect compliance with seat belt use could further lower the already falling highway death rate.

4. The answer is B. Breast cancer is the leading cause of cancer death in persons in the 25- to 44-year age group, an astounding statement, because it applies to both sexes. In fact, breast and prostate cancers are virtually tied for third place as causes of cancer fatalities in individuals of all ages; they each lag well behind lung cancer, the leading cause, and, colorectal cancer, the second leading cause. The incidence of leukemias is much lower than in the four types of cancer. Although the incidence of cervical cancer has increased, it is an unusual cause of death because of the secondary prevention made possible by use of the Papanicolaou (Pap) smear.

5. The answer is B. A 7-mm Hg average drop (6–8 mm) [or more] in the average mean blood pressure of the American population would lead to a significant reduction in the incidence of both coronary artery disease and stroke. Increased surveillance and treatment of even mild-to-moderate hypertension, having already resulted in the prevention of heart disease and strokes, could have an even greater impact.

6. The answer is D. This "common sense" recommendation is based on the assumption that lipids do not change rapidly in individuals in this age group and that, barring other risk factors for atherosclerosis, the implications of development of dyslipidemia during a 5-year

interval are not serious. However, it should be pointed out to patients that a significant weight increase or the development of diabetes may result in rapid progression to dyslipidemia. Furthermore, if other pertinent risk factors develop (e.g., smoking or hypertension), the cholesterol level that corresponds to the overall higher risk status would be lower.

7. The answer is B. The ranking cause of death in the under 40-year adult age group is accidental injury. More than 50% of automobile accidents involve alcohol, and one-third of motorists do not use seat belts, which are 60% effective in preventing fatalities in motor vehicle accidents. Therefore, the most urgent lifestyle modification in this man, who has demonstrated alcohol abuse and other evidence of high-risk behavior, is intercession to control alcohol intake. The wearing of seat belts is less of a lifestyle issue than one of education, and physicians could probably address it while they discuss alcohol abuse.

Smoking is a critical risk factor for vascular disease of all forms, and this patient already has the risk factors of family history and mild hypertension. However, the vascular disease is less likely to cause this man's death in the next 5 years than is the combination of alcohol and motor vehicle use. The physician should take every opportunity to point out the folly of cigarette smoking, but individuals are generally not capable of changing two major features of their lifestyle at the same time. Perhaps in 6–12 months, after the man has dealt with the alcohol abuse, consideration of smoking cessation is more realistic.

Dietary fats is another lifestyle issue that bears on vascular disease. However, over the long run, smoking cessation produces far greater results in preventing vascular disease than does lowering of lipid levels. In this patient, these values are moderately unfavorable but not severely elevated.

8. The answer is C. Although the suicidal "gesture" has become infamous in emergency departments, persons who make such a "gesture" or attempt fall along a spectrum between the extremes of attention-getting and determination. Virtually all individuals who have gone so far as to "rehearse" the act of suicide have seriously considered taking their own lives.

9. The answer is D. Td immunization is necessary at less than 10-year intervals only in the event of a contaminated skin-breaking injury.

10. The answer is B. It is believed that serious susceptibility to any of these three diseases does not exist after the age of 30 years.

11. The answer is C. Health care workers and recipients of blood products are at risk for hepatitis B. The disease is preventable by avoiding IV drug abuse and homosexual–heterosexual contacts. Travelers should be warned that informal sexual liaisons may be risky.

12. The answer is A. Individuals with chronic medical conditions (e.g., chronic lung disease, chronic heart failure) and elderly persons (> age 75 years) should receive the pneumococcal vaccine. For high-risk individuals, pneumococcal pneumonia may be catastrophic.

13. The answer is A. Influenza is similar to bacterial pneumonia in terms of its implications for individuals who are chronically ill or elderly. (See the answer to question 12.) Tetanus booster need not be given before travel, except to a developing country and if the last booster were longer than 5 years earlier.

BIBLIOGRAPHY

Ferrante JM: Preventive Care of the Young Adult (20–40 Years). In *Family Medicine* (House Officer Series). Edited by Rudy DR, Kurowski K. Baltimore, Williams & Wilkins, 1997, pp 721–728.

US Preventive Services Task Force: Guide to Clinical Preventive Services, 2nd edition. Baltimore, Williams & Wilkins, 1996.

Test 46

Preventive Care of the Middle-Aged Adult (40–65 Years)

DIRECTIONS (Items 1–11): Each of the numbered or incomplete statements in this section is followed by answers or by completions of the statement. Select the ONE lettered answer or completion that is BEST in each case.

1. You are consulting with a 50-year-old man at the time of his first comprehensive physical examination in 15 years. He smokes one package of cigarettes per day, weighs 208 lb (94.5 kg) at a height of 5′10″ (1.8 m), and has a history of high cholesterol. He expresses a desire to begin preventive health care under your guidance. He fears heart disease and desires a prescription for the newest "statin" (HMG-CoA inhibitor) on the market. You begin by informing him of what percent of premature deaths result from "unhealthy habits." This value is

(A) 10%
(B) 20%
(C) 30%
(D) 40%
(E) 50%

2. During a routine physical examination, a 40-year-old Caucasian woman of northern European ancestry wishes to know how frequently she should return for routine "physicals." A married woman, she is monogamous and has had three negative consecutive annual Papanicolaou (Pap) smears. According to the Guide to Clinical Preventive Services (US Preventive Services Task Force), how often should you recommend she return for pelvic examination and Pap smear?

(A) Every 6 months
(B) Every year
(C) Every 2 years
(D) Every 3 years
(E) Every 4 years

3. You are discussing the frequency of clinical breast examination (CBE) with the woman described in question 2, who has no first-degree relatives with any history of breast cancer. In accordance with most practitioners [as opposed to the conservative view of the Guide to Clinical Preventive Services (US Preventive Services Task Force), 1996], you recommend that she receive routine CBE

(A) every 6 months
(B) every year
(C) every 2 years
(D) every 3 years
(E) not at all until the age of 50 years

4. In the case of the woman in question 2, what is your recommendation regarding the frequency of screening mammography [according to the latest literature regarding mortality in screened versus unscreened populations in the 40- to 49-year age group (not including the conservative Guide to Clinical Preventive Services)]?

(A) Every 6 months
(B) Every year
(C) Every 2 years
(D) Every 3 years
(E) Not at all until the age of 50 years

5. A 45-year-old man, a new patient, visits the office for a complete physical examination. While eliciting his family history, you discover that his father died of colon cancer contracted at the age of 60. He has no other first-degree relatives with colon cancer. Based on the recommendations of the American Cancer Society (ACS), you suggest that this patient have colon cancer screening with

(A) digital rectal examination (DRE) and fecal occult blood testing (FOBT) now; if negative, repeat every 3–5 years
(B) colonoscopy now; if negative, repeat every year
(C) FOBT every year
(D) DRE, FOBT, and flexible sigmoidoscopy every year for 2 years; if negative, repeat every 3–5 years
(E) flexible sigmoidoscopy and barium enema every 2 years

6. If the patient in question 5 were 35 years of age, had no symptoms, and had no family history of colon cancer, what recommendation would you make regarding digital rectal examination (DRE) as to a preventive measure for colon cancer?

(A) Every 2 years beginning at 35 years
(B) Every year beginning at 40 years
(C) Every year beginning at 45 years
(D) Every year beginning at 50 years
(E) Every year beginning at 55 years

7. A 35-year-old woman inquires about cholesterol testing. You inform her that the National Cholesterol Education Program recommends cholesterol testing every 5 years starting at age 45 in women until the age of 65 and 35 years in men until the age of 65. This testing consists of

    (A) total cholesterol (TC)
    (B) total lipid profile [TC, high-density lipoprotein (HDL) cholesterol, low-density lipoprotein (LDL) cholesterol, and triglyceride level]
    (C) TC and HDL cholesterol
    (D) lipoprotein electrophoresis (LPE)
    (E) TC and serum triglycerides

8. A 50-year-old man, a municipal bus driver who smokes, is 5′6″ (1.7 m) tall and weighs 180 lb (81.8 kg). Which one of the following conditions is least exacerbated by sedentary lifestyle, thus aggravating the role of other risk factors?

    (A) Coronary heart disease
    (B) Diabetes
    (C) Osteoporosis
    (D) Osteoarthritis
    (E) Hypertension

9. The 50-year-old male bus driver (see question 8), with whom you are discussing immunizations, mentions tuberculosis (TB), alert to the appearance of articles about a resurgence of the disease in the United States. He wonders if he should have a TB skin test at this time. He has no history of positive TB skin tests; is not a resident in a homeless shelter, nursing home, or corrective institution; was born of American-born parents in the United States; and denies abuse of alcohol or drugs. Which of the following constitutes another high-risk category for TB and an indication for TB skin testing?

    (A) Obesity
    (B) Smoking history
    (C) Atopic allergies complicated by frequent attacks of asthmatic bronchitis
    (D) Chronic renal failure and maintenance on dialysis
    (E) Age over 50 years

10. For which of the following conditions is obesity a protective factor?

    (A) Coronary heart disease
    (B) Diabetes
    (C) Osteoporosis
    (D) Osteoarthritis
    (E) Hypertension

11. You are discussing immunizations with a 60-year-old Caucasian man who has a 35-pack-year smoking history. He has a chronic "smoker's" cough and a reduced forced expiratory volume in 1 second (FEV_1). His occupation is that of an insurance broker. He had a tetanus-diphtheria (Td) booster 7 years ago during a simple laceration repair. Which of the following vaccine combinations would you order at this time?

    (A) Pneumococcal and influenza vaccines
    (B) Influenza and *Haemophilus influenzae* type b (Hib) vaccines
    (C) Td and influenza vaccines
    (D) Hepatitis B, Td, and pneumococcal vaccines
    (E) Hepatitis B, Td, and Hib vaccines

ANSWERS AND EXPLANATIONS

1. The answer is E. Approximately one-half of all premature deaths result from "unhealthy habits" [*Family Medicine* (House Officer Series)]. At the top of the list, experts all agree, is tobacco smoking; it contributes to the prevalence of vascular diseases and many cancers (overall, the two ranking causes of death) [see Test 39]. Second is obesity, a prevalent condition that aggravates dyslipidemia, hypertension, and insulin resistance. Third is alcohol consumption, because of its contribution to fatalities from motor vehicle accidents in individuals from 15 to 45 years, followed closely by drug abuse. Lack of exercise completes the list. Not only does it contribute substantially to obesity and hence to the increasing prevalence of type II diabetes, but it may also lead to hypertension and osteoporosis, which is now in epidemic proportions as the female population ages.

2. The answer is D. Papanicolaou (Pap) smears can be performed at the reduced frequency of every 3 years, provided the patient has no significant risk factors. Three consecutive negative Pap smears, whether separated by intervals of several weeks or 1 year, have a sensitivity of over 90% for cervical carcinoma. The time of evolution from a precancerous lesion discoverable on Pap smear until invasive carcinoma is 5–10 years.

This answer is in accord with the Guide to Clinical Preventive Services (US Preventive Services Task Force). Until recently, most gynecologists and obstetricians recommended Pap smears every 6 months. At this time, the American College of Obstetrics and Gynecology, the National Cancer Institute (NCI), the American Cancer Society (ACS), and the American Academy of Family Physicians all recommend annual Pap smears for sexually active women who are 18 years of age or older.

3. The answer is B. Most physicians recommend that women with no special risk status undergo clinical breast examination (CBE) annually beginning at age 30. The Guide to Clinical Preventive Services (US Preventive Services Task Force) is conservative and does not recommend for or against CBE in the 40 to 50 year age group. However, the Guide recommends mammography with or without CBE in the 50 to 69 year age group.

4. The answer is B. As the question suggests, there has been recent controversy regarding mammographic screening recommendations in women in the 40- to 49-year age group. Until 1996, no study had been conducted to show reduced mortality in this population as a result of routine screening mammography, although it has long been accepted that annual screening mammography has led to reduced mortality from breast cancer in women over 50 years of age. Recent information suggests that the reason the results may not have been as favorable in younger patients may relate to the increased aggressiveness of breast cancers in younger women. Perhaps screening should take place more frequently than the previously recommended every 2 years. Finally, the views of the National Cancer Institute (NCI) and the American Cancer Society (ACS) have begun to converge; they recommend annual screening mammography from the ages of 40–49 because of recent studies supporting the concept of decreased mortality if screening frequency is increased.

5. The answer is D. For individuals over 50 years of age with no special risk status for colorectal cancer or individuals 40 years or older with family history of colon cancer or adenomatous polyps, the American Cancer Society (ACS) recommends digital rectal examination (DRE), fecal occult blood testing (FOBT), and flexible sigmoidoscopy every year for 2 years at intervals of 3–5 years if two consecutive screens are negative. In this man, and in any individual with a first-degree relative with colon cancer (or adenomatous polyps), annual FOBT and DRE are not adequate.

Even given the family history, colonoscopy, if visualization is complete, need not occur annually. Many practitioners recommend colonoscopy in a case such as this, but the procedure need be repeated no more often than every 3 years because of the long "dwell time" of colorectal cancers. For patients with no special risk factors, annual FOBT, FOBT combined with flexible sigmoidoscopy every 5 years, fecal occult double-contrast barium enema every 5 years, colonoscopy every 10 years, and flexible sigmoidoscopy combined with double-contrast barium enema every 5 years are each well-accepted screening methods. If these procedures are executed faithfully and correctly, they are each more or less equivalent in terms of years of life saved, although the combination of flexible sigmoidoscopy and double-contrast barium enema appears to have a statistical edge. Using this particular method, computer models project a 77% reduction in deaths from colorectal cancer.

6. The answer is B. Digital rectal examinations (DREs) should be initiated on an annual basis at 40 years of age, according to most medical organizations. The best reasons are, perhaps first, detection of prostate cancer (suspected when encountering asymmetry or nodularity, especially pebble-sized nodules that are stony hard) and second, the chance of detecting perhaps 10% of colorectal cancers. It can thus be inferred that DRE alone is inadequate as a screening tool for colorectal cancer (see the answer to question 5).

7. The answer is C. According to the National Cholesterol Education Program, cholesterol testing should measure total cholesterol (TC) and high-density lipoprotein (HDL) cholesterol. In women, the TC:HDL ratio should be less than or equal to 4.0, and in men, the TC:HDL ratio should be less than or equal to 4.5. Many practitioners favor using a complete lipid profile and hope for a low-density lipoprotein (LDL):HDL ratio of 2.5 or less. The total profile allows assessment of the triglycerides, which become elevated with many cases of obesity and uncontrolled diabetes.

8. The answer is D. A sedentary lifestyle is least likely to aggravate osteoarthritis. Inactivity predisposes an individual to all the other conditions listed. Sedentary habits are characterized by a tendency for obesity that may precipitate diabetes; aggravate hypertension; promote osteoclastic in excess of osteoblastic activity (thus, osteoporosis); increase total cholesterol (TC); and decrease high-density lipoprotein (HDL) cholesterol. All of these except osteoporosis are risk factors for coronary artery disease. Sedentary occupations and lifestyles worsen osteoarthritis, unless it is argued that resultant obesity predisposes to osteoarthritis of weight-bearing joints.

9. The answer is D. Chronic renal failure and maintenance on dialysis are high risk factors for tuberculosis (TB). Obesity, age, atopic asthma, and smoking history are not among the high risks for this disease [see Chapter 46, *Family Medicine* (House Officer Series)].

10. The answer is C. Obesity does not aggravate osteoporosis; in fact, obesity helps prevent osteoporosis in two ways. One, increased weight-bearing stimulates osteoblastic activity. Two, in women, adipose tissue is a storage site for estrogen, which is the most powerful protective factor against osteoporosis.

11. The answer is A. Pneumococcal and influenza vaccines are recommended because of the patient's smoking status and apparent chronic bronchitis. Immunization for hepatitis B is not necessary, because the patient is not in a high-risk category for the disease. Tetanus-diphtheria (Td) is needed only every 10 years, barring a skin wound, and *Haemophilus influenzae* type b (Hib) vaccine is not indicated in adults.

BIBLIOGRAPHY

Kerlikowske K, Grady D, Barclay J: Effects of age, breast density, and family history on the sensitivity of first screening mammography. *JAMA* 276:33–38, 1996.

Marwick C: Other voices weigh in on mammography decision. Medical news and perspectives. *JAMA* 277:1027–1028, 1997.

Miller KE: Preventive Care of the Middle-Aged Adult (40–65 Years). In *Family Medicine* (House Officer Series). Edited by Rudy DR, Kurowski K. Baltimore, Williams & Wilkins, 1997, pp 729–740.

US Preventive Services Task Force: Guide to Clinical Preventive Services, 2nd edition. Baltimore, Williams & Wilkins, 1996.

Winawer SJ, Fletcher RH, Miller L, et al: Colorectal cancer screening: clinical guidelines and rationale. *Gastroenterology* 112:594–642, 1997.

Test 47

Preventive Care of the Older Adult (> 65 Years)

DIRECTIONS (Items 1–10): Each of the numbered or incomplete statements in this section is followed by answers or by completions of the statement. Select the ONE lettered answer or completion that is BEST in each case.

1. Which of the following is the most sensitive method for determining the existence of alcohol abuse in an elderly individual?

   (A) Asking how much the particular individual drinks
   (B) Checking cerebellar function on physical examination
   (C) Using standardized screening questions for alcoholism
   (D) Checking serum aminotransferase (AST)
   (E) Looking for spider angiomas on the skin

2. An active 75-year-old woman who has no complaints is being seen for a general physical examination. Twenty years ago she had a complete hysterectomy for benign uterine fibroids, and she has not had a Papanicolaou (Pap) smear since then. She had a normal cholesterol level 2 years ago. Her physical examination is unremarkable. Her lungs are clear. Her breasts have no masses. There are no abdominal masses. Her rectal examination indicates no masses and is negative.

   Two years ago she had a screening flexible sigmoidoscopy, with a normal result. Last year she had a normal mammogram. Two months ago she had an influenza vaccination and 5 years ago, a pneumonia vaccination. Which of the following preventive measures is now indicated?

   (A) Repeat pneumonia vaccination
   (B) Stool guaiac for occult blood times 3
   (C) Mammogram
   (D) Pap smear
   (E) Lipid profile

3. You make a house call to visit an 78-year-old woman, a new patient. You are assessing the possibility of her falling. Which of the following increases the risk of falls?

   (A) Cervical spine osteoarthritis
   (B) Cigarette smoking
   (C) Decreased abilities in one of the activities of daily living (ADLs)
   (D) History of osteoporosis
   (E) Postural hypotension

4. What percentage of 80-year-old individuals have at least mild dementia?

   (A) 5%
   (B) 10%
   (C) 20%
   (D) 30%
   (E) 40%

5. Which of the following tasks is an instrumental activity of daily living (ADL)?

   (A) Ability to get up and out of a bed or chair and ambulate around the home
   (B) Ability to prepare meals
   (C) Ability to dress oneself
   (D) Ability to use the bathroom
   (E) Ability to feed oneself

6. In the United States, who is most likely to abuse an elderly individual?

   (A) A spouse
   (B) A hired caregiver
   (C) A son
   (D) A daughter
   (E) A stranger who has broken into the home

7. Which of the following is the most prevalent severe mental illness in the elderly?

   (A) Depression
   (B) Bipolar disorder
   (C) Delirium
   (D) Dementia
   (E) Schizophrenia

8. An elderly couple asks several questions about living wills while you are updating their health history. Which of the following statements about living wills is correct?

   (A) They are not usually honored by courts.
   (B) They are only appropriate for the terminally ill to communicate desires regarding specific life support measures.
   (C) The do not take legal precedence over the wishes of immediate family members.
   (D) They allow individuals to communicate desires about specific life support measures (i.e., for or against their use) when their health status makes them unable to do so.
   (E) They must be prepared by attorneys.

9. A self-analysis of your group practice has shown poor physician compliance with preventive care recommendations in elderly patients. Which of the following actions is most likely to improve future compliance?

(A) Conscientiously devoting initial visits to all preventive services

(B) Focusing on patient desires for specific preventive services to gain patient compliance

(C) Establishing a flow sheet on each patient's chart to track and date what services have been performed

(D) Follow the recommendations of the American Cancer Society (ACS) to avoid confusion with recommendations of other organizations

(E) Target screening toward nutritional interventions, because they have been shown to have the greatest effect on mortality

10. Which of the following is a common cause of nutritional deficits in very elderly individuals in the United States?

(A) Increased basal metabolic rate

(B) Decreased basal metabolic rate

(C) Increased tendency for isolated systolic hypertension

(D) Depression

(E) Decreased sensitivity to angiotensin-converting enzyme (ACE) inhibitors

ANSWERS AND EXPLANATIONS

1. The answer is C. The use of standardized alcoholic screening questions is a more sensitive indicator than just asking about alcohol consumption. The CAGE questionnaire, which concerns Cutting down, Annoyance on the part of others, Guilt about drinking, and the need for an Eye opener) provides important information.

Regarding the other answer choices: Impairment of cerebellar function may be subtle and only manifests with acute intoxication. Individual propensities for development of alcoholic hepatitis and telangiectasias vary, even for a particular amount and period of alcohol consumption. Elevated aspartate aminotransferase (AST), a nonspecific indicator of hepatocellular damage, is not necessarily present in alcoholism. Spider angiomas, if seen in moderate numbers, are a physical sign of chronic liver disease. Alcoholic or postinflammatory cirrhosis may be the cause. However, many alcoholics never develop cirrhosis.

2. The answer is B. Fecal occult blood testing (FOBT) is recommended every year after the age of 50. This screening test (along with colonoscopies every 3 years) begins at age 40 if the patient has ulcerative colitis or a family history of familial polyposis. (For other acceptable screening programs for colorectal cancer, see Test 46, question 5.) Pneumococcal vaccine is effective for at least 6 or 7 years in immunocompetent individuals. Mammography is not necessary; the generally accepted upper age cutoff point for screening mammography is 70–75 years (although some advocate extended screening for patients with long life expectancies). The woman's hysterectomy was for benign disease, and she does not need Papanicolaou (Pap) smears. A lipid profile is not particularly relevant. For a 75-year-old individual, a change in the lipid profile, with drugs or diet, is not likely to alter life expectancy.

3. The answer is E. Postural hypotension, which occurs with moving from a sitting to an erect, standing position, leads to falls because of decreased cerebral perfusion. Arthritis would not increase the risk of falls unless a functional loss in a weight-bearing joint occurs or neurologic sequelae affecting gait (e.g., a spinal stenosis) develops. Falls increase with alcohol use, not cigarette smoking, and if patients have diminished abilities in at least two activities of daily living (ADLs). Osteoporosis increases the risk that the woman would sustain a fracture if she did fall, but it would not increase her risk of falling.

4. The answer is C. Although 20% of 80-year-old individuals have mild dementia, only 5% of 65-year-olds demonstrate clinical dementia. There appears to be a "normal" degree of cognitive impairment with advancing age beyond 65 years. Organic events (e.g., urinary infection, pneumonia, anemia) may precipitate delirium with increasing probability with age beyond 65 in individuals who can be diagnosed with dementia.

5. The answer is B. Being able to prepare meals is an instrumental activity of daily living (ADL), and the other listed choices all represent more basic ADLs. Basic ADLs involve near-vegetative self-care (e.g., eating, voiding, dressing, bathing). Instrumental ADLs such as shopping, using the telephone, preparing meals, housekeeping, and doing laundry involve integrative and organizational skills.

6. The answer is A. Relatives, especially spouses, are most likely to engage in abuse, which may be active or passive. They are the most trapped in the situation without visible means of escape. In contrast, hired caregivers can leave job responsibilities at work.

7. The answer is D. An effort to determine the cause of dementia must be made even though most cases are secondary to Alzheimer's disease. Depression can present as a "pseudodementia," that is, an event or illness in an aging person that can precipitate delirium [an acute organic brain syndrome (see the answer to question 4)]. In people who can be diagnosed with Alzheimer's disease, depression may be such an illness.

8. The answer is D. Living wills have been honored by courts and do not require the use of an attorney. Although catastrophic illness that leaves an individual unable to communicate can occur to anyone, it is particularly likely in elderly persons. Living wills give them a mechanism to convey their wishes. Because living wills are civil, not statutory, matters, no assumptions regarding their legal impact can be made. However, it is highly unlikely that the desires of immediate family members would prevail over a living will that has been clearly written by a competent person.

9. The answer is C. Making a flow chart for each patient is useful, and assignment of an office staff member to track preventive services is also effective. It is not always practical to try to perform all preventive services on the first visit. Even if this is accomplished, follow-up preventive services in the geriatric population will again be necessary. Focusing on the patient's desires alone would be quite limited as to preventive care. Following the guidelines of the American Cancer Society (ACS) is not likely to be helpful. Lack of approved guidelines is not a significant barrier to physician compliance. A practitioner may check lipid levels in elderly individuals, but nutritional fine-tuning is not likely to make a difference, and restriction to this narrow focus misses other aspects of preventive care.

10. The answer is D. Depression frequently hampers good nutrition in elderly individuals for three reasons: (1) its significant prevalence and incidence, (2) its often undiagnosed status, and (3) its causal role in affecting competence for activities of daily living (ADLs) [even basic ADLs when presenting as pseudodementia]. Although hyper- and hypometabolism may interfere with nutrition and often are not recognized in older persons, these conditions are not common. Isolated systemic hypertension is common, but it does not interfere with nutrition until a complication occurs. Reduced sensitivity to angiotensin-converting enzyme (ACE) inhibitors, commensurate with decreasing activity of the renin–angiotensin system with increasing age, does not affect nutrition.

BIBLIOGRAPHY

Bross MH, Tryon AF: Preventive Care of the Older Adult (> 65 Years). In *Family Medicine* (House Officer Series). Edited by Rudy DR, Kurowski K. Baltimore, Williams & Wilkins, 1997, pp 741–750.

Test 48

Travel Medicine

DIRECTIONS (Items 1–17): Each of the numbered or incomplete statements in this section is followed by answers or by completions of the statement. Select the ONE lettered answer or completion that is BEST in each case.

1. Of the 30 million individuals who travel from the United States to other countries, only slightly more than one-fourth visit developed nations. This has significant health implications, because travelers from the United States who spend at least 1 month in a developing country have a 60% chance of becoming ill and a 1% chance of being admitted to hospital. Which of the following diseases most commonly affects US travelers?

    (A) Diarrhea
    (B) Pneumonia
    (C) Malaria
    (D) Skin rash
    (E) Viral hepatitis

2. Which of the following conditions is the most significant travel-related medical problem in terms of both frequency and severity?

    (A) Diarrhea
    (B) Pneumonia
    (C) Sunburn
    (D) Skin rash
    (E) Viral hepatitis

3. Which of the following traveling experiences constitutes the highest health risk for young adults?

    (A) Staying in small hotels on an African safari for 4–8 weeks
    (B) Camping and rural travel in India for 1–3 weeks
    (C) Staying with family or friends in Central America for 3–6 months
    (D) Backpacking in South America for 6 months
    (E) A cruise in the Caribbean for 1–3 weeks with guided day tours

4. Many immunizations are recommended before travel simply because it is believed that travelers should remain current in terms of all routine immunizations. Other immunizations are recommended for reasons specific to the place(s) to be visited. Which of the following immunizations is recommended 1–3 months before travel to any developing country?

    (A) Tetanus-diphtheria (Td)
    (B) Influenza
    (C) Polio
    (D) Rabies
    (E) Japanese encephalitis

5. A 25-year-old man plans to travel to an area where malaria is endemic. The plasmodium species that occurs there is resistant to the usual medication used for malaria prophylaxis. Which of the following agents is the best choice to prescribe for prophylaxis before, during, and after travel?

    (A) Chloroquine phosphate
    (B) Chloroquine hydrochloride
    (C) Halofantrine
    (D) Mefloquine
    (E) Sulfadoxine (500 mg)-pyrimethamine (25 mg)

6. Traveler's diarrhea is caused by bacteria in 80% of cases, mostly *Escherichia coli* but also *Shigella, Salmonella,* and *Campylobacter*. Which of the following statements about traveler's diarrhea is correct?

    (A) Prophylactic antibiotics are generally recommended routinely before travel to areas where the potability of water is questionable, regardless of length of stay.
    (B) Bismuth subsalicylate tablets (262 mg, 2–4 times per day) while in an endemic area is a safe prophylactic measure under all medical conditions.
    (C) Bismuth subsalicylate (2–4 times per day) while in an endemic area is virtually 100% effective for prevention.
    (D) For travel to south Asia, in special circumstances where antibacterial prophylaxis is used, trimethoprim-sulfamethoxazole is used routinely.
    (E) Antibiotic/antibacterial prophylaxis is best used in anticipation of short stays in certain areas and with diabetes or chronic diarrhea. In such situations, it is 90% successful in prevention of disease.

7. A female patient consults you about health-related concerns when traveling abroad. Eventually you introduce the topic of typhoid because you know that one of her planned destinations is a country for which typhoid vaccination is recommended. Which of the following countries or regions is on this woman's itinerary?

    (A) Canada
    (B) Israel
    (C) Europe
    (D) Australia
    (E) New Zealand

8. A 25-year-old pregnant woman solicits your opinion about the advisability of travel. Which of the following statements regarding travel during pregnancy is correct?

(A) Travel is best done in the first trimester.
(B) Most airlines require a physician's permission for air travel by a pregnant woman.
(C) Travel to areas where the risk of malaria is high should be avoided.
(D) For symptomatic treatment of upper respiratory infections (URIs) in the first trimester, astemizole or terfenadine may be used.
(E) For diarrhea during the first or second trimester, sulfamethoxazole, erythromycin, and loperamide should be avoided.

9. Alveolar PO_2, which is normally about 100 mm Hg in a healthy person at sea level, falls to what level at an altitude of 10,000 feet?

(A) 46 mm Hg
(B) 47 mm Hg
(C) 61 mm Hg
(D) 79 mm Hg
(E) 87 mm Hg

10. A 25-year-old man is mountain climbing. On the second day he develops nausea, headache, inability to concentrate, and 1–2+ ankle edema. Significant numbers of travelers who have not adjusted to high altitude in advance may begin to experience these symptoms above what altitude?

(A) 2000 feet
(B) 6500 feet
(C) 8000 feet
(D) 12,500 feet
(E) 15,000 feet

11. The most serious symptoms that may occur with mountain sickness are pulmonary edema [high-altitude pulmonary edema (HAPE)] and cerebral edema [high-altitude cerebral edema (HACE)]. At what altitude do HAPE and HACE become significant possibilities for travelers who are unadjusted to altitude?

(A) 2000 feet
(B) 6500 feet
(C) 8000 feet
(D) 12,500 feet
(E) 15,000 feet

12. What is the normal maximum altitude limit for passenger conveyance in unpressurized aircraft?

(A) 2000 feet
(B) 5000 feet
(C) 10,000 feet
(D) 20,000 feet
(E) 40,000 feet

13. Which one of the following conditions is a contraindication to air travel?

(A) Three months status post-acute myocardial infarction (MI) [stable]
(B) Hypercapnea
(C) Diabetes mellitus
(D) Chronic renal failure
(E) Uncomplicated pregnancy

14. A 36-year-old woman consults you in August after 1 week of onset of rhinitis symptoms because she is planning a trip by a commercial air carrier to Nova Scotia. She has a history of atopic diseases consisting of seasonal rhinitis (spring and fall), without asthma. Once, while recovering from a cold, she suffered severe ear pain. Which of the following statements regarding secretory otitis media of flight ("barotitis" or "aerotitis") is correct?

(A) It occurs most frequently during ascent in flight.
(B) It is most frequently caused by the bacterial organism *Streptococcus pneumoniae*.
(C) It can be prevented if air can be forced into the middle ears through the eustachian tubes during descent by the modified Valsalva maneuver.
(D) It is evident physically as a bulging tympanic membrane seen at otoscopy.
(E) A similar problem may occur during scuba diving, requiring the diver to delay ascent to control symptoms and "clear the ears."

15. Which of the following statements regarding jet lag is correct?

(A) Rapid west-to-east travel across time zones often results in somnolence inappropriate to local time at the destination.
(B) Rapid east-to-west travel often results in difficulty in sleep onset relative to local time at the destination.
(C) Anti–jet lag diets have proven effective in preventing symptoms of jet lag.
(D) Paradoxical hypovolemia in the face of fluid retention plays a significant role in the pathophysiology of jet lag.
(E) Cabin altitudes of 5000 feet play a significant role in the pathophysiology of jet lag.

16. Post-travel evaluation is an emerging concept in travel medicine. Which of the following measures would be a logical part of evaluation of an asymptomatic returning traveler who had been in a tropical area?

(A) Liver function tests
(B) Tuberculosis (TB) skin testing
(C) Weil-Felix test (i.e., for Rocky Mountain spotted fever)
(D) Sigmoidoscopy for schistosomiasis
(E) Stool for ova and parasites

17. In a man returning from a tropical locale, which of the following conditions is the most likely cause of fever within the weeks following return?

(A) Typhoid fever
(B) Lassa fever
(C) Prostatitis
(D) Amebic liver abscess
(E) Neurocystocercosis

DIRECTIONS (Items 18–20): The incomplete statements in this section are negatively phrased, as indicated by the capitalized words such as EXCEPT or NOT. Select the ONE lettered answer or completion that is BEST in each case.

---

18. A 25-year-old man who is planning to go mountain climbing in the French Alps seeks your medical advice regarding altitude-related health problems. In a discussion of acute mountain sickness, you advise him to take any of the following measures to prevent these conditions EXCEPT

(A) at the end of a day's climb, plan to descend for sleeping
(B) stay warm, dry, and rested
(C) travel and climb in pairs
(D) exercise early in the trip at moderate altitudes to increase oxygen uptake by the tissues
(E) maintain adequate caloric intake

19. An individual has planned a trip that involves air travel from the United States to Europe and a group tour with several changes of hotels over a 2-week period. To which of the following patients would you NOT give medical clearance for such a trip?

(A) A 57-year-old Caucasian man with stable angina pectoris
(B) A 37-year-old Caucasian woman 3 weeks after an uncomplicated myocardial infarction (MI)
(C) A 60-year-old woman with chronic lung disease who is able to climb two flights of stairs and who is able to walk two blocks without stopping to rest
(D) A 62-year-old African-American man with hypertension (blood pressure: 150/95 mm Hg) who is receiving treatment with hydrochlorothiazide-triampterene and who denies symptoms of dyspnea, orthopnea, and peripheral edema
(E) A 28-year-old woman in her second trimester of an uncomplicated pregnancy

20. Immunization for yellow fever is NEITHER required NOR recommended prior to travel to which of the following countries?

(A) Bolivia
(B) French Guiana
(C) Egypt
(D) Kenya
(E) Nigeria

DIRECTIONS (Items 21–24): For each numbered medication, select the lettered remedial action used in agents for high-altitude cerebral edema (HACE) and high-altitude pulmonary edema (HAPE).

(A) Increase ventilatory drive by direct action

(B) Reduce pulmonary arterial pressure

(C) Increase in ventilation though induction of metabolic acidosis

(D) Increase PaO_2, especially during sleep

(E) Reduction in cerebral edema

21. Dexamethasone

22. Acetazolamide

23. Nifedipine

24. Prochlorperazine

ANSWERS AND EXPLANATIONS

1. The answer is A. Traveler's diarrhea is the most common medical problem among visitors to developing countries [see *Family Medicine* (House Officer Series)]. Although it is possible that other problems are more common in travel, they do not come to the attention of medical professionals.

2. The answer is E. Of those conditions mentioned, viral hepatitis is the most serious common medical problem encountered in travel. Travelers not only experience this commonly, but the condition can be particularly disabling in travel situations.

3. The answer is D. Travel conditions are quantitatively rated in direct proportion to potential health risks [see Table 48.1 in *Family Medicine* (House Officer Series)]. Travel can be classified in four ways: by country visited; by degree of "independence" (e.g., backpacking at one extreme, full-time shipboard oversight at the other); by length of stay; and by the individual's epidemiologic status (e.g., age, underlying medical conditions). Each category is graded from 1 to 3, with increasing risk in the first three categories and up to 8 in the third category for an 80-year-old individual with immunologic deficiency and three chronic conditions.

A total of more than 8 points constitutes possible high risk of illness and warrants advice concerning pre- and post-travel physical examinations, a list of clinics available in the area, and instructions regarding health problems encountered in the country to be visited. Backpacking in South America for 6 months rates 9 points. Staying in small hotels on an African safari for 4–8 weeks scores 7 points; camping and rural travel in India for 1–3 weeks scores 6 points; staying with family or friends in Central America for 3–6 months scores 7 points; and a Caribbean cruise with guided day tours scores 2 points.

4. The answer is B. Influenza vaccination is recommended 1–3 months before travel to all developing countries. In addition, tetanus-diphtheria (Td) immunization should also be current before travel to developing countries. Although "current" means having had a tetanus booster within the past 10 years, it has been redefined to mean having had a Td booster less than 5 years previously (in the event of a skin-breaking wound). It is best to be prepared for this eventuality before traveling. [In Table 48.3 of *Family Medicine* (House Officer Series), the omission of a Td recommendation for Egypt is inadvertent.]

5. The answer is D. Mefloquine is the best choice to prescribe for prophylaxis before, during, and after travel to an area where plasmodium is resistant to chloroquine, the standard antimalarial medication. Halofantrine, another alternative, is associated with cardiac toxicity and is contraindicated in the presence of prolonged QT interval and in pregnancy. The sulfadoxine–pyrethamine combination may occasionally cause serious or fatal cutaneous reaction.

6. The answer is E. Antibiotic/antibacterial prophylaxis against traveler's diarrhea is best used in certain situations; in such instances, it is 90% successful. Regions in which antibiotics might well be used (before, during, and 2 days after returning), even for healthy travelers, are those in which water used in food preparation is suspect. Such areas include Mexico, the Caribbean, most of Latin America, Africa, and southern Asia. In general, prophylactic antibiotics are not recommended. Bismuth subsalicylate is not necessarily a safe prophylactic measure under all circumstances, and it is only about 65% effective in preventing traveler's diarrhea. Because this medication is a salicylate, care must be taken to avoid its use in the presence of influenza or varicella to avoid Reye's syndrome. For travel to non-Caribbean parts of Mexico, trimethoprim-sulfamethoxazole (two standard tablets, one every other day until 2 days out of the region) should be taken. For travel to all other areas, the best antidiarrhetic regimen is a quinolone such as norfloxacin 400 mg/day, ciprofloxacin 500 mg/day, or ofloxacin 200 mg/day.

7. The answer is B. Israel, surprisingly and perhaps unnecessarily, is the one region mentioned among the choices where typhoid vaccination is recommended. Canada, Europe, Australia, and New Zealand are among the very few regions for which typhoid vaccination is not recommended.

8. The answer is C. Pregnant women should avoid traveling to areas where the risk of malaria is high, especially areas noted for chloroquine resistance. Malaria has a more malignant course in pregnancy, and the toxicity of alternative treatment methods used in chloroquine-resistant malaria is increased, even in nonpregnant patients.

The best time for pregnant women to travel is during the second trimester. Only after 35 or 36 weeks' gestation do most airlines require a physician's permission for air travel by a pregnant woman. Ampicillin is safe in pregnancy, but astemizole and terfenadine should not be used in the first trimester. For diarrhea during pregnancy, trimethoprim-sulfamethoxazole, erythromycin, and loperamide are safe to use, except in the third trimester.

9. The answer is C. Remember, at best, alveolar PO_2 is the *ambient* PO_2 minus the partial pressure of alveolar CO_2 and H_2O (the latter is constant at 47 mm Hg). Regarding the other answer choices: 46 mm Hg is the alveolar PO_2 at an altitude of 15,000 feet; 47 mm Hg is the constant partial pressure of water vapor at all ambient pressures; 79 mm Hg is the *ambient* PO_2 at 18,000 feet, the altitude beneath which lies one-half of the atmosphere; and 87 mm Hg represents the total atmospheric pressure at 50,000 feet. Oxygen flow across the alveoli ceases because the combined alveolar PCO_2 and water vapor pressure are offset by the atmosphere.

10. The answer is B. Above 6500 feet, symptoms of mountain sickness occur in 25% of travelers. The incidence increases to 50% as altitude rises to 10,000 feet. Symptoms are likely to be classified as mild, consisting of headache, dysphoria, nausea, peripheral edema, unexpected sighing, and nocturnal Cheyne-Stokes breathing. Resting at altitude for 1–2 days nearly always results in abatement of mild symptoms of altitude sickness.

11. The answer is D. High-altitude pulmonary edema (HAPE) and high-altitude cerebral edema (HACE) are the most serious symptoms that may occur with mountain sickness. Onset of HAPE may be delayed. Symptoms, which are increasingly likely and worse if ascent is rapid, consist of tachycardia, tachypnea, severe dyspnea, frothy or blood-tinged sputum, and weakness. Symptoms of HACE include undue drowsiness, unsteadiness, irritability, hallucinations, and focal neurologic symptoms and signs.

12. The answer is C. Above 10,000 feet, oxygen supplementation must be supplied. (An altitude of 5000 feet approximately corresponds to the elevation of the city of Denver, Colorado.) At 20,000 feet, supplemental oxygen must be given at 100% concentration. At 40,000 feet, oxygen must be at pressures exceeding the atmosphere. In commercial aircraft, cabin pressurization solves the problem of oxygen supplementation.

13. The answer is B. Hypercapnea, like other conditions characterized by compromised oxygen exchange (e.g., $PAO_2 < 50$ mm, diffusing capacity $< 50\%$ of predicted), is a contraindication to air travel. All other conditions listed, assuming no complications, allow for safe travel by commercial air.

14. The answer is C. This presupposes that the underlying cause [e.g., viral upper respiratory infection (URI) or atopic symptoms] of the otitis media is not so severe as to preclude the preventive measure (i.e., eustachian tubes may be so obstructed even before descent that they cannot be opened). Bacterial organisms are not involved in barotitis media. The physical evidence of this form of secretory otitis media is a retracted tympanic membrane. This entity occurs during scuba diving, likewise during descent; the definitive treatment is simply to return to the surface, along with clearing the ears.

15. The answer is D. Cabin altitudes of 8000 feet, not 5000 feet, for prolonged periods may play a significant part in the pathophysiology. (Resting in a seat at 5000 feet has little effect on healthy persons.) Rapid east-to-west travel often results in difficulty in staying awake appropriate to local time, whereas west-to-east travel leads to sleep onset relative to local time at destination (the opposite to the statements presented in the question). Anti–jet lag diets have not proven effective in preventing symptoms of jet lag. Helpful preventive measures include generous hydration, minimizing alcohol intake, moving around frequently during long (particularly transoceanic) flights, and use of gentle over-the-counter sedatives such as diphenhydramine to assist in sleeping on an airplane at times appropriate to the port of origin.

16. The answer is E. Stool for ova and parasites should be checked as appropriate for asymptomatic travelers who have returned from tropical locations. The other listed tests, except for the tuberculosis (TB) skin test, are aimed at symptomatic conditions. With TB testing, although conversion may occur without symptoms, skin testing is recommended only in symptomatic cases [see Chapter 48 in *Family Medicine* (House Officer Series).] There is no need to test for Rocky Mountain spotted fever, because it is not a tropical disease. In addition, many experts recommend a malaria smear, complete blood count (CBC) with attention to eosinophils, urinalysis, and serologic tests for syphilis, HIV, and schistosomiasis.

17. The answer is C. Of these conditions, prostatitis is the most likely cause of fever within weeks following return. Most of the time, a nonexotic condition is the cause of problems in travelers returning from exotic locations.

18. The answer is D. Engaging in significant exercise during the first 2 days at altitude to prevent altitude sickness is the wrong advice. It is not known whether light exercise is beneficial. All other choices are correct. The phrase "climb high, sleep low" is a guide to prevention of high-altitude pulmonary edema (HAPE) and high-altitude cerebral edema (HACE). Risk is significant in individuals who have not adjusted to high altitudes and who remain too long at altitudes above 8000 feet during the first few days.

19. The answer is B. Any individual, regardless of age or gender, who is status less than 4 weeks post-myocardial infarction (MI) should not travel. Reasons involve the lowered threshold for dysrhythmias and increased susceptibility to development of ventricular aneurysms and papillary muscle rupture when exposed to increased physical demands and tensions before scar tissue has formed well.

The man with stable angina pectoris may travel without fear, assuming he has his medication with him, knows how to use it, and is aware of the situations that may precipitate attacks and knows how to avoid them. The man with uncomplicated controlled hypertension can also be approved for travel. If he had symptoms of nocturnal dyspnea and orthopnea or other symptoms of congestive heart failure, he should not be allowed to travel because of the unpredictability of available medical care while he is on a tour. The woman with chronic lung disease may travel because her exercise tolerance exceeds one flight of stairs and one block walking before stopping to rest. The woman may with the uncomplicated pregnancy may travel unless she is in her third trimester and wishes to travel more than 100 miles from home by automobile.

20. The answer is C. Yellow fever, which is essentially a viral hepatitis, can be severe and involve gastrointestinal (GI) hemorrhage. Approximately one-fifth to one-twentieth of infected individuals develop jaundice; of those, 20% die. The disease is caused by a flavivirus (family Flaviviridae, formerly group B arboviruses) that is carried by the mosquito *Aedes aegypti,* which inhabits moist areas. Egypt does not contain such environments. All the other countries mentioned and some 15 others around the world share the characteristics of underdevelopment and humid climates with much moisture, which supports the growth of the mosquito. Each country requires immunization before permission to enter from abroad is granted.

21. The answer is E. Dexamethasone effects a reduction in cerebral edema, of particular application in high-altitude cerebral edema (HACE). Initially, 8 mg are given, followed by 4 mg every 6 hours until descent has been achieved.

22. The answer is C. Acetazolamide increases ventilation through induction of metabolic acidosis, resulting in beneficial affects that counterbalance the unfavorable shift along the oxygen dissociation curve attendant to acidosis.

23. The answer is B. As a calcium channel blocker, nifedipine theoretically acts to reduce pulmonary arterial pressure.

24. The answer is A. Prochlorperazine, in ordinary antiemetic doses (e.g., 5 mg every 6 hours), increases ventilatory drive by direct action. This is intuitively puzzling, because prochlorperazine is a tranquilizer.

Choice D, increase in PaO_2, especially during sleep, is the aim of oxygen therapy at altitude and is not a suitable choice for any of the lettered agents.

BIBLIOGRAPHY

Gross Z, Rudy DR: Travel Medicine. In *Family Medicine* (House Officer Series). Edited by Rudy DR, Kurowski K. Baltimore, Williams & Wilkins, 1997, pp 751–770.

SECTION **XV**

Behavior and Psychology in Family Practice

Test 49

Counseling Methods in Family Practice: Cognitive Strategies

DIRECTIONS (Items 1–2): Each of the numbered or incomplete statements in this section is followed by answers or by completions of the statement. Select the ONE lettered answer or completion that is BEST in each case.

1. A 24-year-old male college student has just been informed that he has been rejected for admission by his graduate school of choice. He consults you, his primary physician, because he is depressed, and he says that he is a total failure and would like to be referred to a psychiatrist. Although he has had some sleep-onset difficulties, once he falls asleep, he has been able to remain so until the alarm sounds. He denies suicidal ideation. You decide you can manage this case with a few sessions of rational emotive therapy. Which of the following statements of "self talk" in this young man typify irrational inward statements that result in neurotic or psychophysiologic responses?

    (A) "I act fallibly"
    (B) "This situation causes me a lot of inconvenience"
    (C) "I behave idiotically"
    (D) "I will change my approach to that situation to avoid that catastrophic outcome next time"
    (E) "I am worthless"

2. In the patient described in question 1, which of the following statements of "self talk" would typify the rational inward statements that allow for healthy adaptations in both behavior and psychophysiology?

    (A) "I am worthless"
    (B) "I prefer to have others approve of things that I do"
    (C) "This situation is catastrophic"
    (D) "I must be loved by others"
    (E) "I am wonderful"

DIRECTIONS (Items 3–7): For each numbered description of events in the cognitive-rational emotive model presented in Chapter 49 of *Family Medicine* (House Officer Series), select the letter of the best matching stage in the "ABCDE" system proposed by Albert Ellis to describe dynamic interrelationships among events.

QUESTIONS 3–7

You have followed a 55-year-old salesman with hypertension for 3 years. The man's height is 5'10" (1.8 m), and his weight is 168 lb (76.4 kg). Until last month, his condition had been well controlled on sustained-release verapamil 240 mg twice daily and a no-salt-added diet. Last month, the man's blood pressure was 160/110 mm Hg. Following the initiation of captopril 12.5 mg tid, it was 155/100 mm Hg after 2 weeks, and it is 160/95 mm Hg today. In response to your queries about pressures at work, the patient says that all the agents in his insurance office have been experiencing slow sales, but that his boss asked him 5 weeks ago about his (the patient's) sales record over the previous 5 months. Since then, the man believes he is under scrutiny and feels that his job security is threatened.

    (A) Stage A
    (B) Stage B
    (C) Stage C
    (D) Stage D
    (E) Stage E

3. Physiological response

4. Perceived outside occurrence

5. Interpretation of significance of the outside occurrence

6. Emotional response

7. Behavioral response

DIRECTIONS (Item 8): The numbered statement in this section is followed by five answers. Select the ONE lettered answer or completion that is BEST.

8. You have counseled the man described in questions 3–7 four times, each visit lasting 20 to 30 minutes. He now understands that several factors contributed to his flagging sales record over the previous 7 months, including the vagaries of the economy and the loss of a major client through no fault of his own. He has also discovered that other agents whose sales records depended heavily on the same major client have also suffered downturns in their sales records.

At your urging, the man approached his boss, the sales manager, and asked him directly what the boss has felt about the changes in the patient's sales record for the previous 7 months. His boss expressed surprise that the man felt defeated about his sales record; he readily attributed the difficulties to the previously mentioned factors.

On the man's fifth visit, his blood pressure has subsided to 120/80 mm Hg without any change in medication. He realizes that his perception of the event—failure to deliver sales at the desired pace—need not have led to such negative thoughts, which in turn resulted in the physiologic response of elevated blood pressure. You instruct him not to take the most recent addition to his drug therapy, captopril, and to return in 1 week. On the sixth visit, you take the man's blood pressure before the counseling session and find it to be 115/75 mm Hg. Over the next several weeks, you find that you are able to reduce the verapamil to one 240-mg tablet per day without finding a blood pressure level higher than 125/82 mm Hg. Which of the following describes best the pathophysiology of this hypertension?

(A) Syndrome X, with hyperinsulinemia
(B) Salt-sensitive essential hypertension
(C) High-renin essential hypertension
(D) Primary aldosteronism
(E) Pheochromocytoma

ANSWERS AND EXPLANATIONS

1. The answer is E. "I am worthless" typifies the irrational statements to self that result in neurotic or psychophysiologic responses. Such irrational statements involve generalities, absoluteness, superlatives, and immutability as opposed to specific details, relativeness (i.e., evaluation of the desirability and undesirability as relative ranges on a continuum), and changeability. Thus, irrational statements tend to use the verb "to be" and categorize the whole self as opposed to an isolated action or deed done by the self. It works exactly as in fair fighting (i.e., adversaries address each other regarding specific acts and relative positions, instead of mutual assumptions of stubborn positions and mutual character assassination). The result is mutual exchange of information. Instead of constructive, realistic criticism or praise, the self is labeled or castigated categorically. Thus, the self-statements "I am worthless" or "I am wonderful" are equally unrealistic and overgeneralizing and tend to paint the sayer into a corner. The result on the receiving side (the hearing self) is variations on stress response and defensiveness. A psychophysiologic response such as coronary arteriospasm or bronchospasm is possible. On the other hand, a behavioral response may occur, which may be exaggerated (and socially negative or unconstructive) or unnecessarily inhibited, leading to still other physiologic responses such as raising of blood pressure.

2. The answer is B. "I prefer to have others approve of things that I do" is an example of a rational statement that allows for healthy adaptations in both behavior and in psychophysiology (see the answer to question 1).

3.–7. The answers are: 3-D; 4-A; 5-B; 6-C; 7-E. Following occurrence of an outside event, a person perceives (A) and interprets it (B), based on rational beliefs or irrational beliefs harbored in advance. This produces an emotional or affective response (C), which tends to be neutral if the controlling interpretation is rational (and no bodily harm or other realistic threat is imminent). On the other hand, the affect produced is probably negative if the controlling belief is irrational. This may produce a pathophysiologic response (D) or a self-defeating behavioral response (E).

8. The answer is C. This patient fits the profile of a "hot reactor" in that his hypertension was aggravated by a neurogenic mechanism and has responded to rational therapy. This form of hypertensive patient likely has elevated catecholamines and renin levels higher than appropriate for his sodium intake. He may respond to a variety of behavioral approaches, including biofeedback. He would also likely respond to angiotensin-converting enzyme (ACE) inhibitors as opposed to diuretics.

Regarding the other answer choices: Syndrome X is the constellation of dyslipidemia, tendency for hypertension, frequent salt sensitivity (diuretic responsiveness), and the tendency for development of type II diabetes mellitus. Eighty percent of patients are obese (see Test 9). Salt-sensitive hypertension often exists in isolation. It responds to diuretics, often as a single drug regimen (e.g., hydrochlorothiazide). Primary aldosteronism is a salt-sensitive hypertension that is characterized by hypokalemia. Pheochromocytoma is caused by autonomous production of epinephrine or norepinephrine, usually by the adrenal medulla. None of the other mechanisms alluded to besides high-renin essential hypertension is caused by nor responsive to neurogenic approaches.

This case illustrates the ABCDE model of Ellis and Harper, as developed further by Tosi. The perception of the event (A) [the sales record] was interpreted irrationally in a most pessimistic manner (B), which produced a negative affect (C) [anxiety and stress]. This led to a psychophysiologic reaction (D) consisting of beta- and alpha-adrenergic discharge. The latter resulted in direct vasoconstriction and secretion of renin, with resultant release of angiotensin II and more powerful vasoconstriction along with angiotensin III, which led to release of aldosterone. The addition of the insult of fluid volume retention to the powerful increased peripheral resistance all effected a critical rise in blood pressure. The physician treated the hypertension nonpharmacologically more by changing the patient's perception of the event than by using biofeedback.

Test 50

Depression

DIRECTIONS (Items 1–14): Each of the numbered or incomplete statements in this section is followed by answers or by completions of the statement. Select the ONE lettered answer or completion that is BEST in each case.

1. The highest incidence of depression occurs in individuals who are

   (A) 5–10 years of age
   (B) 13–20 years of age
   (C) 25–34 years of age
   (D) 35–55 years of age
   (E) > 65 years of age

2. A 34-year-old woman reports that she is depressed after her older sister died unexpectedly of a pulmonary embolism 1 month ago. Although she does not feel like participating in her usual social activities, she has continued to work and take care of her family without difficulty. She has unintentionally lost five pounds over the last month, and she is glad about the weight loss. The woman has expressed some guilt; perhaps if she had spent more time caring for her sister, her death could have been avoided.

   Although the woman has experienced some initial difficulty falling to sleep, once she does, she sleeps through the night. She has not noted episodes of inflated self-esteem and has not been going on spending sprees. She has been taking no medication (including street drugs), has no medical condition to account for her symptoms, and has no personal or family history of psychiatric illness. She denies suicidal ideation, hallucinations, or delusions. According to the criteria in the *Diagnostic and Statistical Manual of Mental Disorders,* 4th ed. (DSM-IV), how would you best classify her symptoms?

   (A) Adjustment disorder with depressed mood or bereavement
   (B) Dysthymic disorder
   (C) Major depressive episode
   (D) Cyclothymic disorder
   (E) Mixed episode

3. Which of the following statements regarding depression and alcoholism is correct?

   (A) Alcoholic men, not women, have a higher incidence of depression.
   (B) If both alcoholism and depression exist together, the alcoholism should be treated first.
   (C) Alcoholic patients who are depressed fail at abstinence unless the depression is treated first.
   (D) Patients with both alcoholism and depression are less likely to attempt suicide.
   (E) Antidepressants should be avoided in alcoholics, even if depression persists after months of abstinence.

4. Patients with which of the following chronic medical diseases have the highest suicide rate?

   (A) Diabetes mellitus
   (B) Chronic obstructive pulmonary disease
   (C) Chronic renal failure
   (D) Prostate carcinoma
   (E) AIDS

5. Which of the following statements regarding postpartum depression is correct?

   (A) It lasts on average as long as major depressive episodes that do not occur in association with childbirth.
   (B) It affects about 3% of new mothers.
   (C) It takes longer for a spontaneous remission to occur than in major depressive episodes that are not associated with childbirth.
   (D) It is characterized by more severe depression, and suicide attempts are more common than with major depressive episodes that are not associated with childbirth.
   (E) It is sometimes considered an adjustment disorder with depressed mood.

6. A 32-year-old woman is seeing you for moderate depression. She reports a 10-pound weight gain over the last month, and her last menstrual period was 3 days ago. At present, she has no interest in leaving her apartment and only forces herself to go to work, where she has difficulty concentrating. She also reports having trouble falling asleep at night. She has had several bouts of depression over the last 8 years but denies any suicidal ideations. In the past, she has not responded well to psychotherapy but does report improvement on medication, although she has been noncompliant with costly medications. She is currently taking no medications and denies smoking or alcoholism. Which of the following agents do you recommend?

   (A) Amitriptyline at bedtime
   (B) Sertraline each morning
   (C) Venlafaxine twice a day
   (D) Short-acting benzodiazepine at bedtime
   (E) Fluoxetine each morning

7. Which of the following side effects is more commonly seen with tricyclic antidepressants (TCAs) than with selective serotonin reuptake inhibitors (SSRIs)?

(A) Nausea and diarrhea
(B) Nervousness and agitation
(C) Tremors
(D) Ejaculatory delay in males
(E) Cardiac dysrhythmias

8. Which of the selective serotonin reuptake inhibitors (SSRIs) listed below is most prone to produce the side effects of dry mouth and sleepiness?

(A) Fluoxetine
(B) Paroxetine
(C) Sertraline
(D) Fluvoxamine

9. Which of the following are blocked by venlafaxine?

(A) Serotonin reuptake only
(B) Serotonin and adrenergic receptors
(C) Serotonin and histaminic receptors
(D) Serotonin and epinephrine reuptake
(E) Serotonin and cholinergic receptors

10. You are selecting an antidepressant for a 60-year-old man. Which of the following antidepressants is associated with the highest incidence of priapism?

(A) Trazodone
(B) Nefazodone
(C) Nortriptyline
(D) Fluoxetine
(E) Desipramine

11. Which of the following antidepressants has been associated with seizures?

(A) Amitriptyline
(B) Imipramine
(C) Fluoxetine
(D) Trazodone
(E) Bupropion

12. You are concerned about the potential for suicide in an 18-year-old teenager whom you are treating for depression. Which of the following patient conditions increases the risk for suicide?

(A) Having a dysthymic disorder
(B) Having a moderate bout of depression, which improves on selective serotonin reuptake inhibitors (SSRIs) after 1 month
(C) Having a major depressive episode
(D) Being an African-American living in an inner city environment
(E) Being frequently asked about suicidal thoughts or plans

13. Which of the following is the most common method of suicide attempt in teenagers?

(A) Self-inflicted gunshot
(B) Carbon monoxide inhalation
(C) Overdose with alcohol and barbiturates
(D) Overdose with tricyclic antidepressants (TCAs)
(E) Overdose with selective serotonin reuptake inhibitors (SSRIs)

14. A 40-year-old man has major depression that proved refractory to your treatment. The psychiatrist to whom you referred this patient has placed him on tranylcypromine. Which of the following substances could this man safely take while receiving this antidepressant?

(A) Tricyclic antidepressants (TCAs)
(B) Cheese
(C) Over-the-counter pseudoephedrine
(D) Fluoxetine
(E) Benzodiazepines (e.g., diazepam)

ANSWERS AND EXPLANATIONS

1. The answer is C. Depression remains a common diagnosis at all ages, however. The condition is often overlooked in elderly individuals, and the suicide rate among older persons is high. Although marriage reduces the risk of depression in men, it increases the risk in women. The occupation of physicians also increases the risk for depression. In addition, the risk is doubled in individuals who have a first-degree relative with depressive illness when compared with controls.

2. The answer is A. According to the *Diagnostic and Statistic Manual of Mental Disorders,* 4th ed. (DSM-IV), this woman has adjustment disorder with depressed mood or bereavement. Although she has some symptoms of a major depressive episode, they are temporally related to the recent loss of a loved one. Note also that she is basically functioning well and without impairment. She has had no manic or euphoric episodes to suggest a mixed disorder. Dysthymic and cyclothymic disorders are both characterized by long-term (> 2 years), mild mood alterations without sustained remissions. In dysthymia, patients have a chronically depressed mood of varying but milder intensity. In cyclothymia, episodes of elevated mood alternate with periods of depression.

3. The answer is B. Alcoholism should be treated first if the two diagnoses exist together. However, the depression is also treated if it persists after 1 month of alcohol abstinence. Incidence of depression is increased in both alcoholic men and women. When both alcoholism and depression coexist, there is a rise in the incidence of attempted and successful suicides.

4. The answer is E. In individuals with AIDS, the risk of suicide is approximately 66 times greater than normal. In dialysis patients, the risk of suicide is 50 times greater than expected, and in persons with cancer and with chronic respiratory disease, the risk is 10 times greater than expected.

5. The answer is E. Postpartum depression, which affects about 10% of new mothers, is sometimes considered an adjustment disorder with depressed mood. It tends to be milder with a shorter time period for spontaneous remission and is less likely to be characterized by suicidal attempts.

6. The answer is A. Amitriptyline before bedtime is appropriate. In this case, the insomnia is a feature of the depression. Among antidepressant drugs, amitriptyline has known sedative properties, and it ameliorates the insomnia even before it acts to elevate mood. In addition, amitriptyline is much less expensive than the other listed antidepressants.

The woman would probably develop tolerance to chronic benzodiazepines, and this would not alleviate her other symptoms. Furthermore, benzodiazepines are mood-sedating and may aggravate depression.

7. The answer is E. The association of cardiac dysrhythmia with tricyclic antidepressants (TCAs) is the major reason why quantities of these drugs should be limited for potentially suicidal patients. The selective serotonin reuptake inhibitors (SSRIs) have a better therapeutic index, which is a major reason for their popularity. Nausea and diarrhea, as well as tremors and agitation, are among the most common side effects of SSRIs. Although priapism is associated with the heterocyclic agent trazodone, delayed ejaculation is not listed as a side effect of any of the common drug groups used to treat depression.

8. The answer is B. Paroxetine produces drug mouth as a side effect. Fluoxetine actually tends to produce nervousness and insomnia. Sertraline may cause diarrhea, whereas fluvoxamine has no significant listed side effects.

9. The answer is D. Serotonin and epinephrine reuptake are blocked by venlafaxine, just as with the traditional tricyclic antidepressants (TCAs). But unlike the TCAs, the selective serotonin reuptake inhibitor (SSRI) venlafaxine has no effect on adrenergic, histaminic, or cholinergic receptors.

10. The answer is A. Nefazodone might be a better heterocyclic alternative than trazodone, especially in a male patient. Furthermore, it does not tend to produce the orthostatic hypotension associated with trazodone, but both have sedative effects. Neither nortriptyline, fluoxetine, nor desipramine is known to be associated with priapism.

11. The answer is E. Although tricyclic antidepressants (TCAs) have rarely been associated with seizures, as have selective serotonin reuptake inhibitors (SSRIs), bupropion is associated with these attacks in about 0.4% of individuals who take it. A higher dose, history of seizures, central nervous system (CNS) tumor, or head trauma further increases the risk. Neither amitriptyline, imipramine, fluoxetine, nor trazodone is associated with seizures.

12. The answer is C. An individual who is having a major depressive episode is more likely to commit suicide than one who is experiencing a bout of more moderate depression or another related condition such as dysthymic disorder or adjustment disorder with depressed mood. Generally, African-American individuals have a lower risk of suicide compared to the population at large. Although it is important to ask about suicidal ideation and assess risk, this does not increase the rate of suicide; however, this question is important.

13. The answer is D. Although mixed alcohol–drug combinations are the most common drugs in overdoses overall, tricyclic antidepressants (TCAs) are most commonly used by teenagers to commit suicide. The selective serotonin reuptake inhibitors (SSRIs) are much less toxic in overdose than the TCAs.

14. The answer is E. Benzodiazepines (e.g., diazepam) are appropriate. Tranylcypromine is a monoamine oxidase (MAO) inhibitor. With tyramine-rich foods or sympathomimetic amines such as pseudoephedrine, MAO inhibitors can produce a hypertensive crisis, and with tricyclic antidepressants, with TCAs, hyperpyrexia, and with selective serotonin reuptake inhibitors (SSRIs), a serotonergic syndrome.

BIBLIOGRAPHY

Bauman KA: Depression. In *Family Medicine* (House Officer Series). Edited by Rudy DR, Kurowski K. Baltimore, Williams & Wilkins, 1997, pp 791–810.

Test 51

Anxiety, Phobia, and the Undifferentiated Primary Care Syndrome

DIRECTIONS (Items 1–11): Each of the numbered or incomplete statements in this section is followed by answers or by completions of the statement. Select the ONE lettered answer or completion that is BEST in each case.

1. A 32-year-old man, a middle-class patient you have known professionally for 10 years, is troubled by feelings of impending doom and pounding heart, lasting for up to 15 minutes. The college-educated man, who has a stable marriage and two children, is employed as a writer of computer software. His condition began suddenly on a Friday evening after a day of intense discussions when he had drunk more coffee than usual. During the attacks he says that he is "losing my mind." He manifests an intense gaze, with hunched shoulders.

The blood pressure is 115/75 mm Hg, and his pulse is 84 beats/min and regular. What is the most likely category of diagnosis of this patient?

(A) Pheochromocytoma
(B) Carcinoid syndrome
(C) Thyrotoxicosis
(D) Panic/phobic disorder
(E) Schizophrenia

2. What percentage of patients with psychosocial problems seen in primary care are referred to psychiatrists or psychologists?

(A) 1%
(B) 4%–6%
(C) 10%–15%
(D) 20%
(E) 30%

3. Which of the following statements regarding anxiety and depression is correct?

(A) These two conditions usually (i.e., in the majority of cases) occur as clearly defined entities, which are easily distinguished from each other.
(B) Anxiety disorders are seldom confused with medical conditions.
(C) Mixed anxiety and depression is less disabling than "pure" of anxiety or depression.
(D) One important aid in management of mixed anxiety/depression is maintenance of "evenly hovering attention" and delaying diagnostic closure before making a definitive disposition.
(E) Clear diagnosis of anxiety or depression usually obviates the need for further evaluation for organic disease.

4. A 45-year-old housewife and mother complains of a vague chest pain and subjective shortness of breath. Her condition is characterized by a sensation that her lungs are not large enough to satisfy her need for air, although she acknowledges that she feels no sensation of obstruction of respiratory effort. She has no family history of atherosclerotic heart disease and expresses a fear of any heart disease as well as a concern that she may be having a heart attack. She is a nonsmoker.

Her blood pressure is 110/75 mm Hg, her pulse 88 beats/min, and her respiratory rate 24 breaths/min with deep respiratory efforts. Auscultation of the lungs is negative for adventitious sounds, including wheezes. You diagnose hyperventilation syndrome secondary to acute anxiety. Which of the following is the most powerful therapeutic tool at your disposal?

(A) Meditation
(B) Diazepam
(C) Acupuncture
(D) Amitriptyline
(E) You, the physician

5. If the woman in question 4 has free-floating anxiety without a somatic focus, you may decide to treat her with medication as well as assure her that she is suffering from a syndrome that does not affect her mental competence and has a self-limited course. Her anxiety may also well be mixed with depression, which she does not presently appreciate. While interviewing her to confirm depression (e.g., checking possible anhedonia and problems with sleep interruption), you suggest that she take which of the following categories of drugs?

(A) Tricylic antidepressants (TCAs)
(B) Angiotensin-converting enzyme (ACE) inhibitors
(C) Benzodiazepines
(D) Beta-adrenergic blocking agents
(E) Major tranquilizers

6. Which of the following anxiolytic medications has the shortest half-life?

(A) Chlordiazepoxide
(B) Diazepam
(C) Clonazepam
(D) Alprazolam
(E) Phenobarbital

7. A 31-year-old woman complains of attacks consisting of palpitations, dyspnea, facial paresthesias, feelings of impending doom, and sensations of detachment. These attacks, which last 5–10 minutes, occur several times per week. Which of the following statements regarding this disorder is correct?

(A) It is more prevalent among males than females.
(B) It has no identifiable hereditary component.
(C) It may lead to phobic responses.
(D) Onset is virtually never related to events in the patient's life.
(E) Treatment is entirely based on counseling.

8. Which of the following categories of drugs is first-line pharmacologic treatment for prevention of panic attacks?

(A) Benzodiazepines
(B) Selective serotonin reuptake inhibitors (SSRIs)
(C) Barbiturates
(D) Phenothiazines
(E) Angiotensin-converting enzyme (ACE) inhibitors

9. Which of the following approaches in treatment of panic attacks most likely would prevent development of phobic reaction and phobic disorder?

(A) Deep psychoanalysis
(B) Generous approval for "sick days" away from work
(C) Protection from mental and physical stress
(D) Counseling utilizing a medical model in the earliest possible period, combining clear explanation and early use of correct medication
(E) Transactional analysis

10. A 40-year-old woman complains of the obsessional need to check her doors in the morning repeatedly to make certain they are locked before she leaves home for work. In addition, she washes her hands at least ten times per hour. Which of the following categories of drugs holds the most promise for the management of her condition?

(A) Benzodiazepines
(B) Barbiturates
(C) Selective serotonin reuptake inhibitors (SSRIs)
(D) Phenothiazines
(E) Azopirones

11. The patient described in question 10 suffers from chronic worry but no compulsive symptomatology. Which of the following types of drugs is a first-line choice for generalized anxiety disorder?

(A) Benzodiazepines
(B) Barbiturates
(C) Selective serotonin reuptake inhibitors (SSRIs)
(D) Phenothiazines
(E) Azopirones

DIRECTIONS (Item 12): The incomplete statement in this section is negatively phrased, as indicated by the capitalized word NOT. Select the ONE lettered answer or completion that is BEST.

12. A 25-year-old man comes to your office complaining of bouts of palpitations, pounding heart, shortness of breath, and diaphoresis, along with feelings of impending doom. Panic attacks, which can be components of phobic reaction, may mimic many medical conditions. Which of the following conditions would you NOT consider before embarking on a management program?

(A) Thyrotoxicosis
(B) Narcolepsy
(C) Carcinoid syndrome
(D) Pheochromocytoma
(E) Pulmonary embolism

ANSWERS AND EXPLANATIONS

1. The answer is D. Panic or phobic disorder is the most likely diagnosis. Pheochromocytoma is exceedingly rare in comparison with panic/phobia disorder. In the norepinephrine-secreting type of pheochromocytoma, such attacks would not occur, and blood pressure would be elevated in the steady state. In the more common epinephrine-secreting type of disease, elevated blood pressure during attacks would lead one to suspect the diagnosis. Carcinoid syndrome, too, is rare. To diagnose both carcinoid and pheochromocytoma, 24-hour urine collections [5-hydroxyindoleacetic acid for carcinoid; vanillylmandelic acid (VMA), metanephrines, and free catecholamines for pheochromocytoma] are used. Thyrotoxicosis is ruled out by the normal resting pulse. Schizophrenia is unlikely because of the normal premorbid status of the patient as well as his appropriate, albeit anxious, affect.

2. The answer is B. Although 4%–6% of patients with psychosocial problems seen in primary care are referred to psychiatrists or psychologists, nearly 50% of patients in primary care have some degree of anxiety, depression, mixed anxiety/depression, or somatizing symptoms of psychological distress.

3. The answer is D. The maintenance of "evenly hovering attention" and delay of diagnostic closure is important. Mixed anxiety/depression is more common than occurrence of either condition as a separate entity. Anxiety is often confounded with medical conditions diagnostically (e.g., with pheochromocytoma and thyrotoxicosis) and because it often occurs in conjunction with such conditions.

4. The answer is E. The physician is the most effective therapeutic agent in this form of anxiety (i.e., one which has presented in the medical model, when anxiety is manifested with a somatic symptom). Although meditation and acupuncture each demonstrate therapeutic advantages under certain conditions, nothing replaces the increase in patient understanding through counseling. Drugs are of less value than counseling for dealing with hyperventilation as a presenting symptom of panic, especially early in the course before phobias have developed.

5. The answer is A. Because this patient manifests mixed anxiety and depression, the tricyclic antidepressants (TCAs) are a reasonable choice. Examples of TCAs, the oldest category of mood-elevating agents, are amitriptyline, imipramine, and desipramine. Amitriptyline is particularly sedating. Not only does this agent serve as a tranquilizer while blood levels rise to therapeutic levels for depression, but taken characteristically at bedtime, it has a salutary effect on sleep difficulties. Benzodiazepines are tranquilizing without elevating mood; thus, they may aggravate depression. Major tranquilizers (e.g., chlorpromazine) are indicated in psychotic illness, typically schizophrenia, and they do not ameliorate depression. Angiotensin-converting enzyme (ACE) inhibitors and beta-adrenergic blocking agents have no place in the therapy of depression. In fact, some patients experience depression as a side effect of treatment with beta-blockers.

6. The answer is D. Of the anxiolytic drugs mentioned, all except phenobarbital are members of the benzodiazepine category. Alprazolam has the shortest half life (i.e., < 24 hours) [see Table 52.1 in the *Family Medicine* (House Officer Series)]. The other benzodiazepines each has a half-life exceeding 24 hours.

7. The answer is C. The patient clearly has panic disorder, which may lead to phobic responses. Regarding the other distractors: Panic disorder is two times more common in females, and it also has a genetic component (e.g., there is a 50% concordance among twins and 18% among relatives). In addition, the first attack (onset) may be related to events in the patient's life (e.g., a major emotional loss or shocking event such as death of a friend or significant acquaintance). Finally, treatment now rests on pharmacotherapy as much as counseling to reassure affected patients that they are not "going crazy" or are likely to die during an attack. Medications that have been used successfully include the benzodiazepine alprazolam and the selective serotonin reuptake inhibitors (SSRIs).

8. The answer is B. Selective serotonin reuptake inhibitors (SSRIs) are the first line of therapy in panic attacks. However, if symptoms are disabling, benzodiazepines such as clonazepam may be used. Panic attacks once prompted the use of barbiturates, but these agents are not effective unless the point of oversedation is reached. Both phenothiazines used as major tranquilizers and angiotensin-converting enzyme (ACE) inhibitors have no place in the treatment or prevention of panic disorder.

9. The answer is D. Approaching the illness medically in the earliest possible period, with clear explanation and early use of correct medication has the greatest chance of preventing development of phobic conditions. Deep psychoanalysis would probably convey permission for the patient to remain "sick." Approval of sick leave is perhaps the worst possible therapy and would reinforce any tendencies to form phobic reactions. Likewise, protection from mental and physical stress would reinforce phobic tendencies. Although transactional analysis may be useful for certain other outpatient counseling situations, it has not been proposed for prevention of phobic reactions.

10. The answer is C. Selective serotonin reuptake inhibitors (SSRIs) have constituted a breakthrough in the management of obsessive-compulsive disorder. Until these agents were developed, no other medications, including the other categories mentioned as answer choices, had a perceptible beneficial effect on this condition.

11. The answer is E. Azopirones (e.g., buspirone) are recommended as first-line choices for generalized anxiety disorder [see Chapter 51 in *Family Medicine* (House Officer Series)]. The azopirones are the newest anxiolytic/antidepressants. Buspirone was the first azopirone to be developed.

12. The answer is B. Narcolepsy does not mimic anxiety, although individuals with narcolepsy may manifest hypertension and irritability diurnally between sleep attacks. All the other entities mentioned (and several more) [e.g., angina attacks where apprehension may be out of proportion to the otherwise mild chest discomfort, side effects of sympathomimetic drugs] should occur to the physician and be considered before making the diagnosis of anxiety.

BIBLIOGRAPHY

Ronning GF: Anxiety, Phobias, and the Undifferentiated Primary Care Syndrome. In *Family Medicine* (House Officer Series). Edited by Rudy DR, Kurowski K. Baltimore, Williams & Wilkins, 1997, pp 811–828.

Test 52

Somatic Symptoms Without Organic Basis

DIRECTIONS (Items 1–11): Each of the numbered or incomplete statements in this section is followed by answers or by completions of the statement. Select the ONE lettered answer or completion that is BEST in each case.

1. What percentage of symptoms described by patients in a primary care setting has no biomedical basis?

- (A) 5%–10%
- (B) 10%–20%
- (C) 20%–40%
- (D) 40%–60%
- (E) 60%–80%

2. A 35-year-man who has been your patient since childhood complains that he has vague left groin pain. He expresses apprehension about having a hernia and an underlying fear of loss of sexual prowess. For the past 15 years this man has been evaluated for constipation and diarrhea as well as vague difficulty in swallowing, none of which yielded diagnoses on ancillary clinical evaluation. Two months ago he complained of chest pains that were intermittent and "nondescript." He has no present or family history of coronary disease, hypertension, diabetes, or stroke, and he is not a smoker. The recent evaluation was negative for heart disease.

Today, abdominal examination is negative for deep or rebound tenderness except for a probable exaggerated guarding response to deep palpation in the left lower quadrant. From which of the following somatoform disorders does this patient most likely suffer?

- (A) Somatization disorder
- (B) Conversion disorder
- (C) Pain disorder
- (D) Hypochondriasis
- (E) Body dysmorphic disorder

3. A 45-year-old mother has seen you three times for a left upper quadrant abdominal pain that has yielded no historical, physical, radiographic, or laboratory findings suggestive of any organic disease. This woman is convinced that she has cancer of the stomach and cannot be dissuaded despite negative upper gastrointestinal x-rays and upper endoscopy. She most likely suffers from which of the following somatoform disorders?

- (A) Somatization disorder
- (B) Conversion disorder
- (C) Pain disorder
- (D) Hypochondriasis
- (E) Body dysmorphic disorder

4. A 38-year-old man has been complaining of low back pain for 6 months. Ostensibly, the pain began during moderately heavy lifting while he was working as a machinist. The straight-leg raising test is negative on both sides, and no sensory or motor deficit is evident. Neither spinal list nor loss of lumbar lordosis is apparent. X-rays of the lumbosacral spine are unremarkable and specifically negative for osteoblastic or osteolytic disease processes. This man has no conditions such as prostatitis that might cause pain that could be referred to the back. He most likely suffers from which of the following somatoform disorders?

- (A) Somatization disorder
- (B) Conversion disorder
- (C) Pain disorder
- (D) Hypochondriasis
- (E) Body dysmorphic disorder

5. An 18-year-old girl has had numerous seizures that resemble the "grand mal" (tonic-clonic) type. However, no episodes of urinary incontinence, physical injury, or postictal drowsiness have occurred. The apparent seizures have resulted in frequent calls from the college in which she has enrolled, and lately her status at the college has been threatened because of the seizures. You suspect her of manipulative antics to gain your attention. When she is being evaluated as an inpatient, these actions sometimes take the form of bizarre posturing the moment you appear. This girl most likely suffers from which of the following somatoform disorders?

- (A) Somatization disorder
- (B) Conversion disorder
- (C) Pain disorder
- (D) Hypochondriasis
- (E) Body dysmorphic disorder

6. What percentage of patients presenting in a primary care setting display significant degrees of anxiety?

- (A) 10%
- (B) 20%
- (C) 40%
- (D) 60%
- (E) 80%

7. A 48-year-old Caucasian woman complains of shortness of breath without orthopnea, with palpitations, dizziness, and nausea and diarrhea, along with a vague feeling of impending doom. These symptoms have occurred episodically two or three times a day for the past 10 days. Which of the following statements regarding anxiety in a primary care setting is correct?

(A) Anxiety-based somatic symptoms such as chest pain do not easily yield to education and reassurance regarding the feared organic implications of the symptom.

(B) Typical symptoms of somatized anxiety include constipation and fatigue.

(C) Pharmacologic approaches to anxiety in the primary care setting include beta-agonists.

(D) Patients readily express fears regarding the implications of their somatic symptoms such as heart disease in the case of chest pain.

(E) Somatic symptoms brought on by anxiety are entirely without measurable physical or laboratory findings.

8. A 35-year-old man frequently comes to the emergency department doubled over with flank pain, usually with gross blood in his urine. He has been diagnosed with ureterolithiasis and generally given injections of meperidine, prescriptions for codeine, and instructions to strain his urine and to see his family physician. Follow-up intravenous pyelograms (IVPs) have consistently been negative for stones in the kidney, renal pelvis, and ureter. One night in the emergency department, while he is waiting to be seen by a physician, an orderly witnesses the man pricking his finger and dropping some blood into the diagnostic urine cup. Which of the following diagnoses best fits this patient?

(A) Somatization disorder
(B) Factitious disorder
(C) Conversion disorder
(D) Hypochondriasis
(E) Malingering

9. A 35-year-old woman frequently comes to the office complaining of gross blood in the urine. Outpatient intravenous pyelograms (IVPs) have always been negative. Consequently, she has undergone several cystoscopies, one retrograde ureteral catheterization, and two magnetic resonance imaging (MRI) scans of the kidneys. She has never required prescriptions for analgesics, much less parenteral narcotics, for pain. One day, while the woman is waiting to be seen by the physician, the office nurse witnesses her pricking her finger and dropping some blood into the diagnostic urine cup. Which of the following diagnoses best fits this patient?

(A) Somatization disorder
(B) Factitious disorder
(C) Conversion disorder
(D) Hypochondriasis
(E) Malingering

10. A 45-year-old woman complains that just as her son enters his junior year in high school and her daughter begins junior high, with the accompanying need for transport to various school events, her widowed mother develops the early stages of Alzheimer's disease. The younger woman now complains of fronto-occipital headaches as well as alternating constipation, abdominal cramps, and mild diarrhea, although she continues to menstruate regularly. These symptoms, along with peptic ulcer disease, and aggravated angina pectoris and asthma are examples of

(A) somatization disorder
(B) stress disorder
(C) conversion disorder
(D) hypochondriasis
(E) somatic anxiety equivalent

11. Families comprise systems of relating in which children may be imprinted from before their earliest memory with patterns that determine their responses to stresses throughout life. Enmeshment, rigidity, poor conflict resolution, overprotectiveness, and a tendency to "triangulate" children (e.g., place them in the cross-fire of praise under threat of blame, keep them in the role of "bad" or "sick") are characteristics of what type of family dynamics?

(A) Collaborating
(B) "Psychosomatic"
(C) Fight evading
(D) Discouraging of emotion-oriented statements
(E) Cross-cultural

DIRECTIONS (Item 12): The incomplete statement in this section is negatively phrased, as indicated by the capitalized word EXCEPT. Select the ONE lettered answer or completion that is BEST.

12. A 42-year-old man complains of 2–3 weeks of vague chest pain that has been more-or-less constant but not severe. He cannot remember the date or time of pain onset. When asked if he is concerned about the significance of the pain, he is vague while appearing sadly disturbed. He indicates the location of the pain with two fingers softly pressed over the left precordium. All of the following statements regarding this condition of symptoms without an organic basis in the primary care setting are true EXCEPT

    (A) up to 50% of patients with this condition in the primary care presentation do not receive the diagnosis in that setting

    (B) the majority of patients in the primary care setting present with somatic symptoms

    (C) in 25%–50% of patients with chronic diseases such as coronary artery disease, diabetes mellitus, Alzheimer's disease, or stroke, this condition coexists and is often undiagnosed

    (D) patients presenting with this condition typically exaggerate the implications of their somatic symptoms

    (E) this condition is masked in primary care for several reasons, including patients' own denial as well as stigmatization

DIRECTIONS (Items 13–20): For each numbered psychiatric illness, select the best lettered description. Each lettered option may be selected once, more than once, or not at all.

    (A) One or two unexplained, fiercely defended complaints of pain

    (B) One or two complaints of recent onset that are vaguely expressed but amenable to explanation

    (C) One or two motor or sensory complaints, often with neurologic implications

    (D) One or two complaints of recent onset that are vaguely expressed and mild in severity, with understated emotional charge attached

    (E) Lifetime history of multiple complaints

    (F) Somatic symptoms experienced only during bouts of affective distress

    (G) Rampant noncompliance with conscious secondary gain

    (H) Patient focus on fear of disease, not symptoms

13. Anxiety equivalent

14. Depressive equivalent

15. Panic disorder

16. Hypochondriasis

17. Pain disorder

18. Conversion disorder

19. Somatization disorder

20. Malingering

ANSWERS AND EXPLANATIONS

1. The answer is D. Between 40% and 60% of symptoms given by patients in a primary care setting have no biomedical basis. Reasons for presenting with such symptoms vary from straightforward desire for information and alleviation of fears to somatization of anxiety and depression as well as hysterical conversion.

2. The answer is A. This patient, who displays somatization disorder, satisfies the following criteria: (1) multiple system involvement, (2) onset early in life (often adolescence), and (3) absence of abnormalities in ancillary tests. The overlying sexual fear associated with the groin pain is an additional supporting factor.

3. The answer is D. This patient, who has hypochondriasis, has the definitive fixation on a single disease and one persistent symptom. Although hypochondriacs may fixate on different diseases at various times, they do not fear more than one disease at any given time.

4. The answer is C. The hallmark of pain disorder is the persistence of the single pain. This syndrome is often associated with possible secondary gain such as a workman's compensation claim or a civil suit. Somatization disorder differs primarily with regard to its involvement of multiple systems and multiple symptoms (see answer to question 2). Conversion disorder, which usually has its onset between the ages of 10 and 35 years, involves predominantly motor or sensory symptoms. Hypochondriasis focuses on a disease rather than on pain and disability. Body dysmorphic disorder involves a distorted body image, not pain, and is usually associated with anorexia nervosa or depression.

5. The answer is B. This girl has conversion disorder. Her symptoms, which are voluntary manifestations of ostensibly involuntary functions, have apparently been designed for the (albeit dubious) purpose of secondary attention-gaining at college and on the part of her physician. The best treatment is counseling, both tactically (over the short-term) and strategically (over the long-term), to steer the patient in a positive direction; her response to emotional need or stress should occur in honest, constructive, incremental steps. She should not be directly confronted with the invalidity of her symptoms.

6. The answer is B. Approximately 20% of patients presenting in a primary care setting have significant degrees of anxiety, either perceived or submerged and underlying a symptom that constitutes an anxiety equivalent.

7. The answer is D. Patients readily express fears regarding the implications of their somatic symptoms. However, these symptoms generally easily respond to education and reassurance regarding feared organic implications of the symptom. Typical symptoms of somatized anxiety include not constipation or fatigue but palpitations, tachycardia, chest pain, hyperventilation, and perhaps nausea and diarrhea. Pharmacologic approaches to anxiety in the primary care setting include minor sedatives and the selective serotonin reuptake inhibitors (SSRIs). Many symptoms caused by anxiety are entirely organic (i.e., psychophysiologic) such as hyperventilation syndrome (respiratory alkalosis) or asthma and have measurable physical and laboratory findings.

8. The answer is E. This patient, who is deceiving his physician by drawing blood to effect hematuria, is malingering. Clearly, he is seeking the secondary gain of narcotics. Factitious disorder, which is similar to malingering, differs in having a less "rational" goal. A patient who presents with apparent thyrotoxicosis from surreptitious ingestion of thyroid hormone has a much more neurotic (albeit more psychoneurotic) goal than one who seeks a narcotic "high."

9. The answer is B. Although this woman is also deceiving her physician, the mechanism of action is different from that in the answer to question 8. She exhibits factitious disorder. She has undergone several painful and inconvenient procedures for which she achieved no visible secondary gain beyond a bizarre satisfaction from attention-getting when affecting illness.

10. The answer is B. Stress disorder is the classification reserved for psychophysiologically induced organic syndromes such as tension or vascular headaches, irritable bowel syndrome, or worsening of existing organic syndromes such as angina or asthma, all of which are precipitated by stress. These conditions represent the tension of ambivalence-laden conflict combined with time/motion demands such as those in the vignette. The other answer choices are reinforced in questions 13 through 20 [see also Chapter 52 in *Family Medicine* (House Officer Series)]. None of the choices is characterized by organic pathology as a cause of symptoms.

11. The answer is B. "Psychosomatic" type of family dynamics is the term applied to the characteristics of enmeshment, rigidity, poor conflict resolution, overprotectiveness, and a tendency to "triangulate" one of the children. Such dynamics promote psychosomatic responses to stress (symptoms without organic basis). Most of the categories in the other answer choices are fictional, although fight evasion and suppression of emotion-oriented statements are subtypes of mechanisms used in such families. Some cultures may normally discourage feelings expression more than others (i.e., Asian or Anglo-Saxon cultures more than Mediterranean or Latin cultures); this is not to say that this characteristic in itself promotes psychosomatic mechanisms for dealing with stress.

12. The answer is D. This patient has somatic depressive equivalent or somatized depression. Unlike patients with anxiety, those with somatized depression do not typically display exaggerated symptoms. Anxious individuals may tend to be overexcited and fear the implications of a somatic symptom, whereas depressed people exhibit indifferent body language in response to potentially serious symptoms. Patients with somatic depressive equivalent may display body language that indicates they have something of greater concern to them than the ostensible somatic symptoms for which they have visited a physician. Hysterical patients (i.e., those with somatic symptoms of conversion) seem indifferent both to the symptom and the strong emotion; they exhibit the notorious "la belle indifférence."

13. The answer is B. Patients who display somatic anxiety equivalent (somatized anxiety) focus on disease rather than symptoms as in hypochondriasis. However, they are easily reassured by clear explanation.

14. The answer is D. Patients with somatic depressive equivalent (somatized depression) are not focused on a feared diagnosis. Rather, they seem preoccupied and somewhat distant, but not detached, as they explain their complaints.

15. The answer is F. The affective distressed state is the panic attack. See Test 51 for a discussion of both clinical presentation and management.

16. The answer is H. Unlike individuals who have somatic anxiety equivalent, patients with hypochondriasis are very difficult to dissuade from their feared diagnosis.

17. The answer is A. Patients with pain disorder are seen in pain clinics. They are tenaciously focused on the pain rather than the import attached to it.

18. The answer is C. Patients with conversion disorder may exhibit the famous "la belle indifférence." That is, their body and facial language indicates a lack of concern, although the implications of their symptoms may be quite serious.

19. The answer is E. Patients with somatization disorder keep returning to the physician with their complaints. A simple investment in time and a continuing modicum of respect on the part of the physician often keeps them in a stable emotional state.

20. The answer is G. Malingering patients are often sociopathic. Insurance settlements and workman's compensation pirates are typical. Examples include the patient with back or lower limb pain who comes in on crutches but is seen carrying them to his car and perhaps loading or unloading heavy objects before driving away.

BIBLIOGRAPHY

Post DM, Rudy DR: Somatic Symptoms without Organic Basis. In *Family Medicine* (House Officer Series). Edited by Rudy DR, Kurowski K. Baltimore, Williams & Wilkins, 1997, pp 829–842.

Test 53

Family Systems

DIRECTIONS (Items 1–9): Each of the numbered or incomplete statements in this section is followed by answers or by completions of the statement. Select the ONE lettered answer or completion that is BEST in each case.

---

1. A 3-year-old boy with a 2-day history of pain and fullness in the left ear has had three episodes of otitis media in the last year. He has a temperature of 99.8°F (37.7°C). The left tympanic membrane is mildly erythematous and not bulging. Insufflation results in poor tympanic membrane mobility. You prescribe a second-generation cephalosporin. In addition, you convey the risks and benefits of treatment and options of treatment to the boy's parents and the need for a follow-up visit in 2 weeks. What is the level of physician involvement (LPI) in this case?

    (A) LPI-1
    (B) LPI-2
    (C) LPI-3
    (D) LPI-4
    (E) LPI-5

2. The boy discussed in question 1 is back in your office 2 weeks later. The tympanic membrane still shows poor mobility. The mother admits that he only received about half of the prescribed antibiotic dose. On further questioning, you discover that the mother and father have recently become foster parents of a 10-year-old child with cerebral palsy. This child is wheelchair-bound, has contractures, is incontinent of stool and urine, and needs to be fed by hand for about 1 hour for each meal. The mother, who feels distracted by the care needs of this child, often forgets doses of medication for her 2-year-old son. You develop a plan where doses of medication are instead given by the father. What level of physician involvement (LPI) has now occurred?

    (A) LPI-1
    (B) LPI-2
    (C) LPI-3
    (D) LPI-4
    (E) LPI-5

3. Which of the following usually characterizes family boundaries or family system when abusive relationships exist?

    (A) Excessively permeable boundaries
    (B) Enmeshed system
    (C) Rigid boundaries
    (D) Normally permeable boundaries
    (E) An overly dynamic system

4. The parents of a 13-year-old girl with irritable bowel syndrome have been arguing several times per week for months. They have each threatened divorce. During their louder, more protracted arguments, the girl often experiences increasing abdominal pain and cramping. When this occurs, the parents stop arguing, get her medicine, and comfort her. This is an example of

    (A) dyadism
    (B) triangulation
    (C) reframing
    (D) restorying
    (E) externalizing

5. During strategic family therapy, the parents described in question 4 receive insight into how their interactions and responses may actually be exacerbating the manifestations of their daughter's illness. This is an example of

    (A) dyadism
    (B) externalizing
    (C) second-order change within the system
    (D) reframing or restorying
    (E) triangulation

6. Which of the following represents an idiosyncratic constraint in a family structure?

    (A) A mother who has been raised to believe that children should leave a room only if they have asked and received permission from adults
    (B) A hierarchy
    (C) Parents and children with specific roles in a hierarchy
    (D) Parents and children with reciprocal functions
    (E) Parents and children with complimentary functions

7. Which of the following approaches is characterized by focused structural family therapy to produce an alternative outcome to a specific issue presented by the family?

    (A) Psychoanalysis
    (B) Behavioral therapy
    (C) Brief therapy
    (D) Triangulation
    (E) Use of a genogram to examine transgenerational patterns that may be contributing factors

8. Which of the following can be shown on a genogram using standard geometric symbols and coded abbreviations?

(A) Individual attitudes
(B) Personality traits
(C) Current and previous medications
(D) Symptom surveys
(E) Alcoholism

9. Development "tasks" of individuals and families are identified by

(A) structural family therapy
(B) strategic family therapy
(C) life cycle models
(D) eclectic schools of systems therapy
(E) brief therapy

DIRECTIONS (Item 10): The incomplete statement in this section is negatively phrased, as indicated by the capitalized word NOT. Select the ONE lettered answer or completion that is BEST.

10. Family physicians often play a unique role in the categorization of families through their longitudinal contact with family members. Some practitioners use family systems theory to analyze and affect patterns, which may change over time. Which of the following is NOT a part of a family systems framework?

(A) Examining how an adolescent male interacts with his peer group
(B) Addressing the psychological problems of a family member and the responses of other family members
(C) Looking at the health needs of a 2-year-old child
(D) Examining the impact of a newborn child on the relationship among two parents and their two other children
(E) Assessing how relationships within the family change when catastrophic illness affects one of its members

ANSWERS AND EXPLANATIONS

1. The answer is B. With level 2 of physician involvement (LPI-2), medical findings and treatment options are communicated to key family members. In contrast, LPI-1 involves simple diagnosis and treatment, with little real communication. However, in LPI-2, no integration of a psychosocial model occurs. Treatment is totally based on a medical model; in this context, there is no behavioral analysis. No family interaction frameworks are elicited.

2. The answer is C. With level 3 of physician involvement (LPI-3), some underlying family dynamics that contribute to the health problem are involved, and guidance is offered or appropriate family efforts for solution of the problem are suggested. Note that there was no structural therapy and no counseling effort to address dysfunction.

3. The answer is C. Rigid boundaries tend to isolate the victim of abuse within the family and away from outsiders who could recognize the abuse pattern.

4. The answer is B. This behavior is a classic example of triangulation, a tendency on the part of the feuding dyad to involve a third person when the two individuals begin to argue heatedly. The aggravation of the girl's condition provides a basis for "constructive" focus on her, the third person, and for positive reinforcement of an improved behavior pattern (i.e., cessation of parental fighting).

5. The answer is D. Reframing or restorying is the introduction of new information so alternative interaction responses can develop within the system. It is a first-order change (i.e., the interaction changes but the rules do not, and the system remains). The goal is to change the system itself.

6. The answer is A. Individuals who "learn" uncommon behavior patterns from their own family or outside experiences bring idiosyncratic constraints into the system. Thus, the mother has the imprinted belief that children are unfailingly obedient and need permission to take initiative. The other answer choices all represent generic constraints to the family structure.

7. The answer is C. Brief therapy is not only time-limited but also focused solely on single issues that need change. Psychoanalysis, which is anything but brief, focuses on the individual, not the family. Behavioral therapy, which is not psychoanalytic, also focuses on the individual. A genogram is a graphic expression of medical and psychological identities of an extended family.

8. The answer is E. Alcoholism is signified by the symbol " Et" alongside the geometric icon for male (square) or female (circle). In addition, discord, separation, triangulation, and inappropriate boundaries can all be visualized with the genogram, which may provide insight into dysfunctional families [see page 850 in *Family Medicine* (House Officer Series)].

9. The answer is C. When the life cycle model of an individual conflicts with that of the family, dysfunction and illness may result. The following two examples are good illustrations of this principle.

The parents of a constitutionally shy 12-year-old boy, a first-born child, are seventh-generation Anglo-Americans. Their dreams for their son include his becoming a champion athlete, like his father and maternal grandfather. The boy also has an atopic constitution, and his own dream is to become a concert violinist. The family finds itself in crisis over the boy's plans, and the boy develops asthma at times of stress (as opposed to times of peak levels of allergens to which he is known to be responsive).

The parents of a 16-year-old second-generation Chinese-American girl have very high academic expectations of her. An older brother, who is a 22-year-old Ph.D. student and a former National Merit scholar, shares these expectations. The girl desires to pursue a career as a chef in Asian cuisine and begins bringing home "B" grades in her college preparatory high school courses. As the family becomes involved in the situation concerning her grades and career, she develops symptoms of irritable bowel syndrome.

10. The answer is A. Determining how an adolescent interacts with his peer group does not involve the family systems framework. Family systems, which views changes in interaction between family members, is not directly concerned with relationships outside the family. It can be used to see how individuals within the family are affected when one member has a medical or psychologic illness and how relationships alter in response to this change. The following example illustrates this principle.

A 9-year-old girl, long favored by her mother, develops pauciarticular juvenile rheumatoid arthritis (JRA) with mild symptoms that the family physician is treating with acetaminophen after consultation with a rheumatologist. Because of the incidence of anterior uveitis in this disease, the girl must be examined regularly by an ophthalmologist. As a result, she has become the center of family activity and conversation. The mother has become overprotective and hovering. The girl has begun to assume manipulative postures regarding avoiding activities she dislikes, including physical education and presentation of reports to her class. In addition, the 16-year-old sister has begun to feel rejected just at the time when peer pressures present the temptations of cigarette smoking and alcohol. The parents consult the family physician with concerns about the older daughter's peer group activities. If the physician approaches the problem at its root (i.e., the family's patterns of interaction), he or she is analyzing the family systems framework, not the adolescent's individual interactions.

BIBLIOGRAPHY

Schauer RW: Family Systems. In *Family Medicine* (House Officer Series). Edited by Rudy DR, Kurowski K. Baltimore, Williams & Wilkins, 1997, pp 843–854.

NMS Q&A: Family Medicine Answer Sheet

SECTION I Problems of the Head, Eyes, Ears, Nose, and Throat

Test 1. Problems of the Ears, Throat, and Sinuses

1. A B C D E
2. A B C D E
3. A B C D E
4. A B C D E
5. A B C D E
6. A B C D E
7. A B C D E
8. A B C D E
9. A B C D E
10. A B C D E
11. A B C D E
12. A B C D E
13. A B C D E
14. A B C D E
15. A B C D E
16. A B C D E
17. A B C D E
18. A B C D E
19. A B C D E
20. A B C D E
21. A B C D E
22. A B C D E
23. A B C D E
24. A B C D E
25. A B C D E
26. A B C D E
27. A B C D E
28. A B C D E
29. A B C D E

Test 2. Problems of the Oral Cavity

1. A B C D E
2. A B C D E
3. A B C D E
4. A B C D E
5. A B C D E
6. A B C D E
7. A B C D E
8. A B C D E
9. A B C D E
10. A B C D E
11. A B C D E
12. A B C D E
13. A B C D E
14. A B C D E
15. A B C D E

Test 3. Headache

1. A B C D E
2. A B C D E
3. A B C D E
4. A B C D E
5. A B C D E
6. A B C D E
7. A B C D E
8. A B C D E
9. A B C D E
10. A B C D E
11. A B C D E
12. A B C D E
13. A B C D E
14. A B C D E
15. A B C D E
16. A B C D E

Test 4. Problems of the Eye

1. A B C D E
2. A B C D E
3. A B C D E
4. A B C D E
5. A B C D E
6. A B C D E
7. A B C D E
8. A B C D E
9. A B C D E
10. A B C D E
11. A B C D E
12. A B C D E
13. A B C D E
14. A B C D E
15. A B C D E
16. A B C D E

SECTION II Cardiovascular Problems

Test 5. Common Cardiac Problems in Ambulatory Practice

1. A B C D E
2. A B C D E
3. A B C D E
4. A B C D E
5. A B C D E
6. A B C D E
7. A B C D E
8. A B C D E
9. A B C D E
10. A B C D E
11. A B C D E
12. A B C D E
13. A B C D E
14. A B C D E
15. A B C D E
16. A B C D E
17. A B C D E
18. A B C D E
19. A B C D E
20. A B C D E
21. A B C D E
22. A B C D E
23. A B C D E
24. A B C D E
25. A B C D E
26. A B C D E
27. A B C D E
28. A B C D E
29. A B C D E
30. A B C D E
31. A B C D E
32. A B C D E

Test 6. Peripheral Vascular Disease

1. A B C D E
2. A B C D E
3. A B C D E
4. A B C D E
5. A B C D E
6. A B C D E
7. A B C D E
8. A B C D E
9. A B C D E
10. A B C D E
11. A B C D E
12. A B C D E
13. A B C D E
14. A B C D E
15. A B C D E
16. A B C D E
17. A B C D E
18. A B C D E
19. A B C D E
20. A B C D E

Test 7. Cerebrovascular Disease and Brain Injury

1. A B C D E
2. A B C D E
3. A B C D E

4. A B C D E
5. A B C D E
6. A B C D E
7. A B C D E
8. A B C D E
9. A B C D E
10. A B C D E
11. A B C D E
12. A B C D E
13. A B C D E
14. A B C D E
15. A B C D E

Test 8. Cardiovascular Problems in Children

1. A B C D E
2. A B C D E
3. A B C D E
4. A B C D E
5. A B C D E
6. A B C D E
7. A B C D E
8. A B C D E
9. A B C D E
10. A B C D E
11. A B C D E
12. A B C D E
13. A B C D E
14. A B C D E
15. A B C D E
16. A B C D E

Test 9. Hypertension

1. A B C D E
2. A B C D E
3. A B C D E
4. A B C D E
5. A B C D E
6. A B C D E
7. A B C D E
8. A B C D E
9. A B C D E
10. A B C D E
11. A B C D E
12. A B C D E
13. A B C D E
14. A B C D E
15. A B C D E
16. A B C D E

SECTION III Neurology

Test 10. Neurology in Primary Care

1. A B C D E
2. A B C D E
3. A B C D E
4. A B C D E
5. A B C D E
6. A B C D E
7. A B C D E
8. A B C D E
9. A B C D E
10. A B C D E
11. A B C D E
12. A B C D E
13. A B C D E
14. A B C D E
15. A B C D E

SECTION IV Diseases of the Respiratory Tract

Test 11. Pneumonias, Bronchitides, and Chronic Lung Disease

1. A B C D E
2. A B C D E
3. A B C D E

4. A B C D E
5. A B C D E
6. A B C D E
7. A B C D E
8. A B C D E
9. A B C D E
10. A B C D E
11. A B C D E
12. A B C D E
13. A B C D E
14. A B C D E
15. A B C D E
16. A B C D E
17. A B C D E

Test 12. Respiratory Diseases in Infants and Children

1. A B C D E
2. A B C D E
3. A B C D E
4. A B C D E
5. A B C D E
6. A B C D E
7. A B C D E
8. A B C D E
9. A B C D E
10. A B C D E
11. A B C D E
12. A B C D E
13. A B C D E
14. A B C D E

SECTION V Problems of the Gastrointestinal Tract

Test 13. Medical Problems of the Gastrointestinal Tract

1. A B C D E
2. A B C D E
3. A B C D E
4. A B C D E
5. A B C D E
6. A B C D E
7. A B C D E
8. A B C D E
9. A B C D F
10. A B C D E
11. A B C D E
12. A B C D E
13. A B C D E
14. A B C D E
15. A B C D E
16. A B C D E
17. A B C D E
18. A B C D E

Test 14. Surgical Problems of the Gastrointestinal Tract

1. A B C D E
2. A B C D E
3. A B C D E
4. A B C D E
5. A B C D E
6. A B C D E
7. A B C D E
8. A B C D E
9. A B C D E
10. A B C D E
11. A B C D E
12. A B C D E
13. A B C D E
14. A B C D E
15. A B C D E

Test 15. Diseases of the Liver

1. A B C D E

4. A B C D E
5. A B C D E
6. A B C D E
7. A B C D E
8. A B C D E
9. A B C D E
10. A B C D E
11. A B C D E
12. A B C D E
13. A B C D E
14. A B C D E
15. A B C D E
16. A B C D E
17. A B C D E
18. A B C D E

SECTION VI Problems of the Urinary Tract

Test 16. Urinary Tract Infections

1. A B C D E
2. A B C D E
3. A B C D E
4. A B C D E
5. A B C D E
6. A B C D E
7. A B C D E
8. A B C D E
9. A B C D E
10. A B C D E
11. A B C D E
12. A B C D E
13. A B C D E
14. A B C D E
15. A B C D E

Test 17. Noninfectious Diseases of the Urinary Tract

1. A B C D E
2. A B C D E
3. A B C D E
4. A B C D E
5. A B C D E
6. A B C D E
7. A B C D E
8. A B C D E
9. A B C D E
10. A B C D E
11. A B C D E
12. A B C D E
13. A B C D E
14. A B C D E
15. A B C D E

SECTION VII Problems Unique to Females

Test 18. Gynecology in Primary Care

1. A B C D E
2. A B C D E
3. A B C D E
4. A B C D E
5. A B C D E
6. A B C D E
7. A B C D E
8. A B C D E
9. A B C D E
10. A B C D E
11. A B C D E
12. A B C D E
13. A B C D E
14. A B C D E
15. A B C D E
16. A B C D E

Test 19. Problems of the Female Climacteric

1. A B C D E
2. A B C D E
3. A B C D E
4. A B C D E
5. A B C D E
6. A B C D E
7. A B C D E
8. A B C D E
9. A B C D E
10. A B C D E

11. A B C D E
12. A B C D E
13. A B C D E
14. A B C D E
15. A B C D E

Test 20. Diseases of the Breast

1. A B C D E
2. A B C D E
3. A B C D E
4. A B C D E
5. A B C D E
6. A B C D E
7. A B C D E
8. A B C D E
9. A B C D E
10. A B C D E

11. A B C D E
12. A B C D E
13. A B C D E
14. A B C D E
15. A B C D E
16. A B C D E
17. A B C D E

SECTION VIII Problems Unique to Males

Test 21. Genitourinary Problems of the Male

1. A B C D E
2. A B C D E
3. A B C D E
4. A B C D E
5. A B C D E
6. A B C D E
7. A B C D E
8. A B C D E
9. A B C D E
10. A B C D E

11. A B C D E
12. A B C D E
13. A B C D E
14. A B C D E
15. A B C D E
16. A B C D E
17. A B C D E
18. A B C D E

SECTION IX Musculoskeletal and Connective Tissue Problems

Test 22. Musculoskeletal Problems of the Neck and Back

1. A B C D E
2. A B C D E
3. A B C D E
4. A B C D E
5. A B C D E
6. A B C D E
7. A B C D E
8. A B C D E
9. A B C D E
10. A B C D E

11. A B C D E
12. A B C D E
13. A B C D E
14. A B C D E
15. A B C D E

Test 23. Common Problems of the Upper Extremities

1. A B C D E
2. A B C D E
3. A B C D E
4. A B C D E
5. A B C D E
6. A B C D E
7. A B C D E
8. A B C D E
9. A B C D E
10. A B C D E

11. A B C D E
12. A B C D E
13. A B C D E
14. A B C D E
15. A B C D E
16. A B C D E
17. A B C D E

Test 24. Mechanical Problems of the Lower Extremities

1. A B C D E
2. A B C D E
3. A B C D E
4. A B C D E
5. A B C D E
6. A B C D E
7. A B C D E
8. A B C D E
9. A B C D E
10. A B C D E

11. A B C D E
12. A B C D E
13. A B C D E
14. A B C D E
15. A B C D E

Test 25. Approach to the Patient with Rheumatic Disease

1. A B C D E
2. A B C D E
3. A B C D E
4. A B C D E
5. A B C D E
6. A B C D E
7. A B C D E
8. A B C D E
9. A B C D E
10. A B C D E

11. A B C D E
12. A B C D E
13. A B C D E
14. A B C D E
15. A B C D E
16. A B C D E

Test 26. Musculoskeletal Problems in Children

1. A B C D E
2. A B C D E
3. A B C D E
4. A B C D E
5. A B C D E
6. A B C D E
7. A B C D E
8. A B C D E

Test 27. Approach to the Connective Tissue Diseases

1. A B C D E
2. A B C D E
3. A B C D E
4. A B C D E
5. A B C D E
6. A B C D E
7. A B C D E
8. A B C D E
9. A B C D E
10. A B C D E

11. A B C D E

12. A B C D E
13. A B C D E
14. A B C D E
15. A B C D E

SECTION X Sports Medicine

Test 28. Sports Medicine

1. A B C D E
2. A B C D E
3. A B C D E
4. A B C D E
5. A B C D E
6. A B C D E
7. A B C D E
8. A B C D E
9. A B C D E
10. A B C D E

11. A B C D E
12. A B C D E

SECTION XI Other Infectious Diseases Encountered in Primary Care

Test 29. Adult Acquired Immune Deficiency Syndrome

1. A B C D E
2. A B C D E
3. A B C D E
4. A B C D E
5. A B C D E
6. A B C D E
7. A B C D E
8. A B C D E
9. A B C D E
10. A B C D E

11. A B C D E
12. A B C D E
13. A B C D E
14. A B C D E
15. A B C D E
16. A B C D E
17. A B C D E
18. A B C D E

Test 30. Less Common Infectious Diseases in Primary Care

1. A B C D E
2. A B C D E
3. A B C D E
4. A B C D E
5. A B C D E
6. A B C D E
7. A B C D E
8. A B C D E
9. A B C D E
10. A B C D E

11. A B C D E
12. A B C D E
13. A B C D E
14. A B C D E
15. A B C D E
16. A B C D E

SECTION XII Endocrinology in Primary Care

Test 31. Diabetes Mellitus

1. A B C D E
2. A B C D E
3. A B C D E
4. A B C D E
5. A B C D E
6. A B C D E
7. A B C D E
8. A B C D E
9. A B C D E
10. A B C D E

11. A B C D E
12. A B C D E
13. A B C D E
14. A B C D E
15. A B C D E
16. A B C D E
17. A B C D E

Test 32. Thyroid Problems in Primary Care

1. A B C D E
2. A B C D E
3. A B C D E
4. A B C D E
5. A B C D E
6. A B C D E
7. A B C D E
8. A B C D E
9. A B C D E
10. A B C D E

11. A B C D E
12. A B C D E
13. A B C D E
14. A B C D E
15. A B C D E
16. A B C D E
17. A B C D E
18. A B C D E
19. A B C D E
20. A B C D E

21. A B C D E

Test 33. Triage of Problems of the Adrenal Gland

1. A B C D E
2. A B C D E
3. A B C D E
4. A B C D E
5. A B C D E
6. A B C D E
7. A B C D E
8. A B C D E
9. A B C D E
10. A B C D E

11. A B C D E
12. A B C D E
13. A B C D E
14. A B C D E
15. A B C D E
16. A B C D E
17. A B C D E

Test 34. Problems of Growth and Development

1. A B C D E
2. A B C D E
3. A B C D E
4. A B C D E
5. A B C D E
6. A B C D E
7. A B C D E
8. A B C D E
9. A B C D E
10. A B C D E

11. A B C D E
12. A B C D E
13. A B C D E
14. A B C D E
15. A B C D E

SECTION XIII Allergies

Test 35. Atopic and Food Allergies

1. A B C D E
2. A B C D E
3. A B C D E
4. A B C D E
5. A B C D E
6. A B C D E
7. A B C D E
8. A B C D E
9. A B C D E

10. A B C D E

11. A B C D E
12. A B C D E
13. A B C D E
14. A B C D E
15. A B C D E
16. A B C D E

SECTION XIV Preventive Care, Health, and Efficiency

Test 36. Preventive Care, the Patient, and the Doctor

1. A B C D E
2. A B C D E
3. A B C D E
4. A B C D E
5. A B C D E
6. A B C D E
7. A B C D E
8. A B C D E
9. A B C D E
10. A B C D E

11. A B C D E
12. A B C D E
13. A B C D E

Test 37. Preoperative Clearance and Preparation

1. A B C D E
2. A B C D E
3. A B C D E
4. A B C D E
5. A B C D E
6. A B C D E
7. A B C D E
8. A B C D E
9. A B C D E
10. A B C D E

11. A B C D E
12. A B C D E
13. A B C D E
14. A B C D E
15. A B C D E
16. A B C D E
17. A B C D E
18. A B C D E
19. A B C D E
20. A B C D E

21. A B C D E
22. A B C D E
23. A B C D E

Test 38. Obesity and Dyslipidemia

1. A B C D E
2. A B C D E
3. A B C D E
4. A B C D E
5. A B C D E
6. A B C D E
7. A B C D E
8. A B C D E
9. A B C D E
10. A B C D E

11. A B C D E
12. A B C D E
13. A B C D E
14. A B C D E

Test 39. Smoking Cessation

1. A B C D E
2. A B C D E
3. A B C D E
4. A B C D E
5. A B C D E
6. A B C D E
7. A B C D E
8. A B C D E
9. A B C D E
10. A B C D E

Test 40. Exercise and Health

1. A B C D E
2. A B C D E
3. A B C D E
4. A B C D E
5. A B C D E
6. A B C D E
7. A B C D E
8. A B C D E
9. A B C D E
10. A B C D E
11. A B C D E

Test 41. Preventive Care and Triage of the Infant and Newborn

1. A B C D E
2. A B C D E
3. A B C D E
4. A B C D E
5. A B C D E
6. A B C D E
7. A B C D E
8. A B C D E
9. A B C D E
10. A B C D E

Test 42. Preventive Care of the Preschool Child (1–5 Years)

1. A B C D E
2. A B C D E
3. A B C D E
4. A B C D E
5. A B C D E
6. A B C D E
7. A B C D E
8. A B C D E
9. A B C D E
10. A B C D E
11. A B C D E

Test 43. Preventive Care of the Child Through the Latent Years (5–12)

1. A B C D E

2. A B C D E
3. A B C D E
4. A B C D E
5. A B C D E
6. A B C D E
7. A B C D E
8. A B C D E
9. A B C D E
10. A B C D E
11. A B C D E

Test 44. Preventive Care of the Adolescent (12–20 Years)

1. A B C D E
2. A B C D E
3. A B C D E
4. A B C D E
5. A B C D E
6. A B C D E
7. A B C D E
8. A B C D E
9. A B C D E
10. A B C D E

Test 45. Preventive Care of the Young Adult (20–40 Years)

1. A B C D E
2. A B C D E
3. A B C D E
4. A B C D E
5. A B C D E
6. A B C D E
7. A B C D E
8. A B C D E
9. A B C D E
10. A B C D E
11. A B C D E
12. A B C D E
13. A B C D E

Test 46. Preventive Care of the Middle-Aged Adult (40–65 Years)

1. A B C D E

2. A B C D E
3. A B C D E
4. A B C D E
5. A B C D E
6. A B C D E
7. A B C D E
8. A B C D E
9. A B C D E
10. A B C D E
11. A B C D E

Test 47. Preventive Care of the Older Adult (> 65 years)

1. A B C D E
2. A B C D E
3. A B C D E
4. A B C D E
5. A B C D E
6. A B C D E
7. A B C D E
8. A B C D E
9. A B C D E
10. A B C D E

Test 48. Travel Medicine

1. A B C D E
2. A B C D E
3. A B C D E
4. A B C D E
5. A B C D E
6. A B C D E
7. A B C D E
8. A B C D E
9. A B C D E
10. A B C D E
11. A B C D E
12. A B C D E
13. A B C D E
14. A B C D E
15. A B C D E
16. A B C D E
17. A B C D E
18. A B C D E

19. A B C D E
20. A B C D E
21. A B C D E
22. A B C D E
23. A B C D E
24. A B C D E

SECTION XV Behavior and Psychology in Family Practice

Test 49. Counseling Methods in Family Practice: Cognitive Strategies

1. A B C D E
2. A B C D E
3. A B C D E
4. A B C D E
5. A B C D E
6. A B C D E
7. A B C D E
8. A B C D E

Test 50. Depression

1. A B C D E
2. A B C D E
3. A B C D E
4. A B C D E
5. A B C D E
6. A B C D E
7. A B C D E
8. A B C D E
9. A B C D E
10. A B C D E
11. A B C D E
12. A B C D E
13. A B C D E
14. A B C D E

Test 51. Anxiety, Phobia, and the Undifferentiated Primary Care Syndrome

1. A B C D E
2. A B C D E
3. A B C D E

4. A B C D E
5. A B C D E
6. A B C D E
7. A B C D E
8. A B C D E
9. A B C D E
10. A B C D E
11. A B C D E
12. A B C D E

Test 52. Somatic Symptoms Without Organic Basis

1. A B C D E
2. A B C D E
3. A B C D E
4. A B C D E
5. A B C D E
6. A B C D E
7. A B C D E
8. A B C D E
9. A B C D E
10. A B C D E
11. A B C D E
12. A B C D E
13. A B C D E F G H
14. A B C D E F G H
15. A B C D E F G H
16. A B C D E F G H
17. A B C D E F G H
18. A B C D E F G H
19. A B C D E F G H
20. A B C D E F G H

Test 53. Family Systems

1. A B C D E
2. A B C D E
3. A B C D E
4. A B C D E
5. A B C D E
6. A B C D E
7. A B C D E
8. A B C D E
9. A B C D E
10. A B C D E